Surgical Oncology

Surgical Oncology

Editor: Jonah Armstrong

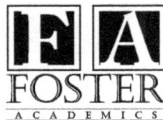

FA
FOSTER
ACADEMICS

www.fosteracademics.com

www.fosteracademics.com

FA
FOSTER
ACADEMICS

Cataloging-in-Publication Data

Surgical oncology / edited by Jonah Armstrong.
    p. cm.
Includes bibliographical references and index.
ISBN 978-1-63242-738-0
1. Cancer--Surgery. 2. Tumors--Surgery. 3. Oncology. I. Armstrong, Jonah.
RD651 .S87 2019
616.994 059--dc23

Foster Academics,
118-35 Queens Blvd., Suite 400,
Forest Hills, NY 11375, USA

ISBN 978-1-63242-738-0 (Hardback)

Contents

Permissions

List of Contributors

Index

Preface

Every book is a source of knowledge and this one is no exception. The idea that led to the conceptualization of this book was the fact that the world is advancing rapidly; which makes it crucial to document the progress in every field. I am aware that a lot of data is already available, yet, there is a lot more to learn. Hence, I accepted the responsibility of editing this book and contributing my knowledge to the community.

Cancer care has evolved significantly in the past few decades with the emergence of varied treatment modalities. The modern standard of cancer cure is a combination of multi-modal therapies and surgery. The field of surgical oncology is concerned with the surgical management of tumors, particularly cancerous tumors. Each surgical procedure targets cancer at a particular site only, such as Whipple procedure or pancreaticoduodenectomy that targets pancreatic cancer, or gastrectomy with extended (D2) lymphadenectomy which targets gastric cancer. There have been significant advances in surgical oncology such as minimally invasive surgical techniques, robotic surgery, reconstructive surgery, intraoperative chemotherapy and radiation therapy, among others. This book includes some of the vital pieces of work being conducted across the world, on various topics related to surgical oncology. It provides significant information of this discipline to help develop a good understanding of clinical principles and practices of this field. For all those who are interested in oncology, this book can prove to be an essential guide.

While editing this book, I had multiple visions for it. Then I finally narrowed down to make every chapter a sole standing text explaining a particular topic, so that they can be used independently. However, the umbrella subject sinews them into a common theme. This makes the book a unique platform of knowledge.

I would like to give the major credit of this book to the experts from every corner of the world, who took the time to share their expertise with us. Also, I owe the completion of this book to the never-ending support of my family, who supported me throughout the project.

Editor

Intraoperative ultrasound in breast cancer surgery—from localization of non-palpable tumors to objectively measurable excision

Natasa Colakovic[1]* , Darko Zdravkovic[2], Zlatko Skuric[1], Davor Mrda[3], Jasna Gacic[2] and Nebojsa Ivanovic[2]

Abstract

Background: The utilization of intraoperative ultrasound (IOUS) in breast cancer surgery is a relatively new concept in surgical oncology. Over the last few decades, the field of breast cancer surgery has been striving for a more rational approach, directing its efforts towards removing the tumor entirely yet sparing tissue and structures not infiltrated by tumor cells. Further progress in objectivity and optimization of breast cancer excision is possible if we make the tumor and surrounding tissue visible and measurable in real time, during the course of the operation; IOUS seems to be the optimal solution to this complex requirement. IOUS was introduced into clinical practice as a device for visualization of non-palpable tumors, and compared to wire-guided localization (WGL), IOUS was always at least a viable, or much better alternative, in terms of both precision in identification and resection and for patients' and surgeons' comfort. In recent years, intraoperative ultrasound has been used in the surgery of palpable tumors to optimize resection procedures and overcome the disadvantages of classic palpation guided surgery.

Objective: The aim of this review is to show the role of IOUS in contemporary breast cancer surgery and its changes over time.

Methods: A PubMed database comprehensive search was conducted to identify all relevant articles according to assigned key words.

Conclusion: Over time, the use of IOUS has been transformed from being the means of localizing non-palpable lesions to an instrument yielding a reduced number of positive resection margins, with a smaller volume of healthy breast tissue excided around tumor, by making the excision of the tumor optimal and objectively measurable.

Keywords: Breast cancer excision, Intraoperative ultrasound, Tumor localization

Background

For a number of years, surgery has been essential in achieving a satisfactory level of locoregional control in patients with breast cancer, especially utilizing radical mastectomy and its modifications. In the last decades, the field of surgical oncology has been striving for a more rational approach, directing its efforts towards removing the tumor entirely, while sparing tissue and structures not infiltrated by tumor cells. This contributes to better functional and esthetic results and, by extension, a better quality of life for the patient.

Two main techniques that highlight the shift from classical to modern breast cancer surgery are breast-conserving surgery and sentinel node biopsy. The former benefits patients esthetically and psychologically, while the latter helps to improve functional results, primarily preventing limited motility and edema of the arm.

The institution of screening programs and the advancement of diagnostic methods significantly increased the percentage of tumors discovered in an early phase while still relatively small in size, effectively allowing for less radical procedures than the overly extensive "quadrantectomy." Another consequence of discovering tumors in an early phase is an increase in the number of non-palpable lesions; the surgeon thereby needing additional tools for the localization and adequate excision of

* Correspondence: colakovicnatasa@yahoo.com
[1]Department of Surgical Oncology, University Medical Center "Bezanijska Kosa", Bezanijska kosa bb, Belgrade 11080, Serbia
Full list of author information is available at the end of the article

such lesions. Two main approaches to this are preoperative (wire- and radio-guided occult lesion localization by mammography: WGL and ROLL) and intraoperative (intraoperative ultrasound: IOUS).

For palpable lesions, localization is easily defined by palpation. However, adequate excision, negative margins with as small excision volume as is possible, may be better achieved if the distance from the tumor border to the resection margin is objectively measured by IOUS, rather than by subjective palpation-guided surgery.

It is clear that palpation-guided surgery cannot improve objectivity and measurability of the resection procedure. If we desire progress in objectivity and optimization of breast cancer excision, we need to make the tumor and the surround tissue visible and measurable during the course of the operation in real time. IOUS seems to be the optimal solution to this complex requirement.

In clinical practice, there are three main purposes of using IUOS in breast surgery: (1) localization of non-palpable lesions, (2) achieving free resection margins, and (3) IOUS-guided surgery in an attempt to obtain optimal excision volume, with negative resection margins and minimal sacrifice of surrounding healthy tissue.

The aim of this review is to highlight the role of IOUS in contemporary breast cancer surgery and its changes over time, from being a tool for the localization of non-palpable lesions, to becoming an instrument that can make tumor excision optimal and even objectively measurable.

Main text

IOUS in localization of non-palpable tumors

The utilization of intraoperative ultrasound in breast cancer surgery is a relatively new concept in this field of surgical oncology. It was introduced into clinical practice as a device for the visualization of non-palpable tumors [1–11]. All studies published thus far, including newly published studies [12–15], have shown an efficacy of almost 100% (Table 1).

The first report was published by Schwartz et al. [1] in 1988 on 92 excised non-palpable breast lesions. They concluded that IOUS had proven effective and accurate, and that in select patients, it may be used in addition to, or instead of, X-ray needle localization for the precise excision of non-palpable breast lesions, excluding calcifications.

The next reports dealing with IOUS appeared more than 10 years later, mostly comparing WGL and IOUS [2, 3, 5]. In two reports [2, 5] with a relatively small number of operated lesions (63 in first study and 49 in the second, the second being a randomized trial) Rahusen et al. showed remarkable difference between IOUS and WGL in the adequacy of resection margins. In the IOUS group, resection margins were negative in 89% in both studies, compared to only 40% and 55% in the WGL group. Snider and Morrison [3] presented their small study on 44 patients, 22 in both IOUS and WGL groups. Both groups had the same number of positive resection margins, but the mean resection volume was

Table 1 Identification rate of a non-palpable breast lesion by IOUS and WGL

Author	Type of the study	IOUS				WGL			
		N° of patients	N° of operations	N° of ident. tumors	Ident. rate (%)	N° of patients	N° of operations	N° of ident. tumors	Ident. rate (%)
Rahusen	prosp	19	20	20	100	43	43	43	100
Snider	retro	22	22	22	100	22	22	22	100
Harlow	retro	62	65	65	100	nd	nd	nd	nd
Smith	retro	81	81	81	100	nd	nd	nd	nd
Rahusen 2	prosp	27	27	27	100	22	22	22	100
Kaufman	prosp	100	101	101	100	nd	nd	nd	nd
Gittleman	retro	15	15	15	100	nd	nd	nd	nd
Beneth	prosp	103	115	115	100	24	24	24	100
Haid	retro	299	299	299	100	61	61	61	100
Potter	retro	32	32	32	100	nd	nd	nd	nd
Ngo	prosp	70	70	67	96	nd	nd	nd	nd
Fortunato	prosp	77	77	77	100	nd	nd	nd	nd
James	retro	96	96	96	100	59	59	59	100
Bouton	retro	28	28	28	100	nd	nd	nd	nd
Berentz	prosp	120	120	120	100	138	138	138	100
Ramos	retro	225	225	224	99	nd	nd	nd	nd

IOUS Intraoperative ultrasound, *WGL* wire-guided localization, *nd* no data, *N°* number, *ident* identified, *ident. rate* identification rate

smaller in the IOUS group (62.6 versus 81.1 cm^3), although mean lesion size was two times larger in the IOUS group than in the WGL group (11 versus 5.5 mm). Smith et al. [4] emphasized that using IOUS avoids the complications of WGL and simplifies the scheduling of surgical procedures. This is a common sentiment among all authors dealing with this topic.

In the following years, very few studies on using IOUS in breast lesion surgery were published. Kaufman et al. [6] reported a series of 101 operations of non-palpable carcinomas in which they had a 100% identification rate. Bennett et al. [7] published a study on 115 resected non-palpable breast lesions of which 42% were malignant. The identification rate for all lesions was 100%. Negative resection margins were achieved in 93% of 48 excised lesions. This was retrospectively compared with hookwire-guided excisions performed by the same author, where negative resection margins were achieved in 83% of cases out of 43 operated malignant lesions. Haid et al. [8] reported 100% efficacy in the identification of occult breast cancer in 299 patients, and the same efficacy was reached in a control WGL group of 61 patients. Potter et al. [9] had the same maximum rate for 32 patients. In a prospective study, Ngo et al. [10] reached a 95.7% identification rate for 70 patients with impalpable lesions. They missed tumors less than 5 mm in diameter in two patients with body mass indexes over 25. In a prospective study, Fortunato et al. [11] achieved a 100%

identification rate for 77 patients (60 malignant and 17 benign). Ramos et al. [14] had a 99.6% identification rate in a retrospective study on 225 invasive breast cancers. Only one tumor smaller than 5 mm could not be located.

IOUS and resection margins

The use of IOUS to guide surgical excision of non-palpable breast carcinoma has also shown that ultrasound-guided breast cancer operations yield a smaller number of positive resection margins [2, 4–8, 15–17]. They also result in a smaller volume of healthy breast tissue excised around the tumor (Table 2).

In a study on 65 breast cancers by Harlow et al. [15], the authors reported only two positive margins with a mean distance of 0.8 cm to the closest margin of excision. Moore et al. [16] reported their prospective study evaluating surgical accuracy and margin status after lumpectomies for palpable breast cancer on two groups of patients. In one group, they used IOUS ($n = 27$) but not in the other ($n = 24$). In the first group, only one patient had a positive margin (1/27 or 3.7%); while in the other group, seven patients had positive margins (7/24 or 29%). The authors concluded that the use of ultrasound-guided surgery optimizes the surgeon's ability to obtain satisfactory margins for breast-conserving techniques in patients with breast cancer and that patient satisfaction with the cosmetic results was excellent. In the Kaufman et al. [6] study, negative margins for invasive

Table 2 Tumor-free resection margins and re-excision rate after IOUS and WGL

Author	Type of the Study	IOUS				WGL			
		N° of pts.	N° of oper	N° of neg. marg.	N° of re-excision	N° of pts.	N° of oper	N° of neg. marg.	N° of re-excision
Rahusen	prosp	19	20	17 (89%)	nd	43	43	17 (40%)	nd
Snider	retro	22	22	18 (82%)	nd	22	22	18 (82%)	nd
Harlow	retro	62	65	63 (97%)	3(4.80%)	nd	nd	nd	nd
Smith	retro	81	81	24/25 mg (96%)	nd	nd	nd	nd	nd
Rahusen 2	prosp	27	27	24 (89%)	nd	22	22	12(55%)	nd
Kaufman	prosp	100	101	90(89%)	9 (9%)	nd	nd	nd	nd
Gittleman	retro	15	15	14(92%)	1(8%)	nd	nd	nd	nd
Beneth	prosp	103	115	39/42 mg (93%)	3(7%)	24	24	19 (83%)	5(17%)
Haid	retro	299	299	242 (81%)	57(19%)	61	61	38 (62%)	23 38%)
Potter	retro	32	32	28(88%)	nd	nd	nd	nd	nd
Ngo	prosp	70	70	66 (94%)	3(4%)	nd	nd	nd	nd
Fortunato	prosp	77	77	75 (97%)	2(3%)	nd	nd	nd	nd
Bouton	retro	28	28	25 (91%)	3(9%)	nd	nd	nd	26%
Berentz	prosp	120	120	112 (93%)	15(13%)	138	138	129(93.5%)	15(11%)
Ramos	retro	225	225	216 (96%)	9(4%)	nd	nd	12(55%)	nd
James	retro	96	96	10(10%)	20(20%)	59	59	52(88%)	18(30%)

N° Number, *IOUS* intraoperative ultrasound, *WGL* wire-guided localization, *nd* no data, *pts.* patients, *prosp* prospective, *retro* retrospective, *neg.marg.* negative margins, *oper* operations

carcinoma were found in 90% of patients; while in the Bennett et al. [7] study, resection margins were adequate in 93% of operations for malignant tumors.

Most authors compared IOUS and WGL in achieving negative resection margins. Haid et al. [8] reported 81% successful operations in IOUS group without metachronous secondary surgery, versus 62% in a WGL group. James et al. [18], in the only study related exclusively to DCIS, reported non-significant differences in resection adequacy between IUOS (96 pts.—10.4% of positive margins) and WGL (59 pts.—11.9% of positive margins). In a retrospective analysis, Bouton et al. [19] found that 28 patients treated by WGL and IOUS (control group was treated by WGL only) had a lower rate of positive margins (9% vs. 26%). Davis et al. [20] in a retrospective study (22 pts. with IOUS and 44 pts. without; tumors were palpable) showed that the IOUS group had significantly less involved margins (9% vs. 41%) and a lower rate of re-excision (9% vs. 34%).

Two studies showed no differences between IOUS and other techniques. In a prospective study on non-palpable tumors, Berentsz et al. [12] compared IUOS and WGL. There were 120 pts. in the IOUS group, and 138 pts. in the WGL group. Tumor-free resection margins were obtained in 93.5% of cases in the WGL group and 93.3% in the IOUS group. It is surprising that in this study, the average diameter of impalpable tumors in the IOUS group was 1.24 cm. Similar results were reported by Fisher et al. [17] in a retrospective analysis comparing resection margins in 73 patients with palpable tumors operated by IOUS-guided surgery and 124 patients operated by palpation guided surgery. Re-excision rates were similar in both groups, 17 (23%) in the IOUS group versus 31 (25%) in the palpation group. Nevertheless, the authors concluded that US guidance provides an excellent tool to aid the breast surgeon.

Eichler et al. [21] had more R0 resections in the IOUS group (84 pts.) than in the control group (without IUOS group 166 pts.), a statistically significant difference. In a retrospective analysis by Yu et al. [13], positive margins were found in only 9.29% of 126 palpable and 255 non-palpable tumors operated by IOUS guidance. In another retrospective analysis of 225 operated non-palpable tumors, Ramos et al. [14] had a re-excision rate of only 4% (9/225) after IOUS-guided surgery.

IOUS-guided surgery

Improved margin status after IOUS-guided surgery for non-palpable tumors have initiated the application of this technique in the surgery of palpable tumors in recent years [12, 13, 17, 20–24], in order to optimize resection procedures and overcome the disadvantages of classic palpation guided surgery. Palpation-guided surgery is a subjective technique, yielding up to 41% of "positive" resection margins according to Krekel et al. [24] while leading to an unnecessary large volume of excision.

All published studies on this topic have unequivocally shown that intraoperative ultrasound improves oncological efficacy and cosmetic outcomes in breast conserving surgery. Olsha et al. [22] concluded that intraoperative ultrasound may help maintain low incidence of reoperation after breast-conserving surgery. In a paper by Davis et al. [20], the authors found that patients who underwent lumpectomies using IOUS were less likely to have an involved margin or to require re-excision. The lumpectomy volumes in the IOUS group were smaller than in the lumpectomy alone group. IOUS can decrease the rate of positive margins and re-excision lumpectomy in patients with palpable breast cancers. Fisher et al. [17] stated that although palpable breast cancers can be excised based on direct palpation or needle localization, ultrasound guidance provides an excellent tool to aid the surgeon. Only 10% of patients in the ultrasound-guided group had a positive margin in final pathology compared to 16% in the palpation-guided group. The re-excision rates were similar for both groups, 23% in the ultrasound-guided group versus 25% in the palpation-guided group. However, the rate of residual disease in re-excision pathology for a positive or close margin was significantly lower for those patients who had an ultrasound-guided lumpectomy than for those who had a palpation-guided lumpectomy.

In the COBALT trial, Krekel et al. [24] showed that the intraoperative use of IOUS for palpable tumors is associated with a 15% reduction in "positive" margins of resection. It also significantly reduced specimen volume when compared to palpation-guided surgery, leading to a more acceptable esthetic result and better quality of life.

Surgical techniques of IOUS guides surgery

The IOUS surgical technique described thus far normally relies on the surgeon to mark the projected tumor margins on the skin of the breast before the first incision is made. The surgeon then inserts the probe into the wound multiple times in an effort to determine the relation between the tumor and the surrounding tissue once surgery proper has started. Once the excision has been completed, the specimen is examined ex vivo (i.e., ultrasound examination of the excised specimen), followed by additional shaving excisions if one of the excision margins if found to be too close to the edge of the tumor. In the COBALT trial, the authors used ultrasound during the entire procedure in order to gauge the distance of the resection line from the edge of the tumor in all directions and the entirety of the volume of the specimen without using any marker inside or around tumor.

Some authors have proposed the use of markers as an anatomical landmark, without any desire for them to aid fine measurements and resection line planning. Kaufman et al. [6] used die and wire needles to mark the position of the tumor. Gittleman [25] described 15 resections in which he had injected the tumor with an ultrasound contrast medium, 9 resections in which he had utilized a radiofrequency localization device (comprising a calibrated shaft with a flexible cutting element to facilitate the positioning of the device and fixing wires that expand radially in order to anchor the device on the target lesion), and 6 cases in which he had opted for an 18G needle as a means of marking the position of the tumor.

Using intraoperative ultrasound in such a "standard" way has been demonstrated by Ivanovic et al. [26, 27] to be fraught with difficulties that interfere with the comfort and precision of the surgical procedure. First, marking the position of the tumor by projecting its margins on the skin is problematic at best, given that the anatomical relations between the tumor and the surrounding tissue changes due to tissue retraction and manipulation normally involved in any type of surgery. Second, once the surgeon starts resecting the tumor, air and fluid in the wound create artifacts that significantly reduce the quality of the ultrasound image, therefore limiting useful interpretation. Third, when the ultrasound probe is inserted into the wound, the surrounding tissue is displaced and compressed which may lead to the surgeon misjudging the distance from the resection line to the edge of the tumor. Fourth, ultrasound refraction which is particularly common when scanning tissue that is irregular in shape, such as a tumor, leads to a discrepancy between the ultrasound-measured size of the tumor and its real size. This is most common in tumors 2 cm or larger. Since documenting this phenomenon, De Jean et al. [28] recommend that an ultrasound contrast medium be inserted into the tumor in relation to which segmental measurements in all directions can be performed.

In the same paper [27], Ivanovic et al. presented an original technique for the optimization of breast cancer excision (both palpable and non-palpable) utilizing IOUS and a specially-constructed needle as a marker for objective measurement. Guided by ultrasound, the needle is inserted into the tumor (the patient lying on the operating table anesthetized) and then used to measure the distance between the line of resection and the needle in all directions. The surgeon then proceeds to do the resection using these measurements while continually measuring the distance of the resection line from the needle, using a sterile ruler.

The preliminary results are encouraging, and it seems that the utilization of the aforementioned technique makes the resection of a breast cancer a measurable and objective undertaking. This should lead to a reduction in the percent of "positive" resection margins, and by extension, relapses. Viewed from a different perspective, one could expect improved conservation of healthy tissue, which should lead to smaller tissue defect and better esthetic results of the surgery. The authors consider the technique to be simple, easy to learn and implement, and comfortable for the surgeon. There is no need to palpate or compress the tumor or the surrounding tissue, and the traction, manipulation, and separation of the tissue is gentler than with palpation-guided surgery. Probably, the only drawback is the extra time needed for measurements before the incision (11 min on average at the moment). However, this time is compensated by the ease with which the resection is done and by the fact that it is done in a more rational and objectively measurable way. One could expect that, with training, the time needed for measurements and the resection itself will be shortened and that the relations (between the desired and achieved size of the tumor specimen) will become more optimal. Nevertheless, we must conclude that conducting a randomized trial is the only way to prove these assumptions.

Discussion

Intraoperative ultrasound in breast cancer is a relatively new technique in this field of surgical oncology. It was introduced into clinical practice as a device for the visualization and localization of non-palpable tumors, and its utility and accuracy for this has always been unequivocally confirmed [1–11]. IOUS-guided surgery improves the accuracy and quality of classical surgery, while at the same time being cheap, time-efficient, simple, and comfortable for both the surgeon and the patient. There is no risk of complications related to the procedure, and thanks to greater precision, it is less likely that subsequent operations will be required.

In addition to being a non-radioactive technique, real-time visualization overcomes the shortcomings of standard preoperative mammography in a number of ways. First, it solves an organizational and technical problem by harmonizing the work of the diagnostics and operating rooms. Second, it reduces pre-surgery psychological stress for the patient, as there is no need for a painful and harsh procedure of breast compression and puncture while conscious. Third, it resolves the inability to check marker position after placement. This is important as there may be a movement of needle marker on the way from the diagnostics room to the operating room, while preparing the operating area before surgery [27].

Data analysis in studies on the use of IOUS to guide surgical excision of non-palpable breast carcinoma has also shown that IOUS-guided breast cancer operations yield a smaller number of positive resection margins [2, 4–7, 15–17]. This effect was unintended and unexpected in some studies [17] but nevertheless pointed to another possibly useful role of IOUS.

Studies comparing IOUS and WGL in achieving negative resection margins [8, 12, 18–20] showed that IOUS is at least equal or more successful than WGL. However, WGL is still a standard approach in the localization of non-palpable breast lesions and is currently irreplaceable when these lesions are invisible to ultrasound. IUOS could be a much better alternative to WGL for ultrasound-visible breast lesions in terms of precision in identification and resection as well as the comfort of patients and surgeons. Knowing this, it is surprising that IOUS-guided surgery is not more commonly used in breast cancer surgery of non-palpable lesions and that WGL is still the method of choice for localization of these lesions. One possible reason could be the lack of surgeons' education in the use of ultrasound [24], which indicates the possible need for workshops and other forms of continuing education. Also, it seems that creating guidelines for optimal tumor excision in breast cancer surgery persuade surgeons to use IOUS more in the future.

The next step in the evolving role of IOUS in breast cancer surgery is "optimal and objectively measurable tumor excision" to achieve two main goals: first, a negative resection margin; and second, minimal sacrifice of surrounding healthy tissue, which improves the esthetic effect of the operation and patients' quality of life. This has been illustrated by contemporary studies where IUOS were used as a means of optimal resection [24, 27], defined as a macroscopic distance of 10 mm in all directions from the tumor to the resection line. This distance is supposed to provide a negative microscopic margin ("no tumor on ink") and minimal sacrifice of healthy tissue. All published studies on this topic have unequivocally shown that IOUS improves oncological efficacy and cosmetic outcomes in breast conserving surgery [17, 20, 22, 24, 27, 29–31].

The authors present a detailed description of surgical techniques of IOUS-guided breast cancer surgery. Basically, there are two main techniques. The first relies on the continuous use of ultrasound during the operation in order to gauge the distance of the resection line from the edge of the tumor in all directions, without using any ultrasound-visible marker inside or around the tumor. The most detailed description of this technique is given by Krekel et al. [24]. The second technique relies on the use of ultrasound-visible markers as an anatomical landmark [6, 25, 27]. The most detailed description of this technique is given by Ivanovic et al. [27].

However, the majority of resections are still performed using classical palpation-guided surgery, where the desired 10 mm distance from the tumor is subjectively approximated. In practice, one cannot help but notice that most surgeons opt for more extensive resections in order to achieve oncological security. However, a significant percentage of "positive" resection margins makes additional surgery or radiotherapy "boosts" a necessity all too often.

Meanwhile, new studies are being published which confirm that IOUS-guided primary tumor resection is associated with a smaller percentage of positive resection lines. This leads to a reduced need for re-excision and mastectomy, with better esthetic effect and consequently improved quality of life. Volders et al. [30] and Haloua et al. [31] report that this is the consequence of an optimal relationship between volume of the tumor and volume of the excised specimen (tumor and surrounding tissue).

Rubio et al. [32] have shown the advantages of IOUS compared to classical WGL techniques after neoadjuvant chemotherapy. The most important advantages were avoiding the placement of a wire, avoiding the need to synchronize work of diagnostic and surgical teams, allowing for intraoperative confirmation of the specimen ("ex vivo" US examination), and excision of less healthy tissue around lesion with the same margin negativity.

In her article, Klimberg [33] claimed that an excised tumor is rarely in the center of the lumpectomy specimen in daily surgical practice and that ultrasound could help in adequate excision, used in vivo or for specimen examination.

Conclusions

Over time, the use of IOUS has been transformed from a means of localizing non-palpable lesions to an instrument yielding a reduced number of positive resection margins, with a smaller volume of healthy breast tissue excided around tumor, making the excision of the tumor optimal and objectively measurable.

It seems that intraoperative real-time imaging of breast tumor resection could be the gold standard in the future, after substantial efforts in the education of surgeons and in creating protocols for optimal breast tumor excision.

Abbreviations
IOUS: Intraoperative ultrasound; WGL: Wire-guided localization

Authors' contributions
NC and DZ prepared the manuscript. ZS, JG, and DM performed research of literature. Conception and manuscript revision was done by NI. All authors read and approved the final manuscript.

Competing interests
The authors declare that they have no competing interests.

Author details
[1]Department of Surgical Oncology, University Medical Center "Bezanijska Kosa", Bezanijska kosa bb, Belgrade 11080, Serbia. [2]Faculty of Medicine, University of Belgrade, Belgrade, Serbia. [3]Department of Radiology, University Medical Center "Bezanijska Kosa", Belgrade, Serbia.

References
1. Schwartz GF, Goldberg BB, Rifkin MD, D'Orazio SE. Ultrasonography: an alternative to X-ray-guided needle localization of nonpalpable breast masses. Surgery. 1988;104:870–3.
2. Rahusen FD, Taets van Amerongen AH, van Diest PJ, Borgstein PJ, Bleichrodt RP, Meijer S. Ultrasound-guided lumpectomy of nonpalpable breast cancers: a feasibility study looking at the accuracy of obtained margins. J Surg Oncol. 1999;72:72–6.
3. Snider H, Morrison D. Intraoperative ultrasound localization of nonpalpable breast lesions. Ann Surg Oncol. 1999;6:308–14.
4. Smith LF, Rubio IT, Henry-Tillman R, Korourian S, Klimberg VS. Intraoperative ultrasound-guided breast biopsy. Am J Surg. 2000;180:419–23.
5. Rahusen FD, Bremers AJ, Fabry HF, van Amerongen AH, BOOm RP, Meijer S, et al. Ultrasound-guided lumpectomy of nonpalpable breast cancer versus wire-guided resection: a randomized clinical trial. Ann Surg Oncol. 2002;9:994–8.
6. Kaufman CS, Jacobson L, Bachman B, Kaufman LB. Intraoperative ultrasonography guidance is accurate and efficient according to results in 100 breast cancer patients. Am J Surg. 2003;186:378–82.
7. Bennett IC, Greenslade J, Chiam H. Intraoperative ultrasound-guided excision of nonpalpable breast lesions. World J Surg. 2005;29:369–74.
8. Haid A, Knauer M, Dunzinger Jasarevic Z, Köberle-Wührer R, Schuster A, et al. Intra-operative sonography: a valuable aid during breast-conserving surgery for occult breast cancer. Ann Surg Oncol. 2007;14:3090–101.
9. Potter S, Govindarajulu S, Cawthorn SJ, Sahu AK. Accuracy of sonographic localisation and specimen ultrasound performed by surgeons in impalpable screen-detected breast lesions. Breast. 2007;16:425–8.
10. Ngô C, Pollet AG, Laperrelle J, Ackerman G, Gomme S, Thibault F, et al. Intraoperative ultrasound localization of nonpalpable breast cancers. Ann Surg Oncol. 2007;14:2485–9.
11. Fortunato L, Penteriani R, Farina M, Vitelli CE, Piro FR. Intraoperative ultrasound is an effective and preferable technique to localize non-palpable breast tumors. Eur J Surg Oncol. 2008;34:1289–92.
12. Barentsz MW, van Dalen T, Gobardhan PD, Bongers V, Perre CI, Pijnappel RM, et al. Intraoperative ultrasound guidance for excision of non-palpable invasive breast cancer: a hospital-based series and an overview of the literature. Breast Cancer Res Treat. 2012;135:209–19.
13. Yu CC, Chiang KC, Kuo WL, Shen SC, Lo YF, Chen SC. Low re-excision rate for positive margins in patients treated with ultrasound-guided breast-conserving surgery. Breast. 2013;22:698–702.
14. Ramos M, Díaz JC, Ramos T, Ruano R, Aparicio M, Sancho M, et al. Ultrasound-guided excision combined with intraoperative assessment of gross macroscopic margins decreases the rate of reoperations for non-palpable invasive breast cancer. Breast. 2013;22:520–4.
15. Harlow SP, Krag DN, Ames SE, Weaver DL. Intraoperative ultrasound localization to guide surgical excision of nonpalpable breast carcinoma. J Am Coll Surg. 1999;189:241–6.
16. Moore MM, Whitney LA, Cerilli L, Imbrie JZ, Bunch M, Simpson VB, et al. Intraoperative ultrasound is associated with clear lumpectomy margins for palpable infiltrating ductal breast cancer. Ann Surg. 2001;233:761–8.
17. Fisher CS, Mushawah FA, Cyr AE, Gao F, Margenthaler JA. Ultrasound-guided lumpectomy for palpable breast cancers. Ann Surg Oncol. 2011;18:3198–203.
18. James TA, Harlow S, Sheehey-Jones J, Hart M, Gaspari C, al SM. Intraoperative ultrasound versus mammographic needle localization for ductal carcinoma in situ. Ann Surg Oncol. 2009;16:1164–9.
19. Bouton ME, Wilhelmson KL, Komenaka IK. Intraoperative ultrasound can facilitate the wire guided breast procedure for mammographic abnormalities. Am Surg. 2011;77:640–6.
20. Davis KM, Hsu CH, Bouton ME, Wilhelmson KL, Komenaka IK. Intraoperative ultrasound can decrease the re-excision lumpectomy rate in patients with palpable breast cancers. Am Surg. 2011;77:720–5.
21. Eichler C, Hubbel A, Zarghooni VThomas A, Gluz O, Stoff-Khalili M, et al. Intraoperative ultrasound: improved resection rates in breast-conserving surgery. Anticancer Res. 2012;32:1051–6.
22. Olsha O, Shemesh D, Carmon M, Sibirsky O, Abu Dalo R, Rivkin L, et al. Resection margins in ultrasound-guided breast-conserving surgery. Ann Surg Oncol. 2011;18:447–52.
23. Krekel NM, Lopes Cardozo AM, Muller S, Bergers E, Meijer S, van den Tol MP. Optimising surgical accuracy in palpable breast cancer with intra-operative breast ultrasound--feasibility and surgeons' learning curve. Eur J Surg Oncol. 2011;37:1044–50.
24. Krekel NM, Haloua MH, Lopes Cardozo AM, de Wit RH, Bosch AM, de Widt-Levert LM, et al. Intraoperative ultrasound guidance for palpable breast cancer excision (COBALT trial): a multicentre randomised controlled trial. Lancet Oncol. 2013;14:48–54.
25. Gittleman MA. Single-step ultrasound localization of breast lesions and lumpectomy procedure. Am J Surg. 2003;186:386–90.
26. Ivanovic N. Intraoperative ehosonography in the surgery of breast tumors. Belgrade: Foundation Andrejevic; 2013.
27. Ivanovic N, Zdravkovic D, Skuric Z, Kostic J, Colakovic N, Stojiljkovic M, et al. Optimization of breast cancer excision by intraoperative ultrasound and marking needle - technique description and feasibility. World Journal of Surgical Oncology. 2015;13:153.
28. DeJean P, Brackstone M, Fenster A. An intraoperative 3D ultrasound system for tumor margin determination in breast cancer surgery. Med Phys. 2010;37:564–70.
29. Karadeniz Cakmak G, Emre AU, Tascilar O, Bahadir B, Ozkan S. Surgeon performed continuous intraoperative ultrasound guidance decreases re-excisions and mastectomy rates in breast cancer. Breast. 2017;33:23–8.
30. Volders JH, Haloua MH, Krekel NM, Negenborn VL, Kolk RH, Lopes Cardozo AM, et al. Intraoperative ultrasound guidance in breast-conserving surgery shows superiority in oncological outcome, long-term cosmetic and patient-reported outcomes: Final outcomes of a randomized controlled trial (COBALT). Eur J Surg Oncol. 2017;43:649–57.
31. Haloua MH, Volders JH, Krekel NM, Lopes Cardozo AM, de Roos WK, de Widt-Levert LM, et al. Intraoperative ultrasound guidance in breast-conserving surgery improves cosmetic outcomes and patient satisfaction: results of a multicenter randomized controlled trial (COBALT). Ann Surg Oncol. 2016;23:30–7.
32. Rubio IT, Esgueva-Colmenarejo A, Espinosa-Bravo M, Salazar JP, Miranda I, Peg V. Intraoperative ultrasound-guided lumpectomy versus mammographic wire localization for breast cancer patients after neoadjuvant treatment. Ann Surg Oncol. 2016;23:38–43.
33. Klimberg S. Intraoperative image-guided breast-conservation surgery should be the gold standard. Ann Surg Oncol. 2016;23:4–5.

2

The combined effect of non-alcoholic fatty liver disease and metabolic syndrome on colorectal carcinoma mortality: a retrospective in Chinese females

Zhou-Feng Chen, Xiu-Li Dong, Qing-Ke Huang, Wang-Dong Hong, Wen-Zhi Wu, Jian-Sheng Wu and Shuang Pan[*]

Abstract

Background: This research aimed to investigate whether metabolic syndrome (MetS) and non-alcoholic fatty liver disease (NAFLD) had both individual and synergistic effects on the prognosis for female colorectal carcinoma (CRC) patients.

Methods: The relationship between CRC prognosis and NAFLD as well as MetS was evaluated in 764 female participants. Based on the NAFLD level, patients were divided into significant NAFLD (SNAFLD), "moderate" and "severe" level, and non-SNAFLD, "non" and "mild" level. All the patients were categorized into four subgroups according to the status of SNAFLD and MetS and then a comparison of CRC prognosis among those four groups was performed.

Results: NAFLD, SNAFLD, and MetS were independent factors for CRC-specific mortality with the adjustment of age and other confounders. The hazard ratio (HR) of CRC-specific mortality in MetS (+) SNAFLD (+) group was significantly higher than that in other three groups. Relative excess risk of interaction (RERI) was 2.203 with 95% CI ranged from 0.197 to 4.210, attributable proportion (AP) was 0.444 with range from 0.222 to 0.667, and synergy index (SI) of 2.256 with 95% CI from 1.252 to 4.065, indicating SNAFLD and MetS had a significant synergic effect on CRC-specific mortality.

Conclusions: SNAFLD and MetS are independent risk factors for CRC-specific mortality in females. Moreover, those two diseases have a synergistic effect on promoting CRC-specific mortality.

Keywords: Non-alcoholic fatty liver, Metabolic syndrome, Colorectal carcinoma, Prognosis

Background

Reports within the past few decades indicate that the incidence of colorectal carcinoma (CRC) has remarkably climbed, making it a worldwide prevalent cancer, including Asia [1]. In China, CRC has been one of the top contributors of cancer-related death, which will lead to poor quality of life in survivors [2–5]. As mentioned in previous literature reviews, the prognosis for CRC can be influenced by a variety of clinicopathological features [5]. Also, previous studies indicate that appropriate postoperative strategies can evidently improve the prognosis for CRC [6, 7]. Therefore, it is of urgent need to determine the adverse outcome-associated predictors for CRC patients.

Non-alcoholic fatty liver disease (NAFLD), a common issue worldwide, is induced by fat accumulation in the liver [8]. Numerous studies have discovered that NAFLD can promote the development of CRC [9]. Nonetheless, few studies are available concerning the association between NAFLD and CRC prognosis. Currently, only four studies have mentioned inconsistent results [10–13]. On the other hand, metabolic syndrome (MetS) is defined as a synergic syndrome involving different metabolic dysfunctions, including central obesity, hypertension, hyperglycemia, and dyslipidemia, which is also considered as a

* Correspondence: psdigestion@outlook.com
Department of Gastroenterology, The First Affiliated Hospital of Wenzhou Medical University, Wenzhou 325000, Zhejiang, People's Republic of China

risk factor of CRC occurrence [14]. However, the relationship between MetS and CRC prognosis remains a source of controversy. Some studies show that MetS will increase the risk of developing CRC and will lead to poor prognosis [9, 15], but other studies demonstrate that MetS exerts no apparent influence on CRC outcomes [16].

Both NAFLD and MetS are important risk factors of CRC, but the individual and synergistic effects of NAFLD and MetS on CRC prognosis remain unclear yet. Recently, NAFLD and MetS are considered to show reciprocal causality, and each singular one has perpetuating or exacerbating effect on the other [17–20]. Specifically, NAFLD is not a simple component of MetS. Besides, the synergetic effect of NAFLD and MetS has been proved in numerous diseases [21–23]. Also, it is shown in a large sample epidemiological investigation that NAFLD can only affect the cancer-specific mortality in females but not in males, indicating that a gender-dependent property may influence disease progression [13]. Therefore, to avoid the influence of gender-dependent features, only the female patients were focused in the present study. This study aimed to evaluate whether NAFLD and MetS had both individual and synergistic effects on the prognosis for female CRC patients.

Methods

Demographic data and laboratory measurements

CRC patients undergoing primary surgical resection from February 2007 to November 2014 at our hospital were collected. All subjects developed no distant metastasis at diagnosis. The patient exclusion criteria were as follows: (1) patients with a past cancer history and (2) those with familial adenomatous polyposis syndrome or hereditary nonpolyposis CRC. The demographic information and clinicopathological data, including body mass index (BMI), triglycerides (TGs), and other related blood parameters, were recorded in the hospital electronic medical system. Additionally, the sixth edition of the American Joint Committee on Cancer Staging Manual was employed to estimate the CRC stage.

Assessments of NAFLD and MetS

The severity of NAFLD was determined through hepatic ultrasound scan (Siemens, Germany) by experienced radiologists who were blinded to the CRC prognosis outcomes. The diagnosis criteria were as follows: patients with mild increase in liver echogenicity, mild attenuation in the penetration of ultrasound signal, and slightly decreased lucidity of the borders of intrahepatic vascular walls and diaphragm, and were identified as mild NAFLD; while those with diffuse increase in liver echogenicity, greater attenuation in the penetration of ultrasound signal

and decrease in the visualization of intrahepatic vascular walls, particularly the peripheral branches, were deemed as moderate NAFLD; and those with gross increase in liver echogenicity, greater reduction in the penetration of ultrasound signal, and poor or no visualization of intrahepatic vascular walls and diaphragm were considered as severe NAFLD [24, 25]. Among them, moderate and severe NAFLD were combined as significant NAFLD (SNAFLD).

MetS was defined with reference to the definition in Diabetes Society of Chinese Medical Association [26]. Specifically, patients presenting at least three of the following items were considered as MetS: (i) BMI of $\geq$ 25 kg/m^2, (ii) patients receiving anti-hypertensive medicine treatment with (or) the systolic blood pressure (SBP) of $\geq$ 140 mmHg or diastolic blood pressure (DBP) of $\geq$ 90 mmHg, (iii) TG of $\geq$ 1.7 mmol/L and (or) HDL of < 0.9 mmol/L (male) or < 1.0 mmol/L (female), and (iv) fasting plasma glucose (FPG) of $\geq$ 6.1 mmol/L or 2-h postprandial glucose of $\geq$ 7.8 mmol/L.

Follow-up

Patients should be reexamined every 3–6 months within the first 2 years after surgery, then every 6 months for the following 5 years, and every 1 year thereafter. During every follow-up, the NAFLD status was re-verified and results in the last follow-up were acquired. Moreover, imaging findings, cytology or biopsy were systematically applied to estimate the recurrence. Moreover, the overall survival (OS) and recurrence-free survival (RFS) were recorded from the date of surgery to the date of CRC-specific death/last follow-up and recurrence/last follow-up date, respectively.

This study was approved by the Ethics Committee of Wenzhou Medical University First Affiliated Hospital, and each subject had signed an informed consent for participation. Additionally, the Helsinki and Strengthening the Reporting of Observational Studies in Epidemiology (STROBE) statement was strictly observed during the whole procedures [27].

Statistics

SPSS 20.0 software (SPSS, Chicago, IL, USA) was employed for statistical analysis. The data were expressed as mean ± standard deviation (SD) or percentages. OS and RFS rates were calculated and compared using the Kaplan-Meier survival curves with log-rank tests. All variables were initially estimated through univariate Cox proportional hazard regression analysis, and only statistically significant variables were incorporated into multivariate Cox analysis. A two-sided p value of < 0.05 was considered as statistically significant.

All subjects were categorized into four subgroups according to the SNAFLD and MetS status. Then, the hazard ratio (HR) was calculated in the multivariate Cox analysis after adjusted age, CEA, stage, tumor location, and tumor differentiation. Additionally, the relative excess risk due to interaction (RERI), attributable proportion (AP), and synergy index (SI) [28] were utilized to estimate the synergistic interactions of SNAFLD and MetS on CRC-specific mortality. The ranges of RERI and AP including 0 or that of SI including 1 indicated no synergistic effect, while a RERI of > 0, AP of > 0, or SI of > 1 suggested the presence of combined biological interaction.

Results

Prognosis related factors

Table 1 showed all the demographic and clinicopathological results. A total of 764 subjects were enrolled, including 196 (25.7%) with MetS and 568 (74.3%) with non-MetS. Specifically, there were 186 (32.7%) and 382 (67.3%) NAFLD and non-NAFLD patients without MetS, respectively. Additionally, there were 130 (66.3%) and 66 (33.7%) MetS subjects with and without NAFLD, respectively.

The mean follow-up duration was 21.3 ± 17.1 months. Meanwhile, 152 (19.9%) and 139 (18.2%) patients had presented CRC-induced death and recurrence, respectively.

The levels of high-density lipoprotein (HDL) cholesterol and low-density lipoprotein (LDL) cholesterol, as well as tumor differentiation and stage were related to mortality in univariate Cox analysis, as shown in Table 2. Additionally, MetS, NAFLD, and moderate/severe NAFLD were also the predictors of mortality in univariate Cox analysis. Subsequently, all significant variables were incorporated into multivariate Cox analysis, the results of which indicated that MetS, NAFLD, and moderate/severe NAFLD were the independent factors associated with mortality. For recurrence, only MetS was the significant predictor in both univariate and multivariate Cox analyses (Table 3).

Synergic effect of SNAFLD and MetS on CRC-specific mortality

The above-mentioned results indicated that "moderate" and "severe" NAFLD had exerted significant positive hazard ratios (HRs) on the CRC-specific mortality, which could not be observed in "mild" NAFLD. Thus, the "non" and "mild" NAFLD were merged into the non-significant NAFLD (non-SNAFLD) group, whereas the other two subgroups, namely, moderate and severe NAFLD, were defined as SNAFLD. Thus, all patients

Table 1 Characteristics of participants categorized by metabolic syndrome and NAFLD status

Characteristics	Metabolic syndrome (−)		Metabolic syndrome (+)	
	NAFLD (−)	NAFLD (+)	NAFLD (−)	NAFLD (+)
Total number	382 (67.3)	186 (32.7)	66 (33.7)	130 (66.3)
Age at diagnosis (years)	50.02 ± 10.31	51.21 ± 11.96	49.92 ± 12.11	51.82 ± 12.31
BMI (kg/m²)	22.42 ± 4.07	22.96 ± 4.26	24.81 ± 3.49	25.92 ± 4.23
SBP (mmHg)	116.67 ± 20.27	120.58 ± 22.32	132.31 ± 20.12	133.32 ± 20.21
DBP (mmHg)	76.62 ± 10.31	74.91 ± 11.31	77.91 ± 9.91	78.31 ± 10.02
Triglycerides (mmol/L)	1.54 ± 1.87	1.62 ± 1.71	2.21 ± 1.55	2.52 ± 1.81
HDL (mmol/L)	1.20 ± 0.312	1.28 ± 0.323	1.32 ± 0.372	1.33 ± 0.298
LDL (mmol/L)	2.52 ± 1.19	2.61 ± 1.21	2.48 ± 1.02	2.50 ± 0.98
Fasting glucose (mmol/L)	5.01 ± 3.11	5.09 ± 2.76	5.39 ± 3.51	5.50 ± 3.42
CEA (ng/ml)	21.0 ± 101.4	22.7 ± 102.1	23.2 ± 98.7	22.7 ± 101.0
Differentiation				
Well/moderate	310 (81.2)	149 (80.1)	55 (83.3)	102 (78.5)
Poorly	72 (18.8)	37 (19.9)	11 (16.7)	28 (21.5)
Stage				
I	68 (17.8)	41 (22.0)	11 (16.7)	21 (16.2)
II	164 (42.9)	87 (46.7)	25 (37.8)	47 (36.2)
III	150 (39.3)	58 (31.2)	30 (45.5)	62 (47.6)
Location				
Ascending, transverse, and descending	102 (26.7)	40 (21.5)	22 (33.3)	36 (27.7)
Sigmoid	108 (28.3)	54 (29.0)	17 (25.8)	32 (24.6)
Rectum	172 (45.0)	92 (49.5)	27 (40.9)	62 (47.7)

NAFLD non-alcoholic fatty livers disease, *BMI* body mass index, *SBP* systolic blood pressure, *DBP* diastolic blood pressure, *HDL* high-density lipoprotein, *LDL* low-density lipoprotein
Data are expressed as mean ± standard deviation and *n* (%)

Table 2 Cancer-specific mortality

Characteristics	Univariable			Multivariable		
	HR	95% CI	p value	HR	95%CI	p value
Age (years)	1.021	0.983–1.111	0.401			
BMI (kg/m²)	0.932	0.821–1.120	0.212			
SBP (mmHg)	1.122	0.913–1.342	0.514			
DBP (mmHg)	0.932	0.821–1.104	0.314			
Triglycerides (mmol/L)	0.915	0.832–1.214	0.423			
HDL (mmol/L)	1.224	1.192–1.913	0.021*	1.201	0.925–1.651	0.312
LDL (mmol/L)	1.231	1.017–1.453	0.015*	1.218	0.941–2.092	0.513
Fasting glucose (mmol/L)	1.011	0.932–1.329	0.614			
CEA (ng/ml)	1.102	0.962–1.322	0.070			
Differentiation	0.912	0.813–0.968	0.010*	0.858	0.771–0.972	0.025*
Location	1.225	0.832–1.564	0.243			
Ascending, transverse, and descending	1.000					
Sigmoid	1.132	0.923–1.231	0.632			
Rectum	1.342	0.831–1.532	0.452			
Stage	1.332	1.024–2.012	0.002*	1.523	1.132–2.432	0.009*
I	1.000			1.000		
II	1.028	0.821–1.223	0.298	1.131	0.882–1.251	0.328
III	2.852	1.852–3.832	0.001*	2.432	1.632–3.212	0.001*
MetS	1.621	1.221–2.133	0.007*	1.558	1.153–2.012	0.012*
NAFLD	1.544	1.031–1.893	0.010*	1.494	1.126–1.961	0.015*
Non	1.000			1.000		
Mild	1.101	0.821–1.231	0.401	1.121	0.901–1.314	0.212
Moderate	1.452	1.113–2.371	0.001*	1.501	1.161–2.481	0.010*
Severe	1.612	1.224–2.471	0.010*	1.631	1.231–2.531	0.005*

NAFLD, non-alcoholic fatty livers disease, *MetS* metabolic syndrome, *BMI* body mass index, *SBP* systolic blood pressure, *DBP* diastolic blood pressure, *HDL* high-density lipoprotein, *LDL* low-density lipoprotein
*represent the p value ≤ 0.05

were categorized into four subgroups according to their MetS and SNAFLD status (Table 4). After adjusting the age, CEA, stage, tumor location, and differentiation, the HRs were 1.845 (95%CI: 1.024–3.323), 1.910 (95%CI: 1.254–2.908), and 4.958 (95%CI: 2.710–9.071) for MetS(+)SNAFLD(−), MetS(−)SNAFLD(+), and MetS(+)SNAFLD(+) compared with MetS(−)SNAFLD(−), respectively. In addition, the OS rates were the lowest in MetS(+)SNAFLD(+) group compared with those in the other three groups during the follow-up period (Fig. 1). On the other hand, RERI was 2.203 (95% CI, 0.197–4.210), suggesting that the synergistic interaction had increased the relative excess risks by 2.203 times. In addition, the AP was 0.444 (95% CI, 0.222–0.667), indicating that 44.4% CRC-specific mortality was resulted from both factors contributing to the combined interaction. Additionally, the SI was 2.256 (95% CI, 1.252–4.065), suggesting that the risk of mortality in both positive patients was 2.256 times as high as the

sum of risks in patients presenting only one singular factor.

Discussion

The underlying interaction between MetS and CRC prognosis has not been fully understandable yet. As mentioned in literature review, MetS is a well-known promoter of CRC [29–32] but is still controversial on prognosis. In our study, MetS is found to be independently associated with the recurrence and CRC-specific mortality in females, which is consistent with some previous researches. MetS is found in studies to be related to CRC mortality in both males and females [33–37]. Also, a strong relationship between MetS and recurrence has been reported in another study in both genders [15]. Moreover, Shen Z et al. [38] indicated that MetS contributed to high mortality and high recurrence in both female and male patients. However, a few results seem to be opposite, which discover that

Table 3 Cox analysis of risk factors associated with recurrence

Characteristics	Univariable			Multivariable		
	HR	95% CI	p value	HR	95%CI	p value
Age (years)	1.105	0.965–1.241	0.314			
BMI (kg/m^2)	1.165	0.823–1.284	0.287			
SBP (mmHg)	1.112	0.963–1.323	0.432			
DBP (mmHg)	1.223	0.932–1.444	0.642			
Triglycerides (mmol/L)	1.013	0.862–1.152	0.426			
HDL (mmol/L)	1.104	1.013–1.324	0.023*	1.312	0.913–1.632	0.452
LDL (mmol/L)	1.342	0.982–1.552	0.313			
Fasting glucose (mmol/L)	1.122	0.951–1.302	0.524			
CEA (ng/ml)	1.123	1.032–1.452	0.014*	1.127	0.972–1.516	0.292
Differentiation	0.882	0.823–0.965	0.009*	0.904	0.832–1.176	0.128
Location	1.302	0.921–1.542	0.392			
Ascending, transverse, and descending	1.000					
Sigmoid	1.242	0.927–1.423	0.542			
Rectum	1.132	0.912–1.402	0.356			
Stage	1.322	1.095–1.932	0.011*	1.522	1.312–1.923	0.008*
I	1.000			1.000		
II	1.092	0.902–1.123	0.223	1.223	0.922–1.433	0.321
III	2.123	1.232–2.873	0.001*	1.923	1.321–2.923	0.001*
MetS	1.722	1.224–2.722	0.020*	1.821	1.164–3.121	0.010*
NAFLD	1.542	0.935–2.226	0.109			
Non	1.000					
Mild	1.097	0.913–1.198	0.312			
Moderate	1.431	0.921–2.216	0.197			
Severe	1.582	0.945–2.368	0.210			

NAFLD, non-alcoholic fatty livers disease, MetS metabolic syndrome, BMI body mass index, SBP systolic blood pressure, DBP diastolic blood pressure, HDL high-density lipoprotein, LDL low-density lipoprotein
*represent the p value ≤ 0.05

there is no association between Mets and CRC prognosis [16]. Typically, our study utilized the Chinese criterion to identify MetS, which is slightly different from the definition in other studies. In addition, most patients in the present study come from southeast China, where the diet and heredity are unique, for example, the high seafood consumption compared to other regions. It is discovered upon literature review that different MetS criteria and races can affect the outcomes [39–41], which may account for the possible explanation for those opposite results.

With regard to NAFLD, only four existing studies have concentrated on the association between NAFLD and

Table 4 Interaction analysis between metabolic syndrome and SNAFLD status on mortality

Subgroup		Case	Total number	HR (95% CI)	p value
MetS(−)SNAFLD(−)		62 (12.4)	500	1.000	
MetS(+)SNAFLD(−)		49 (31.8)	154	1.845 (1.024–3.323)	0.012*
MetS(−)SNAFLD(+)		21 (30.9)	68	1.910 (1.254–2.908)	0.010*
MetS(+)SNAFLD(+)		23 (54.8)	42	4.958 (2.710–9.071)	0.004*
RERI	2.203 (0.197–4.210)				
AP	0.444 (0.222–0.667)				
SI	2.256 (1.252–4.065)				

SNAFLD, significant non-alcoholic fatty livers disease, MetS metabolic syndrome
*represent the p value < 0.05. MetS metabolic syndrome, SNAFLD significant non-alcoholic fatty liver disease

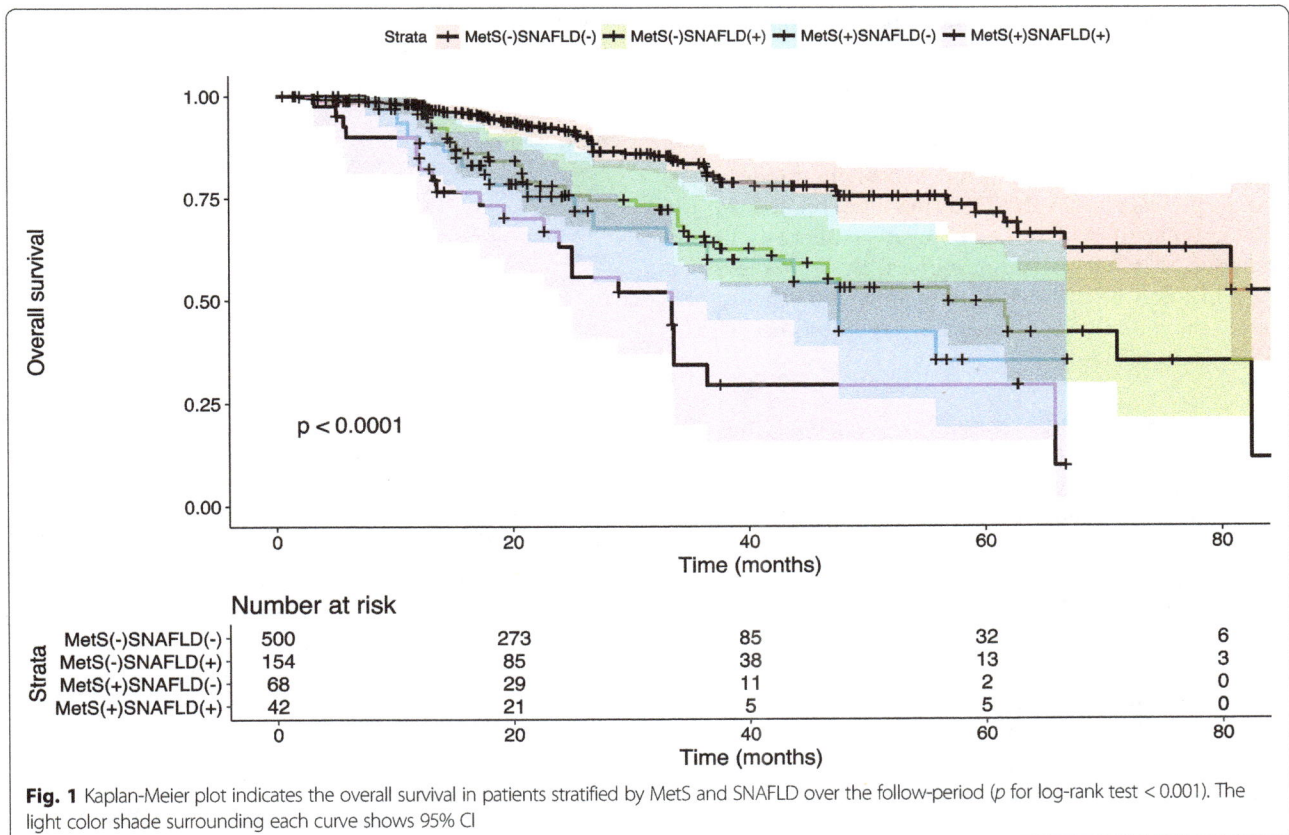

Fig. 1 Kaplan-Meier plot indicates the overall survival in patients stratified by MetS and SNAFLD over the follow-period (*p* for log-rank test < 0.001). The light color shade surrounding each curve shows 95% CI

CRC prognosis. For instance, Min YW et al. [10] indicated that there was no apparent influence of NAFLD on CRC prognosis by investigating 227 male and female participants. Oppositely, You et al. [11] enrolled 1314 male and females CRC patients and found that NAFLD was negatively related to OS. However, another study had collected 953 CRC patients and divided them into two subgroups based on the hepatic fibrosis level rather than NALFD alone. Their results demonstrated that a high hepatic fibrosis level was related to liver metastasis [12]. Additionally, Hwang YC et al. [13] investigated 318,224 Korean subjects and indicated that NAFLD was positively associated with mortality in females but not in males. Our findings indicate that NAFLD is remarkably related to mortality and not recurrence in female CRC patients. Typically, there are several differences between previous and our studies. First of all, most previous studies do not evaluate the gender-dependent issue. Except that, three out of four studies simply classify patients into NAFLD and non-NAFLD, and only one has further categorized NALFD based on the hepatic fibrosis level. By contrast, our study has divided patients into four different levels, including "non," "mild," "moderate," and "severe" NALFD, and the results indicate no difference between "non" and "mild" NAFLD regarding mortality,

which may partially explain the opposite results among different studies. Taken together, our study design is different from the previous ones, which may induce the different results.

The primary results demonstrate no difference between "non" and "mild" NAFLD regarding mortality. Thus, the "moderate" and "severe" NAFLD groups are merged into the SNAFLD group, while the non-SNAFLD consists of "non" and "mild" SNAFLD correspondingly. Accompanied with MetS and non-MetS status, subjects are categorized into four subgroups, and the results demonstrate that there is significant combined effect of those two factors on the CRC-specific mortality. In summary, the results have suggested a powerful synergistic interaction of those two diseases on mortality, which lead to a higher risk than that of either SNAFLD or MetS alone.

Currently, it is difficult to explain this phenomenon, but it may be partly explained by the following hypothesis. As mentioned in the literature review, MetS can induce CRC tumorigenesis and progression through multiple mechanisms, for instance, the inflammatory cytokines [42]. Nonetheless, the pathophysiological link between NAFLD and CRC prognosis remains incompletely understood. NAFLD encompasses a histological process that starts from a simple steatosis (with only fat accumulation in hepatocytes but without inflammation) to moderate and severe forms of NAFLD, such as steatohepatitis, a condition in which hepatic steatosis is accompanied by a necroinflammatory component. Inflammation is attributable to different tumor stages, which may even influence the mortality [43, 44]. Thus, the moderate or severe but not mild NAFLD may be related to the CRC-specific mortality. Taken together, there is an assumption that inflammation, induced by both MetS and SNAFLD, may be the common underlying mechanism affecting the mortality. However, this hypothesis needs to be further studied.

For the first time, this research has evaluated the synergetic influence of SNAFLD and MetS on female CRC-specific mortality. However, there are several limitations in the current study. Firstly, this is an observational study, and no results are available concerning the underlying mechanism. Secondly, the short follow-up period and data collection from only one center may weaken the clinical significance, which should be improved by extending the follow-up duration and implementing in multiple centers. Besides, to avoid gender influence, only females are investigated in the current study. Finally, a Chinese version of MetS definition, which is not worldwide applied, is applied in this study, due to the specific characteristics of patients. But this criterion has been specialized for the Chinese population and has been utilized among various diseases.

Conclusions

It is identified in this study that SNAFLD can affect mortality but not the recurrence in female CRC patients, while MetS can affect both the recurrence and mortality. These results have complemented the field regarding the associations among SNAFLD, MetS, and prognosis in female CRC patients. In addition, the research also suggests a synergistic interaction of those two factors on the CRC-specific mortality. In general, it seems that it is urgently needed to carry out extra postoperative management to control the mortality among Chinese female CRC patients who have both SNAFLD and MetS.

Abbreviations
(HDL) cholesterol: High-density lipoprotein; (LDL) cholesterol: Low-density lipoprotein; AP: Attributable proportion; BMI: Body mass index; CRC: Colorectal carcinoma; DBP: Diastolic blood pressure; MetS: Metabolic syndrome; NAFLD: Non-alcoholic fatty liver disease; OS: Overall survival; RERI: Relative excess risk of interaction; RFS: Recurrence-free survival; SBP: Systolic blood pressure; SI: Synergy index; TGs: Triglycerides

Funding
This study was financed by research grants from the Science and Technology Project of Wenzhou City (2014Y0086).

Authors' contributions
All authors have sufficiently contributed to the study. SP and Z-FC conceived of the study, participated in its design and coordination, and helped to draft the manuscript. Z-FC, X-LD, and Q-KH contributed to the data collection. W-DH, W-ZW, and J-SW conceived of the study, participated in its design, and helped to draft the manuscript. All authors read and approved the final manuscript.

Competing interests
The authors declare that they have no competing interests.

References
1. Ford ES, Giles WH, Dietz WH. Prevalence of the metabolic syndrome among US adults: findings from the third National Health and Nutrition Examination Survey. JAMA. 2002;287:356–9.
2. Fang JY, Dong HL, Sang XJ, Xie B, Wu KS, Du PL, Xu ZX, Jia XY, Lin K. Colorectal cancer mortality characteristics and predictions in China, 1991-2011. Asian Pac J Cancer Prev. 2015;16:7991–5.
3. Wang JW, Sun L, Ding N, Li J, Gong XH, Chen XF, Yu DH, Luo ZN, Yuan ZP, Yu JM. The association between comorbidities and the quality of life among colorectal cancer survivors in the People's Republic of China. Patient Prefer Adherence. 2016;10:1071–7.
4. Li M, Wang S, Han X, Liu W, Song J, Zhang H, Zhao J, Yang F, Tan X, Chen X, et al. Cancer mortality trends in an industrial district of Shanghai, China, from 1974 to 2014, and projections to 2029. Oncotarget. 2017;8:92470–82.
5. Yang J, Du XL, Li S, Wu Y, Lv M, Dong D, Zhang L, Chen Z, Wang B, Wang F, et al. The risk and survival outcome of subsequent primary colorectal cancer after the first primary colorectal cancer: cases from 1973 to 2012. BMC Cancer. 2017;17:783.
6. Pita-Fernandez S, Alhayek-Ai M, Gonzalez-Martin C, Lopez-Calvino B, Seoane-Pillado T, Pertega-Diaz S. Intensive follow-up strategies improve outcomes in nonmetastatic colorectal cancer patients after curative surgery: a systematic review and meta-analysis. Ann Oncol. 2015;26:644–56.
7. Yang KM, Yu CS, Lee JL, Kim CW, Yoon YS, Park IJ, Lim SB, Kim JC. The long-term outcomes of recurrent adhesive small bowel obstruction after colorectal cancer surgery favor surgical management. Medicine (Baltimore). 2017;96:e8316.
8. Dongiovanni P, Stender S, Pietrelli A, Mancina RM, Cespiati A, Petta S, Pelusi S, Pingitore P, Badiali S, Maggioni M, et al. Causal relationship of hepatic fat with liver damage and insulin resistance in nonalcoholic fatty liver. J Intern Med. 2018;283:356–70.
9. Muhidin SO, Magan AA, Osman KA, Syed S, Ahmed MH. The relationship between nonalcoholic fatty liver disease and colorectal cancer: the future challenges and outcomes of the metabolic syndrome. J Obes. 2012;2012:637538.
10. Min YW, Yun HS, Chang WI, Kim JY, Kim YH, Son HJ, Kim JJ, Rhee JC, Chang DK. Influence of non-alcoholic fatty liver disease on the prognosis in patients with colorectal cancer. Clin Res Hepatol Gastroenterol. 2012;36:78–83.
11. You J, Huang S, Huang GQ, Zhu GQ, Ma RM, Liu WY, Shi KQ, Guo GL, Chen YP, Braddock M, Zheng MH. Nonalcoholic fatty liver disease: a negative risk factor for colorectal cancer prognosis. Medicine (Baltimore). 2015;94:e479.
12. Kondo T, Okabayashi K, Hasegawa H, Tsuruta M, Shigeta K, Kitagawa Y. The impact of hepatic fibrosis on the incidence of liver metastasis from colorectal cancer. Br J Cancer. 2016;115:34–9.
13. Hwang YC, Ahn HY, Park SW, Park CY. Non-alcoholic fatty liver disease associates with increased overall mortality and death from cancer,

cardiovascular disease, and liver disease in women but not men. Clin Gastroenterol Hepatol. 2018;16:1131-7. e1135.

14. Stocks T, Lukanova A, Johansson M, Rinaldi S, Palmqvist R, Hallmans G, Kaaks R, Stattin P. Components of the metabolic syndrome and colorectal cancer risk; a prospective study. Int J Obes. 2008;32:304-14.

15. You J, Liu WY, Zhu GQ, Wang OC, Ma RM, Huang GQ, Shi KQ, Guo GL, Braddock M, Zheng MH. Metabolic syndrome contributes to an increased recurrence risk of non-metastatic colorectal cancer. Oncotarget. 2015;6: 19880-90.

16. Yang Y, Mauldin PD, Ebeling M, Hulsey TC, Liu B, Thomas MB, Camp ER, Esnaola NF. Effect of metabolic syndrome and its components on recurrence and survival in colon cancer patients. Cancer. 2013;119:1512-20.

17. Niebergall LJ, Jacobs RL, Chaba T, Vance DE. Phosphatidylcholine protects against steatosis in mice but not non-alcoholic steatohepatitis. Biochim Biophys Acta. 1811;2011:1177-85.

18. Jacobs RL, Zhao Y, Koonen DP, Sletten T, Su B, Lingrell S, Cao G, Peake DA, Kuo MS, Proctor SD, et al. Impaired de novo choline synthesis explains why phosphatidylethanolamine N-methyltransferase-deficient mice are protected from diet-induced obesity. J Biol Chem. 2010;285:22403-13.

19. Shen J, Wong GL, Chan HL, Chan HY, Yeung DK, Chan RS, Chim AM, Chan AW, Choi PC, Woo J, et al. PNPLA3 gene polymorphism accounts for fatty liver in community subjects without metabolic syndrome. Aliment Pharmacol Ther. 2014;39:532-9.

20. Wainwright P, Byrne CD. Bidirectional relationships and disconnects between NAFLD and features of the metabolic syndrome. Int J Mol Sci. 2016;17:367.

21. Russo GI, Cimino S, Castelli T, Favilla V, Gacci M, Carini M, Condorelli RA, La Vignera S, Calogero AE, Motta F, et al. Benign prostatic hyperplasia, metabolic syndrome and non-alcoholic fatty liver disease: is metaflammation the link? Prostate. 2016;76:1528-35.

22. Hong HC, Hwang SY, Ryu JY, Yoo HJ, Seo JA, Kim SG, Kim NH, Baik SH, Choi DS, Choi KM. The synergistic impact of nonalcoholic fatty liver disease and metabolic syndrome on subclinical atherosclerosis. Clin Endocrinol (Oxf). 2016; 84:203-9.

23. Pan S, Hong W, Wu W, Chen Q, Zhao Q, Wu J, Jin Y. The relationship of nonalcoholic fatty liver disease and metabolic syndrome for colonoscopy colorectal neoplasm. Medicine (Baltimore). 2017;96:e5809.

24. Obika M, Noguchi H. Diagnosis and evaluation of nonalcoholic fatty liver disease. Exp Diabetes Res. 2012;2012:145754.

25. Saverymuttu SH, Joseph AE, Maxwell JD. Ultrasound scanning in the detection of hepatic fibrosis and steatosis. Br Med J (Clin Res Ed). 1986;292:13-5.

26. Cooperative Group for the Study of Metabolic Syndrome in Chinese Diabetes Society. Recommendations of Chinese Medical Association Diabetes Society for metabolic syndrome. Chinese Journal of Diabetes. 2004;12(3):156-61.

27. Vandenbroucke JP, von Elm E, Altman DG, Gotzsche PC, Mulrow CD, Pocock SJ, Poole C, Schlesselman JJ, Egger M, Initiative S. Strengthening the reporting of observational studies in epidemiology (STROBE): explanation and elaboration. Epidemiology. 2007;18:805-35.

28. Knol MJ, VanderWeele TJ, Groenwold RH, Klungel OH, Rovers MM, Grobbee DE. Estimating measures of interaction on an additive scale for preventive exposures. Eur J Epidemiol. 2011;26:433-8.

29. Hwang ST, Cho YK, Park JH, Kim HJ, Park DI, Sohn CI, Jeon WK, Kim BI, Won KH, Jin W. Relationship of non-alcoholic fatty liver disease to colorectal adenomatous polyps. J Gastroenterol Hepatol. 2010;25:562-7.

30. Fiori E, Lamazza A, De Masi E, Schillaci A, Crocetti D, Antoniozzi A, Sterpetti AV, De Toma G. Association of liver steatosis with colorectal cancer and adenoma in patients with metabolic syndrome. Anticancer Res. 2015;35:2211-4.

31. Trabulo D, Ribeiro S, Martins C, Teixeira C, Cardoso C, Mangualde J, Freire R, Gamito E, Alves AL, Augusto F, et al. Metabolic syndrome and colorectal neoplasms: an ominous association. World J Gastroenterol. 2015;21:5320-7.

32. Kabat GC, Kim MY, Peters U, Stefanick M, Hou L, Wactawski-Wende J, Messina C, Shikany JM, Rohan TE. A longitudinal study of the metabolic syndrome and risk of colorectal cancer in postmenopausal women. Eur J Cancer Prev. 2012;21:326-32.

33. Jaggers JR, Sui X, Hooker SP, LaMonte MJ, Matthews CE, Hand GA, Blair SN. Metabolic syndrome and risk of cancer mortality in men. Eur J Cancer. 2009; 45:1831-8.

34. Peng F, Hu D, Lin X, Chen G, Liang B, Zhang H, Ji K, Huang J, Lin J, Zheng X, Niu W. Preoperative metabolic syndrome and prognosis after radical resection for colorectal cancer: the Fujian prospective investigation of cancer (FIESTA) study. Int J Cancer. 2016;139:2705-13.

35. Trevisan M, Liu J, Muti P, Misciagna G, Menotti A, Fucci F, Risk F, Life Expectancy Research G. Markers of insulin resistance and colorectal cancer mortality. Cancer Epidemiol Biomark Prev. 2001;10:937-41.

36. Colangelo LA, Gapstur SM, Gann PH, Dyer AR, Liu K. Colorectal cancer mortality and factors related to the insulin resistance syndrome. Cancer Epidemiol Biomark Prev. 2002;11:385-91.

37. Cespedes Feliciano EM, Kroenke CH, Meyerhardt JA, Prado CM, Bradshaw PT, Dannenberg AJ, Kwan ML, Xiao J, Quesenberry C, Weltzien EK, et al. Metabolic dysfunction, obesity, and survival among patients with early-stage colorectal cancer. J Clin Oncol. 2016;34(30):3664.

38. Shen Z, Wang S, Ye Y, Yin M, Yang X, Jiang K, Liu Y. Clinical study on the correlation between metabolic syndrome and colorectal carcinoma. ANZ J Surg. 2010;80:331-6.

39. Esposito K, Chiodini P, Capuano A, Bellastella G, Maiorino MI, Rafaniello C, Panagiotakos DB, Giugliano D. Colorectal cancer association with metabolic syndrome and its components: a systematic review with meta-analysis. Endocrine. 2013;44:634-47.

40. National Cholesterol Education Program Expert Panel on Detection E, Treatment of High Blood Cholesterol in A. Third report of the National Cholesterol Education Program (NCEP) Expert Panel on Detection, Evaluation, and Treatment of High Blood Cholesterol in Adults (Adult Treatment Panel III) final report. Circulation. 2002;106:3143-421.

41. Aykan AC, Gul I, Kalaycioglu E, Gokdeniz T, Hatem E, Mentese U, Yildiz BS, Yildiz M. Is metabolic syndrome related with coronary artery disease severity and complexity: an observational study about IDF and AHA/NHLBI metabolic syndrome definitions. Cardiol J. 2014;21:245-51.

42. Hursting SD, Hursting MJ. Growth signals, inflammation, and vascular perturbations: mechanistic links between obesity, metabolic syndrome, and cancer. Arterioscler Thromb Vasc Biol. 2012;32:1766-70.

43. Crawford S. Anti-inflammatory/antioxidant use in long-term maintenance cancer therapy: a new therapeutic approach to disease progression and recurrence. Ther Adv Med Oncol. 2014;6:52-68.

44. Wang S, Liu Z, Wang L, Zhang X. NF-kappaB signaling pathway, inflammation and colorectal cancer. Cell Mol Immunol. 2009;6:327-34.

3

Safflower polysaccharide inhibits the development of tongue squamous cell carcinoma

Haiyan Zhou[1,2†], Jing Yang[3†], Chuhan Zhang[2], Yuwei Zhang[3], Rui Wang[4], Xiao Li[1,2*] and Shuainan Zhang[5*]

Abstract

Background: Safflower polysaccharide (SPS) is one of the most important active components of safflower (*Carthamus tinctorius* L.), which has been confirmed to have the immune-regulatory function and antitumor effect. This study aimed to explore the effects of safflower polysaccharide (SPS) on tongue squamous cell carcinoma (TSCC).

Methods: HN-6 cells were treated with 5 µg/mL cisplatin and various concentrations of SPS (0, 0.02, 0.04, 0.08, 0.16, 0.32, 0.64, and 1.28 mg/mL), and cell proliferation was measured. After treatment with 5 µg/mL cisplatin and 0.64 mg/mL SPS, the induction of apoptosis and the protein and mRNA expression of Bax, Bcl-2, COX-2, and cleaved caspase-3 in HN-6 cells were quantified. In addition, HN-6 cells were implanted into mice to establish an in vivo tumor xenograft model. Animals were randomly assigned to three groups: SPS treatment, cisplatin treatment, and the model group (no treatment). The body weight, tumor volume, and tumor weight were measured, and the expression of the above molecules was determined.

Results: SPS treatment (0.02–0.64 mg/mL) for 24–72 h inhibited HN-6 cell proliferation. In addition, 0.64 mg/mL SFP markedly induced apoptosis in HN-6 cells and arrested the cell cycle at the G0/G1 phase. Compared with the control group, the expression of Bcl-2 and COX-2 was markedly reduced by SPS treatment, whereas the expression of Bax and cleaved caspase-3 was increased. Moreover, SPS significantly inhibited the growth of the tumor xenograft, with similar changes in the expression of Bcl-2, COX-2, Bax, and cleaved caspase-3 in the tumor xenograft to the in vitro analysis.

Conclusions: Our results indicated that SPS may inhibit TSCC development through regulation of Bcl-2, COX-2, Bax, and cleaved caspase-3 expression.

Keywords: Safflower polysaccharide, Tongue squamous cell carcinoma, Apoptosis, Bcl-2, COX-2, Bax, Cleaved caspase-3

Background

Tongue squamous cell carcinoma (TSCC) is a primary malignant tumor of the tongue, with the highest incidence rate (approximately 39.95%) among oral cancers [1]. With early detection, TSCC can be cured with proper treatment; however, after tumor metastasis, the 5-year overall survival rate is below 50% [2–4]. Therefore, the research and development of effective drugs and methods for the treatment of TSCC would have far-reaching consequences.

* Correspondence: Sherley_Li656@hotmial.com; laurahoney@163.com
†Haiyan Zhou and Jing Yang contributed equally to this work.
[1]Department of Cleft Palate Speech, The First Affiliated Hospital of Harbin Medical University, Harbin 150001, People's Republic of China
[5]Department of Pharmacy, Guiyang University of Chinese Medicine, Guiyang 550025, People's Republic of China
Full list of author information is available at the end of the article

Safflower (*Carthamus tinctorius* L.) is a herbaceous plant of the Asteraceae family, containing various active constituents, including flavonoids, quinochalcones, alkaloids, and safflower polysaccharides (SPS) [5]. Safflower exerts various biological effects, including antioxidant [6], anti-inflammatory [7], and antibacterial [8] activities, and is reported to be beneficial for the improvement of acute cerebral infarction [9] and ischemic stroke [10]. SPS is one of the most important active components of safflower, and accumulating evidences have supported the immuno-regulatory function and antitumor effect of SPS [11–13]. In breast cancer, SPS is shown to inhibit the MCF-7 cell proliferation and metastasis [14]. SPS is also found to inhibit proliferation of human hepatic cancer SMMC-7721 cells through the regulation of the expression of cell cycle-related genes [15]. Moreover, SPS is confirmed to affect cell growth and apoptosis in non-small cell lung cancer [16], gastric cancer [17–19], and colorectal cancer [20]. However, the role of SPS in the development of TSCC remains unexplored.

In this study, we detected the effect of SPS on HN-6 cell proliferation and apoptosis. Moreover, HN-6 cells were implanted into mice to establish an in vivo tumor xenograft model for the assessment of the effect of SPS on tumor growth. The present study investigated the roles and regulatory mechanism of SPS in TSCC to provide new strategies for TSCC therapy.

Methods

SPS preparation

The crude drug containing SPS was purchased from Shiyitang Co., Ltd. (Harbin, PR China), and voucher specimens (No. HLJ-2015008) were deposited at College of Basic Medical Science, Heilongjiang University of Chinese Medicine. The crude drug was dried at 60 °C in a vacuum oven for 24 h and extracted four times in boiling water with agitation for 1 h. The extracts were filtered, concentrated, and precipitated with four volumes of 95% ethanol at 4 °C for 24 h. The mixture was centrifuged, and the sediment was dried at 60 °C in a vacuum oven. The protein contaminants were extracted with Sevage reagent (a 4:1 (v/v) mixture of chloroform to n-butyl alcohol) and removed by centrifugation; this process was repeated 10 times. The water phase was then precipitated in four volumes of 95% ethanol. The sediments were oven-dried at 60 °C to produce SPS, a light-yellow powder, at yield of 0.382% (w/w). SPS was composed of D-glucose in a weight ratio of 97.06%.

Cell culture

The TSCC cell line, HN-6, was obtained from the Laboratory of Oncological Biology of the Ninth Hospital Affiliated to Shanghai Jiao Tong University (Shanghai, PR China). HN-6 cells were then maintained in Dulbecco's modified Eagle medium (DMEM; pH 7.2; Sigma-Aldrich, Shanghai, PR China) supplemented with 10% fetal bovine serum (FBS; Sigma-Aldrich) in a 37 °C incubator with a humidified atmosphere of 5% CO_2.

CCK-8 assay

For the detection of cell proliferation, the Cell Counting Kit-8 (CCK-8) kit (Dojindo, Shanghai, PR China) was used in accordance with the manufacturer's instructions. HN-6 cells were seeded in a 96-well plate (6.0×10^6 cells/well) and cultured in DMEM supplemented with 10% FBS at 37 °C for 24 h. SPS and cisplatin (Qilu Pharmaceutical Co., Ltd., Jinan, PR China) were dissolved in DMEM prior to use. Subsequently, 5 μg/mL cisplatin and various concentrations of SPS (0, 0.02, 0.04, 0.08, 0.16, 0.32, 0.64, and

1.28 mg/mL) were added to each well of HN-6 cells separately and incubated at 37 °C for 24, 48, and 72 h. Optical density (OD) at 450 nm was determined. The inhibitory rate (IR) of cell proliferation was calculated from the following equation: IR = 1 – (OD of treated group/OD of control group) × 100%.

Apoptosis analysis

Apoptosis was analyzed by acridine orange/ethidium bromide (AO/EB) double staining. Briefly, HN-6 cells were seeded in a 6-well plate and incubated with DMEM supplemented with 10% FBS at 37 °C for 48 h. Subsequently, 5 μg/mL cisplatin and 0.64 mg/mL SPS were added separately and incubated with the cells for 24, 48, and 72 h. After this, 5 μL dye mixture (500 mg/mL AO and 500 mg/mL EB in distilled water) was added to each well. Cell apoptosis was then examined by an inverted phase-contrast microscope (Olympus IX70, Hamburg, Germany) at × 400 magnification.

Cell cycle analysis

Cell cycle analysis was performed using a Cell Cycle Detection Kit (NanJing KeyGen Biotech Co., Ltd., Nanjing, JiangSu, China). Briefly, HN-6 cells were seeded in a 6-well plate and incubated with DMEM supplemented with 10% FBS at 37 °C for 48 h. Then, 5 μg/mL cisplatin and 0.64 mg/mL SPS were added to each well and incubated with the cells for 48 h. The cells were harvested, fixed with 75% ice-cold ethanol, and stained with 400 μL propidium iodide (PI) for 45 min in the dark. The cell cycle analysis after different drug treatments was then conducted using a FACSCalibur flow cytometer (BD, USA).

qRT-PCR

Total RNA was extracted using the Trizol kit (Invitrogen, Carlsbad, CA, USA), reverse transcription was then performed using an M-MLV RTase kit (Promega, USA), and qRT-PCR was then performed using One Step SYBR®PrimeScript® RT-PCR Kit (Takara, PR China) and an ABI-7500 PCR machine (Applied Biosystems, USA). The amplification procedure comprised 95 °C for 15 s, followed by 40 cycles of 95 °C for 10 s and 60 °C for 30 s. The forward and reverse primer sequences, respectively, for the amplification of targets were as follows: Bax, 5′-GGCC CTTTTGCTTCAGGGTT-3′ and 5′-GGAAAAAGACCT CTCGGGGG-3′; Bcl-2, 5′-CTTTGAGTTCGGTGGGGT CA-3′ and 5′-GGGCCGTACAGTTCCACAAA-3′; CO X-2, 5′-TTTGCATTCTTTGCCCGC-3′ and 5′-GGGA GGATACATCTCTCCATCAAT-3′; cleaved caspase-3, 5′-AGCAATAAATGAATGGGCTGAG-3′ and 5′-GTAT GGAGAAATGGGCTGTAGG-3′; and GAPDH, 5′-CGCT GAGTACGTCGTGGAGTC-3′ and 5′-GCTGATGATCT TGAGGCTGTTGTC-3′. The relative expression of these

Table 1 The effect of SPS on HN-6 cell proliferation

Group	Concentration (mg/mL)	OD value (24 h)	IR%	OD value (48 h)	IR%	OD value (72 h)	IR%
SPS	0.02	0.816 ± 0.028	1.73	0.798 ± 0.033*	10.82	0.649 ± 0.023*	27.71
	0.04	0.811 ± 0.054	4.74	0.760 ± 0.022*	16.24	0.643 ± 0.036*	31.43
	0.08	0.772 ± 0.033	12.41	0.659 ± 0.012*	20.18	0.622 ± 0.019*	35.33
	0.16	0.677 ± 0.028	18.13	0.619 ± 0.015*	35.41	0.582 ± 0.052*	38.62
	0.32	0.628 ± 0.056	33.33	0.496 ± 0.033*	42.53	0.321 ± 0.031*	47.78
	0.64	0.488 ± 0.027	46.72	0.309 ± 0.031*	51.29	0.266 ± 0.058**	64.95
	1.28	0.53 ± 0.081	42.63	0.451 ± 0.042*	48.12	0.306 ± 0.036*	56.32
Cisplatin	5×10^{-3}	0.461 ± 0.034	58.66	0.283 ± 0.011**	75.59	0.308 ± 0.032**	72.09
Control	0.00	0.822 ± 0.021	-	0.850 ± 0.023	-	0.996 ± 0.012	-

SPS safflower polysaccharide, OD optical density, IR inhibitory rate. *P <0.05 and **P < 0.01

target genes were normalized to GAPDH and then calculated using the $2^{-\Delta\Delta CT}$ method.

Western blot analysis

Total protein was extracted in lysis buffer containing PMSF (Pierce; Rockford, IL). The proteins were separated in a 10% SDS-PAGE and immunoblotted onto polyvinylidene fluoride (PVDF) membranes (Millipore, Boston, USA). Non-specific binding to the membranes was blocked by incubation with 5% nonfat dried milk for 1–2 h, and the membranes were probed separately with rabbit anti-human Bax, Bcl-2, COX-2, cleaved caspase-3, and GAPDH antibodies (1:100, Invitrogen) overnight at

4 °C, followed incubation with the appropriate horseradish peroxidase-conjugated secondary antibody (1:10000, Invitrogen) for 1 h; GAPDH was used as the internal control. The protein bands were visualized by the application of 4-chloronaphthol (Sigma-Aldrich) and analyzed by Gel-Pro 4.0 software (Media Cybernetics, Inc., USA).

In vivo tumor xenograft model

Twenty female BALB/cnu/nu nude mice (4–6 weeks old) were purchased from Beijing Vital River Laboratory Animal Technology Co., Ltd. (Beijing, China). These mice were housed in a room at constant temperature (27 °C ± 1 °C) and humidity (50% ± 10%) and a 12-h light/dark

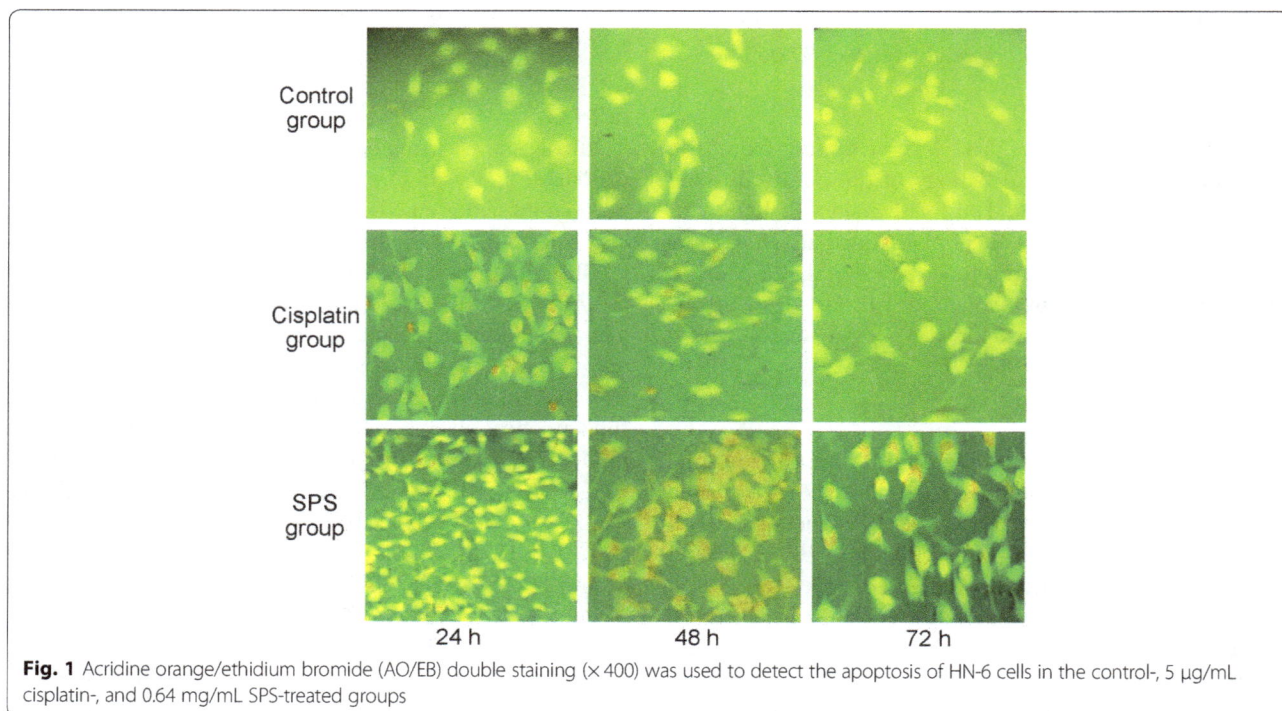

Fig. 1 Acridine orange/ethidium bromide (AO/EB) double staining (× 400) was used to detect the apoptosis of HN-6 cells in the control-, 5 μg/mL cisplatin-, and 0.64 mg/mL SPS-treated groups

Table 2 The effect of 0.64 mg/mL SPS on HN-6 cell cycle

Groups	G0/G1 (%)	S	G2/M
Control	10.71	52.42	36.87
SPS	25.76*	50.49	23.75*
Cisplatin	14.51	47.99	37.50

SPS safflower polysaccharide. *$P < 0.05$

cycle for 1 week. HN-6 cells (4×10^7) were subcutaneously injected into the flanks of mice to establish the in vivo tumor xenograft model. When the volumes of the xenografts reached 100–300 mm³, the animals were randomly divided into three groups: SPS ($n = 8$), cisplatin ($n = 8$), and model ($n = 4$). Throughout the 15 days of treatment, the mice in the SPS group were injected with 40 mg/kg SPS once a day, and the mice in cisplatin and model groups were injected with 0.8 mL/day cisplatin and normal saline every 3 days, respectively. The animal experiments were approved by the Animal Care and Use Committee of China Medical University (Taichung, Taiwan).

During treatment, the body weight of the tumor-bearing mice and the tumor size (length and width) were measured every 3 days. The tumor volume was estimated from the following equation: tumor volume = $0.5ab^2$, where a is the length of the tumor and b is the width of the tumor. The animals were sacrificed at the end of the study, and the tumors were removed and weighed. Tumor xenografts were used for the analysis of the expression of COX-2, Bcl-2, Bax, and cleaved caspase-3 by qRT-PCR and western blot analysis.

Statistical analysis

All measurement data from multiple experiments were presented as the mean ± standard deviation. One-way ANOVA was performed to analyze the significance of differences among groups, followed by a Tukey post hoc test for further between-group comparisons. Statistical software SPSS 17.0 (SPSS Inc., Chicago, IL, USA) was applied, and statistical significance was accepted at $P < 0.05$.

Results

SPS inhibited HN-6 cell proliferation

The effect of SPS on HN-6 cell proliferation was evaluated by a CCK8 assay. The results indicated that SPS inhibited HN-6 cell proliferation in a dose- and time-dependent manner within a certain dose range (0.02–0.64 mg/mL) and time (24–72 h) (Table 1). Among these concentrations of SPS (0.02–1.28 mg/mL), 0.64 mg/mL SPS exhibited the strongest IR on HN-6 cell proliferation at different time points (Table 1), and this concentration was therefore selected for subsequent experiments.

SPS induced the apoptosis of HN-6 cells

AO/EB double staining showed that the morphologies of HN-6 cells in the control group had intact structure and green-stained nuclei (Fig. 1). After treatment with cisplatin or 0.64 mg/mL SPS, shrinkage, chromatin condensation, membrane blebbing, and the formation of apoptotic bodies were identified in HN-6 cells (Fig. 1), indicating that SPS induced apoptosis in HN-6 cells.

SPS arrested cell cycle in the G0/G1 phase

The effect of SPS on the cell cycle was also examined. Compared with the control group, the percentage of HN-6 cells in the G0/G1 phase was significantly increased after treatment with 0.64 mg/mL SPS for 48 h, whereas the percentage of HN-6 cells in the G2/M phase was markedly decreased (Table 2), which indicated that SPS arrested the cell cycle of HN-6 cells in the G0/G1 phase. The percentage of HN-6 cells in different cell cycle stages was not significantly different in the control and cisplatin groups (Table 2).

Analysis of mRNA and protein expression of Bcl-2, COX-2, Bax, and cleaved caspase-3 in HN-6 cells after treatment

To investigate the regulatory mechanism of SPS, the mRNA and protein expression of Bcl-2, COX-2, Bax, and cleaved caspase-3 were detected. The results showed that, compared with the control group, the expression of Bcl-2

Table 3 The relative expression of target mRNAs in the control, cisplatin, and 0.64 mg/mL SPS groups

Groups	Bcl-2	COX-2	Bax	Cleaved caspase-3
Control (24 h)	0.713 ± 0.031	0.638 ± 0.048	0.185 ± 0.043	0.262 ± 0.081
Control (48 h)	0.720 ± 0.196	0.592 ± 0.005	0.166 ± 0.121	0.321 ± 0.021
Control (72 h)	0.693 ± 0.232	0.799 ± 0.923	0.203 ± 0.056	0.301 ± 0.044
Cisplatin (24 h)	0.585 ± 0.055	0.513 ± 0.023*	0.481 ± 0.011*	0.477 ± 0.021*
Cisplatin (48 h)	0.451 ± 0.060*	0.416 ± 0.019*	0.566 ± 0.035*	0.681 ± 0.046*
Cisplatin (72 h)	0.281 ± 0.026*	0.264 ± 0.032*	0.762 ± 0.055*	0.872 ± 0.065*
SPS (24 h)	0.423 ± 0.055*	0.408 ± 0.023*	0.314 ± 0.011*	0.585 ± 0.034*
SPS (48 h)	0.345 ± 0.060*	0.222 ± 0.019*	0.426 ± 0.035	0.822 ± 0.081*
SPS (72 h)	0.201 ± 0.026*	0.118 ± 0.032*	0.582 ± 0.055*	1.031 ± 0.092*

SPS safflower polysaccharide. *$P < 0.05$ compared with the control group

Table 4 The relative expression of the target proteins in the control, cisplatin, and 0.64 mg/mL SPS groups

Groups	Bcl-2	COX-2	Bax	Cleaved caspase-3
Control (24 h)	0.723 ± 0.121	0.918 ± 0.095	0.282 ± 0.164	0.464 ± 0.091
Control (48 h)	0.719 ± 0.196	0.922 ± 0.132	0.283 ± 0.053	0.460 ± 0.021
Control (72 h)	0.733 ± 0.198	0.899 ± 0.210	0.290 ± 0.026	0.465 ± 0.018
Cisplatin (24 h)	0.442 ± 0.113*	0.661 ± 0.066*	0676 ± 0.103*	0.679 ± 0.093*
Cisplatin (48 h)	0.393 ± 0.045*	0.458 ± 0.072*	0.867 ± 0.064*	0.863 ± 0.123*
Cisplatin (72 h)	0.107 ± 0.062	0.237 ± 0.069	0.916 ± 0.093*	0.991 ± 0.133*
SPS (24 h)	0.513 ± 0.101*	0.795 ± 0.135*	0.740 ± 0.0858	0.602 ± 0.076*
SPS (48 h)	0.392 ± 0.083*	0.590 ± 0.099*	0.920 ± 0.083*	0.764 ± 0.063*
SPS (72 h)	0.206 ± 0.106*	0.435 ± 0.021*	1.832 ± 0.925*	0.948 ± 0.089*

SPS safflower polysaccharide. *$P < 0.05$ compared with the control group

and COX-2 mRNA and protein was significantly decreased after SPS or cisplatin treatment in a time-dependent manner, whereas that of Bax and cleaved caspase-3 was obviously increased (Tables 3 and 4).

SPS inhibited the growth of tumor xenograft

The in vivo tumor xenograft model was established to explore the effects of SPS. The tumor weights in the model, SPS, and cisplatin groups were $2.236 ± 0.063$, $1.145 ± 0.210$, and $0.963 ± 0.049$ g, respectively. Moreover, compared with the model group, the tumor volume of the SPS and cisplatin groups were markedly decreased after 2 weeks of intervention ($P < 0.05$, Fig. 2). However, there were no significant differences in the body weight of mice in the different groups (data not shown).

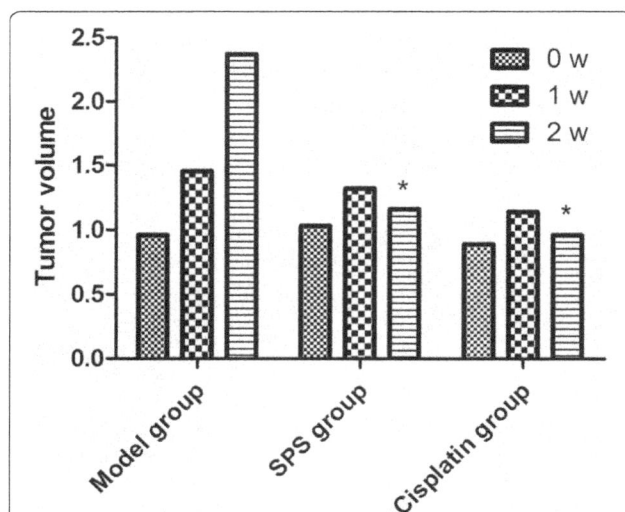

Fig. 2 The tumor volume of mice in the model, SPS, and cisplatin groups after intervention for 1 and 2 weeks. The data are presented as the mean ± standard deviation. *$P < 0.05$ compared with the model group after the same treatment time

Analysis of mRNA and protein expression of Bcl-2, COX-2, Bax, and cleaved caspase-3 in tumor xenograft model after different treatments

Consistent with the expression changes in HN-6 cells after different treatment, Bcl-2 and COX-2 expression in the tumor xenografts from the SPS or cisplatin groups was significantly lower than those from the model group, and the expression of Bax and cleaved caspase-3 was increased (Fig. 3).

Discussion

The present study illustrated that SPS markedly inhibited HN-6 cell proliferation, induced apoptosis, and arrested the cell cycle of HC-6 cells in the G0/G1 phase. Bcl-2 and COX-2 expression was significantly decreased after SPS treatment, whereas Bax and cleaved caspase-3 was significantly increased. Moreover, SPS significantly inhibited growth of the in vivo tumor xenografts, and the changes in the expression of the above molecules in tumor xenograft model after SPS intervention were consistent with previous results.

Apoptosis is an important mechanism involved in cancer progression, involving a series of active death process after the stimulation of many types of death signals [21, 22]. Bcl-2 families, such as Bax and Bcl-2, are regarded as a key mediator of cell apoptosis [23]. The ratio of Bcl-2 to Bax is shown to affect cellular sensitivity to the apoptotic signals. A previous study has confirmed that the mechanism of cantharidin in the promotion of apoptosis in TSCC may be associated with the suppression of the Bcl-2/Bax signaling pathway [24]. Moreover, Bcl-2 inhibition and Bax activation are thought to be promising approaches for cancer therapy [25, 26]. Notably, safflower injection resulted in an increase in the Bax/Bcl-2 ratio [27], which prompted us to speculate that SPS may inhibit TSCC development through the regulation of the Bcl-2/Bax expression ratio. In addition, caspase-3 is also considered to be a key mediator of

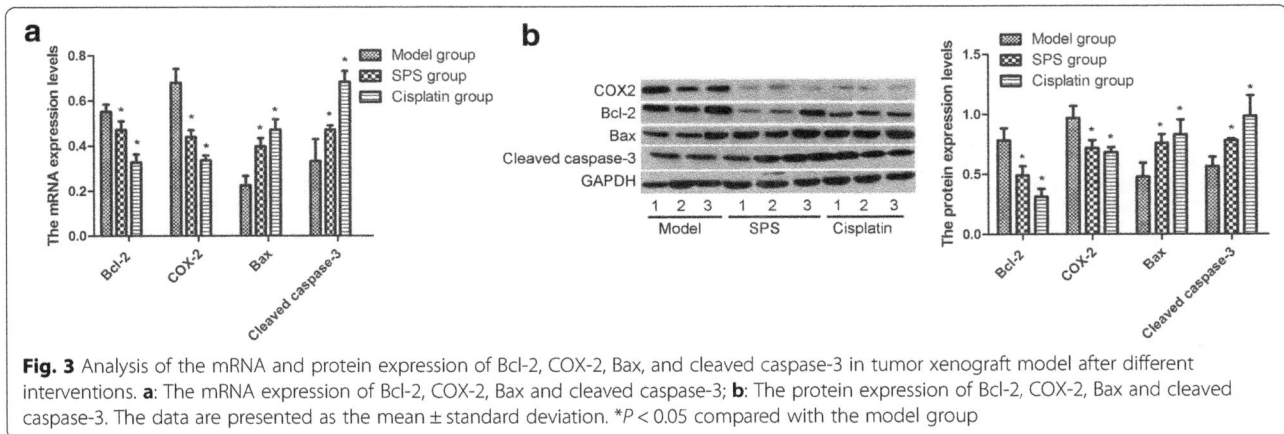

Fig. 3 Analysis of the mRNA and protein expression of Bcl-2, COX-2, Bax, and cleaved caspase-3 in tumor xenograft model after different interventions. **a**: The mRNA expression of Bcl-2, COX-2, Bax and cleaved caspase-3; **b**: The protein expression of Bcl-2, COX-2, Bax and cleaved caspase-3. The data are presented as the mean ± standard deviation. $*P < 0.05$ compared with the model group

mitochondrial apoptosis [28]. Cleaved caspase-3 can induce apoptosis through blocking the contact between the cell and its surroundings [29, 30]. Importantly, the activation of caspase-3 can induce apoptosis in TSCC [31]. In this study, we found that SPS induced apoptosis in HN-6 cells. Moreover, the Bax/Bcl-2 ratio and the expression of cleaved caspase-3 were increased after SPS treatment. Therefore, SPS may promote cell apoptosis in TSCC through an increase in the Bax/Bcl-2 ratio and the expression of cleaved caspase-3.

Furthermore, we also found that the expression of COX-2 was significantly decreased after SPS treatment. COX-2 is an inducible enzyme implicated in the transformation of arachidonic acid to prostaglandin and other eicosanoids [32]. An accumulation of evidence supports the overexpression of COX-2 in various tumor tissues and cells and a close relationship with tumor development [33]. Cao et al. demonstrated that miR-26b regulated cell proliferation and metastasis in TSCC through the regulation of COX-2 [34]. Moreover, COX-2 inhibition suppresses angiogenesis and tumor growth, potentiating antiangiogenic cancer therapy [35]. Consistent with a previous study, in which the dried aqueous extracts of safflower petal attenuated COX-2 protein expression and protected against lipopolysaccharide-induced inflammation [36], we found that SPS treatment resulted in a decrease in the expression of COX-2. Given the key role of COX-2 in tumor development, we speculated that SPS may inhibit TSCC development through a decrease in the expression of COX-2.

Conclusions

In conclusion, our results indicated that SPS may inhibit TSCC development through the regulation of the expression of Bcl-2, COX-2, Bax, and cleaved caspase-3. However, as this study is preliminary, further experiments are required to explore the possible mechanism of SPS in the prevention of TSCC development.

Funding

This work was supported by the National Natural Science Foundation of China (Program No. 81603418), the Natural Science Foundation of Heilongjiang Province (Program No. H2016062), and the University Nursing Program for Young Scholars with Creative Talents in Heilongjiang Province (Program No. UNPYSCT-2016075), and the First Affiliated Hospital of Harbin Medical University Science Research Funds (Program No. 2017Y014).

Authors' contributions

HZ contributed to the conception and design of the research. RW contributed to the acquisition of the data. CZ contributed to the analysis and interpretation of the data. YZ contributed to the statistical analysis. JY helped in obtaining the funding. XL helped in drafting the manuscript. SZ contributed to the revision of the manuscript for important intellectual content. All authors gave final approval of the manuscript.

Competing interests

The authors declare that they have no competing interests.

Author details

[1]Department of Cleft Palate Speech, The First Affiliated Hospital of Harbin Medical University, Harbin 150001, People's Republic of China. [2]Department of Oral and Maxillofacial Surgery, The First Affiliated Hospital of Harbin Medical University, No. 23 Youzheng Road, Nangang District, Harbin 150001, Heilongjiang Province, People's Republic of China. [3]Department of Basic Medical Science, Heilongjiang University of Chinese Medicine, Harbin 150040, People's Republic of China. [4]Department of Pharmacy, Heilongjiang University of Chinese Medicine, Harbin 150040, People's Republic of China. [5]Department of Pharmacy, Guiyang University of Chinese Medicine, Guiyang 550025, People's Republic of China.

References

1. Li H, Zhang Y, Chen SW, Li FJ, Zhuang SM, Wang LP, Zhang J, Song M. Prognostic significance of Flotillin1 expression in clinically N0 tongue squamous cell cancer. Int J Clin Exp Pathol. 2014;7:996–1003.
2. Cannon TL, Lai DW, Hirsch D, Delacure M, Downey A, Kerr AR, Bannan M, Andreopoulou E, Safra T, Muggia F. Squamous cell carcinoma of the oral cavity in nonsmoking women: a new and unusual complication of chemotherapy for recurrent ovarian cancer? Oncologist. 2012;17:1541–6.
3. Dibble EH, Alvarez ACL, Truong M-T, Mercier G, Cook EF, Subramaniam RM. 18F-FDG metabolic tumor volume and total glycolytic activity of oral cavity and oropharyngeal squamous cell cancer: adding value to clinical staging. J Nucl Med. 2012;53:709–15.
4. Trotta BM, Pease CS, Rasamny JJ, Raghavan P, Mukherjee S. Oral cavity and oropharyngeal squamous cell cancer: key imaging findings for staging and treatment planning. Radiographics. 2011;31:339–54.
5. Wakabayashi T, Hirokawa S, Yamauchi N, Kataoka T, Woo J-T, Nagai K. Immunomodulating activities of polysaccharide fractions from dried safflower petals. Cytotechnology. 1997;25:205–11.

6. Ali Sahari M, Morovati N, Barzegar M, Asgari S. Physicochemical and antioxidant characteristics of safflower seed oil. Curr Nutr Food Sci. 2014;10:268–74.

7. Toma W, Guimarães LL, Brito AR, Santos AR, Cortez FS, Pusceddu FH, Cesar A, Júnior SL, Pacheco MT, Pereira CD. Safflower oil: an integrated assessment of phytochemistry, antiulcerogenic activity, and rodent and environmental toxicity. Revista Brasileira de Farmacognosia. 2014;24:538–44.

8. Sabah FS, Saleh AA. Evaluation of antibacterial activity of flavonoid and oil extracts from safflower (Carthamus tinctorius L). Evaluation. 2015;5:41–44.

9. Li L-J, Li Y-M, Qiao B-Y, Jiang S, Li X, Du H-M, Han P-C, Shi J. The value of safflower yellow injection for the treatment of acute cerebral infarction: a randomized controlled trial. Evid Based Complement Alternat Med. 2015; 2015:478793.

10. Fan S, Lin N, Shan G, Zuo P, Cui L. Safflower yellow for acute ischemic stroke: a systematic review of randomized controlled trials. Complement Ther Med. 2014;22:354–61.

11. Ando I, Tsukumo Y, Wakabayashi T, Akashi S, Miyake K, Kataoka T, Nagai K. Safflower polysaccharides activate the transcription factor NF-κB via Toll-like receptor 4 and induce cytokine production by macrophages. Int Immunopharmacol. 2002;2:1155–62.

12. Shi X, Ruan D, Wang Y, Ma L, Li M. Anti-tumor activity of safflower polysaccharide (SPS) and effect on cytotoxicity of CTL cells, NK cells of T739 lung cancer in mice. Zhongguo Zhong yao za zhi= Zhongguo zhongyao zazhi=China journal of Chinese materia medica. 2010;35:215–8.

13. Xi SY, Zhang Q, Wang C, Zhang JJ, Gao XM. Discussion of safflower inhibiting tumor in application and its mechanism of action. Ch inese Archives of Traditional Chinese Medicine. 2008;26:1916–7.

14. Luo Z, Zeng H, Ye Y, Liu L, Li S, Zhang J, Luo R. Safflower polysaccharide inhibits the proliferation and metastasis of MCF-7 breast cancer cell. Mol Med Rep. 2015;11:4611–6.

15. SUN Y, YANG J, ZHANG Q-q, WANG X, XU F, LI M-z, WANG Y-x: Mechanism investigation of cell cycle arrest in hepatic cancer cell induced by safflower polysaccharide Chinese J Experimental Traditional Medical Formulae 2014; 13:046.

16. Li J-Y, Yu J, Du X-S, Zhang H-M, Wang B, Guo H, Bai J, Wang J-H, Liu A, Wang Y-L. Safflower polysaccharide induces NSCLC cell apoptosis by inhibition of the Akt pathway. Oncol Rep. 2016;36:147–54.

17. Xinbo M, Zhenzuo Z, Rufei G, Xue-kui S, Lin S, An-wen Z, Hai-guang S, Shen Y, Ya-xian W. The pilot study on the inhibition of safflower polysaccharide to human gastric carcinoma cell line SGCY7901. Guangxi Medical J. 2012;34:1444Y6.

18. Wang T, Shi X, Sun Y, WANG Y-x: Experimental study on morphologic effect of safflower polysaccharide on the apoptosis of gastric carcinoma cell line SGC-7901. Information Traditional Chinese Medicine 2015; 32:19–21.

19. Tao J, Li QW, Shi XK, Liang Y, Wang YX: Safflower polysaccharide inhibit PI3K/Akt signaling pathway induces apoptosis of human gastric cancer cells. Practical oncology Journal 2012; 26:119–124.

20. Liang A, Jianghong Z, Taijun Z, Xiaoqing L, Qiong Z, Jun C. Analysis of the inhibitory effect of safflower polysaccharide on HT29 colorectal cancer cell proliferation and its relevant mechanism. Biomed Res. 2017;28:2966–70.

21. Porter AG, Janicke RU. Emerging roles of caspase-3 in apoptosis. Cell Death Differ. 1999;6:99–104.

22. Hockenbery DM, Oltvai ZN, Yin XM, Milliman CL, Korsmeyer SJ. Bcl-2 functions in an antioxidant pathway to prevent apoptosis. Cell. 1993;75:241–51.

23. Risso A, Mercuri F, Quagliaro L, Damante G, Ceriello A. Intermittent high glucose enhances apoptosis in human umbilical vein endothelial cells in culture. Am J Physiol Endocrinol Metab. 2001;281:E924–E30.

24. Tian X, Zeng G, Li X, Wu Z, Wang L. Cantharidin inhibits cell proliferation and promotes apoptosis in tongue squamous cell carcinoma through suppression of miR-214 and regulation of p53 and Bcl-2/Bax. Oncol Rep. 2015;33:3061–8.

25. Xin M, Li R, Xie M, Park D, Owonikoko TK, Sica GL, Corsino PE, Zhou J, Ding C, White MA. Small-molecule Bax agonists for cancer therapy. Nat Commun. 2014;5:4935.

26. Souers AJ, Leverson JD, Boghaert ER, Ackler SL, Catron ND, Chen J, Dayton BD, Ding H, Enschede SH, Fairbrother WJ. ABT-199, a potent and selective BCL-2 inhibitor, achieves antitumor activity while sparing platelets. Nat Med. 2013;19:202–8.

27. LIU J, XU X f, YANG W j, Guo C y: Effect of safflower injection on proliferation, apoptosis, and expression of bcl-2/bax gene in hepatic stellate cell in vitro [J]. Chinese Traditional and Herbal Drugs 2009; 8:030.

28. Lakhani SA, Masud A, Kuida K, Porter GA, Booth CJ, Mehal WZ, Inayat I, Flavell RA. Caspases 3 and 7: key mediators of mitochondrial events of apoptosis. Science. 2006;311:847–51.

29. Pan JA, Ullman E, Dou Z, Zong WX. Inhibition of protein degradation induces apoptosis through a microtubule-associated protein 1 light chain 3-mediated activation of caspase-8 at intracellular membranes. Mol Cell Biol. 2011;31:3158–70.

30. Huang Q, Li F, Liu X, Li W, Shi W, Liu FF, O'Sullivan B, He Z, Peng Y, Tan AC, et al. Caspase 3-mediated stimulation of tumor cell repopulation during cancer radiotherapy. Nat Med. 2011;17:860–6.

31. Coutinho-Camillo CM, Lourenço SV, Nishimoto IN, Kowalski LP, Soares FA. Caspase expression in oral squamous cell carcinoma. Head & neck. 2011;33: 1191–8.

32. Khan Z, Khan N, P Tiwari R, K Sah N, Prasad G, S Bisen P. Biology of Cox-2: an application in cancer therapeutics. Curr Drug Targets. 2011;12:1082–93.

33. Song X, Lin HP, Johnson AJ, Tseng PH, Yang YT, Kulp SK, Chen CS. Cyclooxygenase-2, player or spectator in cyclooxygenase-2 inhibitor-induced apoptosis in prostate cancer cells. J Natl Cancer Inst. 2002;94:585–91.

34. Cao J, Guo T, Dong Q, Zhang J, Li Y. miR-26b is downregulated in human tongue squamous cell carcinoma and regulates cell proliferation and metastasis through a COX-2-dependent mechanism. Oncol Rep. 2015;33: 974–80.

35. Xu L, Stevens J, Hilton MB, Seaman S, Conrads TP, Veenstra TD, Logsdon D, Morris H, Swing DA, Patel NL. COX-2 inhibition potentiates antiangiogenic cancer therapy and prevents metastasis in preclinical models. Sci Transl Med. 2014;6:242–ra84.

36. Wang CC, Choy CS, Liu YH, Cheah KP, Li JS, Wang JTJ, Yu WY, Lin CW, Cheng HW, Hu CM. Protective effect of dried safflower petal aqueous extract and its main constituent, carthamus yellow, against lipopolysaccharide-induced inflammation in RAW264. 7 macrophages. J Sci Food Agric. 2011;91:218–25.

4

Association between dietary protein intake and prostate cancer risk

Ye Mao, Yan Tie and Jing Du[*]

Abstract

Background: Many studies were conducted to explore the relationship between dietary protein intake and risk of prostate cancer, obtaining inconsistent results. Therefore, this study aims to comprehensively explore the predicted role of dietary protein intake for risk of prostate cancer.

Methods: Databases of Web of Knowledge, PubMed, Chinese National Knowledge Infrastructure (CNKI), and Wan Fang Med Online were searched up to August 30, 2017. Eligible studies were included based on our definite inclusion criteria. Summarized relative risk (RR) and corresponding 95% confidence interval (CI) were pooled with a random effects model. Sensitive analysis and publication bias were performed.

Results: At the end, a total of 12 articles comprising 13,483 prostate cancer cases and 286,245 participants were included. The summary RR and 95%CI of the highest protein intake compared to those with the lowest protein intake on prostate cancer risk were 0.993 (95%CI = 0.930–1.061), with no between-study heterogeneity found ($I^2 = 0.0\%$, $P = 0.656$). Moreover, the association was not significant on prostate cancer risk with animal protein intake [RR = 1.001, 95%CI = 0.917–1.092] or vegetable protein intake [RR = 0.986, 95%CI = 0.904–1.076]. The results were not changed when we conducted subgroup analysis by study design, cancer type, or geographic locations. We did not detect any publication bias using Egger's test ($P = 0.296$) and funnel plot.

Conclusion: Our study concluded that protein intake may be not associated on prostate cancer.

Keywords: Dietary, Protein intake, Prostate cancer, Meta-analysis

Background

Prostate cancer is one of the most common cancer among men, and nearly a million new cases are diagnosed worldwide [1]. In total, the incidence rate of prostate cancer in western countries is higher than that in other countries [2, 3]. The reason for this status may be the differences in dietary intake [3, 4]. In western countries, they usually eat foods rich in calories, saturated fats, as well as animal protein, and so on. However, lower intake of fruits, vegetables, and whole grains lead to diet imbalance. Therefore, these western diets are not only related to prevalence of obesity [5] but also can directly change the known parameters to promote the growth of prostate cancer [6].

Protein is macromolecules made of amino acids and have basic functions in all known biologic processes. As we all know, protein contains 22 known amino acids. Of these, 9 essential amino acids could not be synthesized in the body [7]. Therefore, humans must eat some levels of foods which are rich in protein, to obtain the essential amino acid that is required for new protein synthesis. The protein usually comes from animal meats, plants such as soy, and dairy products [7]. Many publications were performed to assess the association about prostate cancer with high-protein intake. However, the effect on prostate cancer from different studies remains to be controversial. To address this question, we sought to perform this comprehensive meta-analysis to reflect the current totality of evidence on the subject.

* Correspondence: du___jing@163.com
Cancer Center, West China Hospital, West China Medical School Sichuan University, No. 37, Guoxue Alley, Chengdu 610041, Sichuan Province, China

Methods
Literature search
Articles were searched from the electronic searches of Web of Knowledge, PubMed, Chinese National Knowledge Infrastructure (CNKI), and Wan Fang Med Online, with the strategy of 'protein' OR 'nutrition' OR 'diet' AND 'prostate cancer' OR 'prostate oncology' as recent as August 30, 2017. Moreover, the bibliographies of searched publications were cross-referenced in order to identify additional articles.

Inclusion and exclusion criteria
The inclusion criteria in this meta-analysis were (1) observational studies or experimental studies; (2) studies assessing the association about prostate cancer with protein intake; (3) the relative risk (RR) with the corresponding 95% confidence interval (CI) in the relation was available, or could be calculated basing on relevant data; (4) reporting the studies on humans; and (5) studies published in English language or Chinese language.

By contrast, the studies were excluded if they (1) reported on animal studies or cell studies; (2) were reviews, letter to the editors, or comments; and (3) contained insufficient data for statistical analysis.

Data extraction
The following required data were abstracted according to a predefined standardized form: the first author's last name; publication years; prostate cancer type; protein (total protein, animal protein, or vegetable protein); region for the study; study type; mean age or age range; follow-up duration; cases and participants; RR with 95%CI for the association between dietary protein intake and risk of prostate cancer; and adjustment for covariates. Two independent individuals extracted the data and the disagreements were resolved by a third reviewer.

Statistical analysis
RR with the corresponding 95%CI was combined to calculate the summary results [8]. A chi-square test I^2 statistic was used to assess the heterogeneity [9], and $I^2 < 25\%$, $I^2 = 25–50\%$, $I^2 > 50\%$ suggested low, moderate, and high heterogeneity [10]. All the analysis used random effects model as pooled results. Sensitivity analysis was performed to find if some single study affected the overall results or not. Egger's test [11] and Begg's funnel plots [12] were utilized to examine the publication bias. Stata 12.0 software (STATA, College Station, TX, USA) was used to carry out the statistical analyses. $P < 0.05$ defined statistical significance.

Results
Search results and characteristics of studies
Figure 1 shows the flow diagram. The initial screening identified 43,921 articles from Web of Knowledge,

61,591 articles from PubMed, 341 articles from Chinese National Knowledge Infrastructure (CNKI), and 412 articles from Wan Fang Med Online. After the duplicated publications from different databases were excluded and the title and abstract reviewed, 41 articles were further reviewed for full text. There are 2 additional articles that were searched from the references of reviewed articles. Eleven articles that did not obtain RR and 95%CI, 12 review articles, 6 animal or cell articles, and 2 letters to the editors were further excluded. Therefore, 12 articles [13–24] were left for this study. Eight studies were cohort design, 5 studies were case-control design, and the remaining 1 study was RCTs. Six studies came from Europe, 5 from America, and 1 from Asia. All of the suitable studies included 13,483 prostate cancer cases and 286,245 participants. The characteristics of the included studies are summarized in Table 1.

Meta-analysis
In the overall analysis, the summary RR and 95%CI of the highest protein intake compared to those with the lowest protein intake on prostate cancer risk were 0.993 (95%CI = 0.930–1.061), with no between-study heterogeneity found ($I^2 = 0.0\%$, $P = 0.656$) (Fig. 2).

In the stratified analysis by protein type, the association was significant on prostate cancer risk neither in animal protein intake [RR = 1.001, 95%CI = 0.917–1.092] nor in vegetable protein intake [RR = 0.986, 95%CI = 0.904–1.076]. There is no significant association found either in cohort studies [RR = 1.080, 95%CI = 0.964–1.209] or in case-control studies [RR = 0.960, 95%CI = 0.874–1.055]. The summary RRs (95%CI) of the highest protein intake compared to the lowest protein intake were 1.263 (95%CI = 0.953–1.674) on prostate cancer localized-stage disease risk and 0.973 (95%CI = 0.745–1.272) on prostate cancer advanced-stage disease. The results in the subgroup analysis by geographic locations were not changed. Detailed results are showed in Table 2.

Begg's funnel plots (Fig. 3) and Egger's test ($P = 0.296$) indicated that no publication was found in overall analysis. The sensitivity analysis (Fig. 4) showed that there is no single study that had potential effects on the overall result while removing a study at a time.

Discussion
The overall analyses suggested that high intake of protein were not related to the risk of prostate cancer. The association was significant on prostate cancer risk neither with animal protein intake nor with vegetable protein intake. We did not find any relationship between geographic locations and study design and prostate cancer risk.

43921 articles found from Web of Knowledge
61591 articles found from PubMed
341 articles found from CNKI
412 articles found from Wan Fang Med Online

72163 articles screened after excluding duplicates

72122 articles excluded on screening of title/abstract

41 relevant articles identified for further review

2 article from reference list

43 articles reviewed in full text

Articles (n=31) excluded because:
11 did not report RR and 95%CI
12 reviews
6 animal or cell studies
2 letters to the editors

12 articles included in this meta-analysis
Cohort: (n=8)
Case-control: (n=3)
RCT: (n=1)

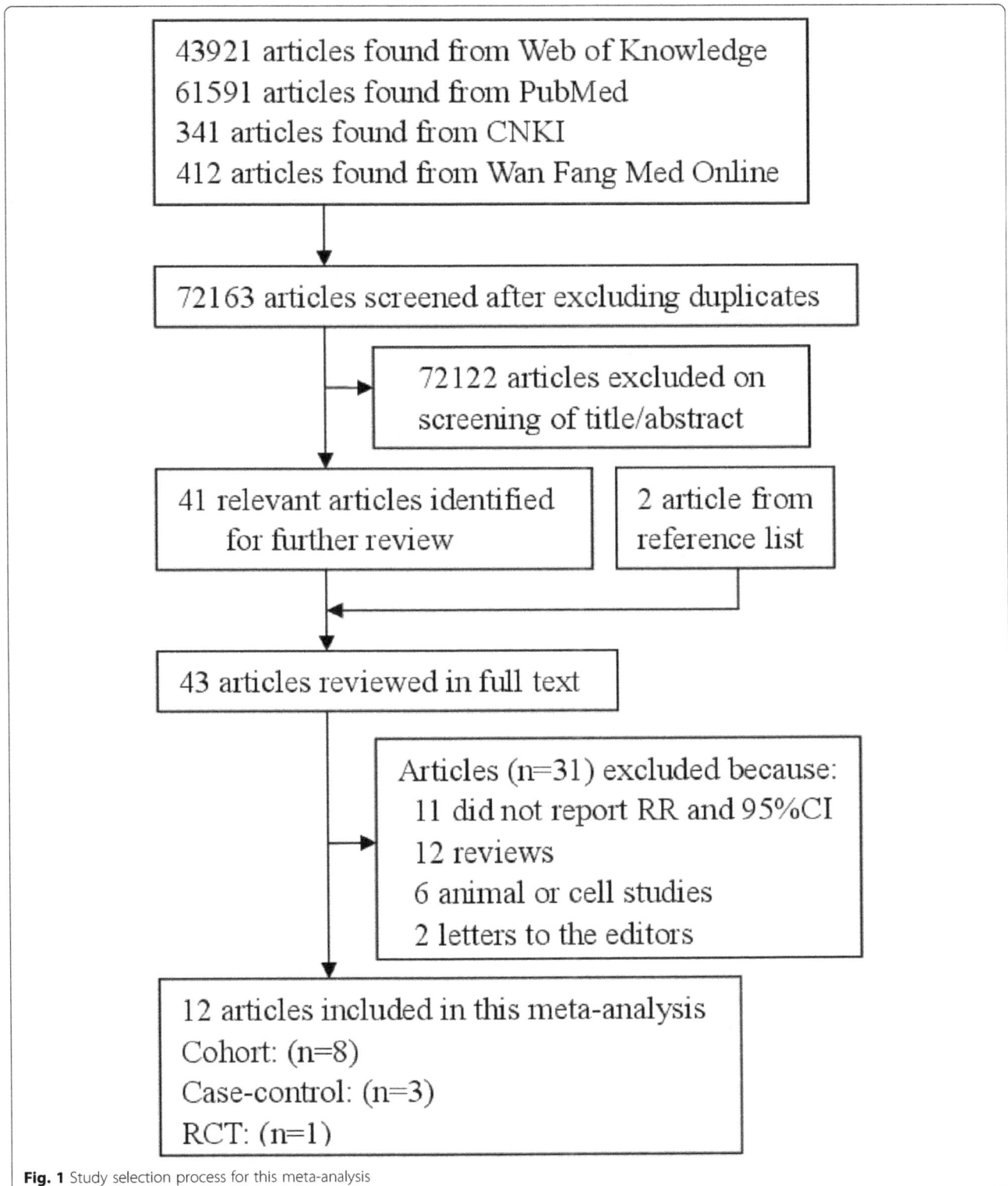

Fig. 1 Study selection process for this meta-analysis

Protein is an important nutrient for the human body, which is essential for body growth and development, as well as the transport of many important substances.

Protein deficiency can lead to growth retardation, nutritional edema, or may even endanger life [25]. Meat is an important source of protein. A previous publication of

Table 1 Characteristics of the included studies about the association of dietary protein intake on prostate cancer risk

Study, year	Design	Age	Participants; cases	Country	Follow-up duration	Protein type	Category	RR (95%CI)	Adjustment
Allen NE, 2008	Cohort	60.3 ± 6.7	142,251; 2727	European countries	8.7	Total protein	Total protein	Total protein	Adjusted for education, marital status, height, weight, and energy intake
						Animal	80 g/day	1	
						Vegetable	90 g/day	0.93 (0.82–1.05)	
							98 g/day	0.90 (0.78–1.04)	
							105 g/day	1.00 (0.85–1.18)	
							121 g/day	1.17 (0.96–1.44)	
							Animal	Animal	
							47 g/day	1	
							59 g/day	0.88 (0.77–1.00)	
							64 g/day	0.84 (0.73–0.97)	
							69 g/day	0.99 (0.86–1.15)	
							80 g/day	0.97 (0.81–1.15)	
							Vegetable	Vegetable	
							29 g/day	1	
							33 g/day	1.09 (0.96–1.22)	
							36 g/day	1.04 (0.91–1.19)	
							38 g/day	1.08 (0.93–1.26)	
							47 g/day	1.01 (0.82–1.23)	
Andersson SO, 1996	Case-control	70.7 ± 5.9	1056; 524	Sweden	NA	Total protein	Quartile 1	1	Adjusted for age and energy
							Quartile 2	0.90 (0.63–1.28)	
							Quartile 3	1.10 (0.78–1.55)	
							Quartile 4	1.07 (0.76–1.50)	
Berndt SI, 2002	Cohort	46–92	454; 69	USA	3.5	Animal	36.8 g/day	1	Adjusted for age and energy
							48.0 g/day	0.94 (0.49–1.82)	
							62.8 g/day	1.06 (0.56–2.01)	
Chan JM, 2000	Cohort	50–69	27,062; 184	Finland	8	Total protein	82 g/day	1	Adjusted for supplementation group, education, and quintiles of age, body mass index, energy, and number of years as a smoker
							94 g/day	0.9 (0.6–1.3)	
							102 g/day	0.6 (0.4–1.0)	
							107 g/day	0.8 (0.5–1.3)	
							117 g/day	1.0 (0.7–1.6)	
Deneo-Pellegrini H, 1999	Case-control	40–89	408; 175	Uruguay	NA	Total protein	Quartile 1	1	Adjusted for age, residence, urban/rural status, education, family history of prostate
							Quartile 2	1.1 (0.6–1.0)	

Table 1 Characteristics of the included studies about the association of dietary protein intake on prostate cancer risk *(Continued)*

Study, year	Design	Age	Participants; cases	Country	Follow-up duration	Protein type	Category	RR (95%CI)	Adjustment
							Quartile 3	1.7 (0.9–1.3)	cancer, body mass index and total energy intake
							Quartile 4	1.0 (0.6–1.8)	
Kristal AR, 2010	RCT	63.6 ± 5.6	9559; 1703	USA and Canada	NA	Total protein	Quartile 1	1	Adjusted for age, race/ethnicity, treatment arm, and body mass index
							Quartile 2	1.00 (0.86–1.17)	
							Quartile 3	0.96 (0.82–1.12)	
							Quartile 4	0.93 (0.79–1.08)	
Lane JA, 2017	Cohort	63.0 ± 6.5	5245; 1717	UK	13.3	Total protein	Quartile 1	1	Adjusted for age, BMI, socioeconomic, smoking and marital status, diabetes and energy intake
							Quartile 2	1.00 (0.82–1.23)	
							Quartile 3	1.16 (0.95–1.42)	
							Quartile 4	1.02 (0.83–1.25)	
							Quartile 5	1.03 (0.83–1.29)	
Mills PK, 1989	Cohort	74	14,000; 180	USA	6	Vegetable	< 1 serving/week	1	Adjusted for age
							1–4 serving/week	0.83 (0.59–1.16)	
							> 4 serving/week	0.67 (0.40–1.12)	
Schuurman AG, 1999	Cohort	63.9 ± 3.8	58,279; 642	Netherlands	6.3	Total protein	Total protein	Total protein	Adjusted for age, family history of prostate cancer, socioeconomic status and total energy intake
						Animal	62 g/day	1	
						Vegetable	69 g/day	1.04 (0.76–1.43)	
							75 g/day	1.12 (0.82–1.53)	
							81 g/day	1.35 (0.98–1.84)	
							90 g/day	1.10 (0.81–1.51)	
							Animal	Animal	
							34 g/day	1	
							42 g/day	1.29 (0.92–1.81)	
							47 g/day	1.16 (0.80–1.68)	
							53 g/day	1.52 (1.01–2.30)	
							64 g/day	1.32 (0.76–2.29)	
							Vegetable	Vegetable	
							22 g/day	1	
							25 g/day	0.86 (0.63–1.17)	
							27 g/day	1.00 (0.74–1.36)	
							30 g/day	0.83 (0.61–1.14)	
							35 g/day	0.90 (0.66–1.23)	

Table 1 Characteristics of the included studies about the association of dietary protein intake on prostate cancer risk (*Continued*)

Study, year	Design	Age	Participants; cases	Country	Follow-up duration	Protein type	Category	RR (95%CI)	Adjustment
Severson, RK 1989	Cohort	NA	7999; 174	Japanese	18	Total protein	0–74.9 g	1	Adjusted for age
							75.0–99.9 g	1.54 (1.07–2.22)	
							100.0+ g	1.13 (0.76–1.67)	
Smit E, 2007	Cohort	45–64	9777; 167	Puerto Rico	12	Total protein	Total protein	Total protein	Adjusted for age, education, body mass index, living, physical activity, smoking and residual energy intake. Calories not adjusted for energy intake
							≤61 g	1	
							62–82 g	0.94 (0.60–1.48)	
							83–103 g	1.02 (0.64–1.63)	
							≥104 g	1.32 (0.81–2.17)	
						Animal	Animal	Animal	
							≤13 g	1	
							14–23 g	0.78 (0.49–1.24)	
							24–40 g	0.91 (0.55–1.51)	
							≥41 g	1.01 (0.52–1.96)	
						Vegetable	Vegetable	Vegetable	
							≤16 g	1	
							17–23 g	1.27 (0.82–1.96)	
							24–31 g	1.07 (0.66–1.75)	
							≥32 g	1.19 (0.66–2.13)	
Tsilidis KK, 2013	Case-control	67.3 ± 5.4	10,155; 5221	European countries	NA	Total protein	Total protein	Total protein	Adjusted for continuous age at blood draw, continuous body mass index and energy consumption
							Tertile 1	1	
							Tertile 2	0.96 (0.87–1.06)	
							Tertile 3	0.95 (0.86–1.05)	
						Animal	Animal	Animal	
							Tertile 1	1	
							Tertile 2	1.05 (0.95–1.16)	
							Tertile 3	1.00 (0.90–1.11)	
						Vegetable	Vegetable	Vegetable	
							Tertile 1	1	
							Tertile 2	0.98 (0.89–1.09)	
							Tertile 3	1.00 (0.90–1.11)	

Abbreviation: RR relative risk, CI confidence intervals, RCT randomized controlled trial, NA not available

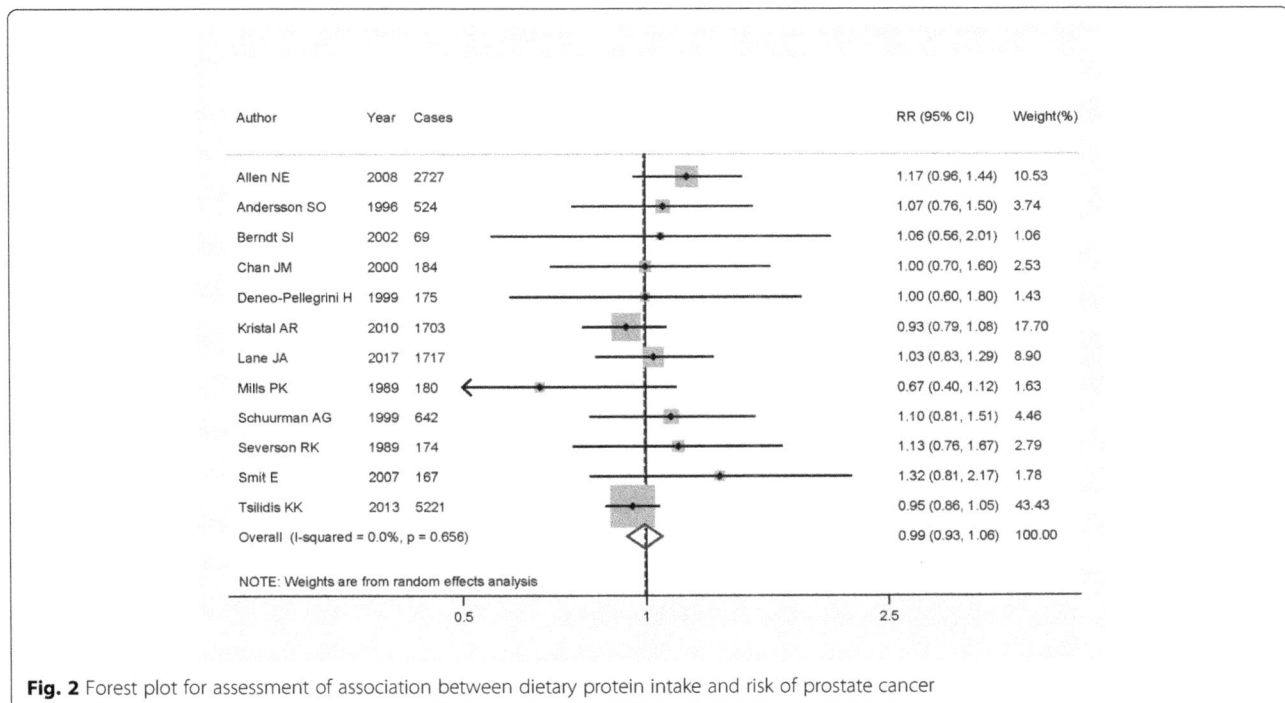

Author	Year	Cases		RR (95% CI)	Weight(%)
Allen NE	2008	2727		1.17 (0.96, 1.44)	10.53
Andersson SO	1996	524		1.07 (0.76, 1.50)	3.74
Berndt SI	2002	69		1.06 (0.56, 2.01)	1.06
Chan JM	2000	184		1.00 (0.70, 1.60)	2.53
Deneo-Pellegrini H	1999	175		1.00 (0.60, 1.80)	1.43
Kristal AR	2010	1703		0.93 (0.79, 1.08)	17.70
Lane JA	2017	1717		1.03 (0.83, 1.29)	8.90
Mills PK	1989	180		0.67 (0.40, 1.12)	1.63
Schuurman AG	1999	642		1.10 (0.81, 1.51)	4.46
Severson RK	1989	174		1.13 (0.76, 1.67)	2.79
Smit E	2007	167		1.32 (0.81, 2.17)	1.78
Tsilidis KK	2013	5221		0.95 (0.86, 1.05)	43.43
Overall (I-squared = 0.0%, p = 0.656)				0.99 (0.93, 1.06)	100.00

NOTE: Weights are from random effects analysis

0.5   1   2.5

Fig. 2 Forest plot for assessment of association between dietary protein intake and risk of prostate cancer

meta-analysis was performed to explore the association on dietary meat intake for prostate cancer risk. No significant relationships were found on prostate cancer either in total red meat consumption or fresh red meat consumption, while higher processed meat consumption could increase the risk of prostate cancer [26]. In our studies, we did not obtain a positive result for prostate cancer with animal protein intake, which is consistent with the above result. Soy food is another source of protein. A study of meta-analysis suggested that soy food consumption could decrease the risk of prostate cancer [27]. The reason for this result may be that soy foods contain many fibers and phytoestrogens that block the cell cycle, induce apoptosis, and inhibit angiogenesis.

Table 2 Summary RR and 95%CI of the association between dietary protein intake and prostate cancer risk

Subgroups	Number of studies	RR	95%CI	P for trend	Heterogeneity test	
					P	I^2 (%)
Overall	12	0.993	0.930–1.061	0.841	0.656	0.0
Protein type						
Animal protein	5	1.001	0.917–1.092	0.988	0.891	0.0
Vegetable protein	5	0.986	0.904–1.076	0.753	0.556	0.0
Study design						
Cohort	8	1.080	0.964–1.209	0.184	0.670	0.0
Case-control	3	0.960	0.874–1.055	0.399	0.797	0.0
RCT	1	–	–	–	–	–
Cancer type						
Localized-stage disease	2	1.263	0.953–1.674	0.103	0.508	0.0
Advanced-stage disease	3	0.973	0.745–1.272	0.843	0.703	0.0
Geographic locations						
Europe	6	1.005	0.931–1.085	0.899	0.566	0.0
America	5	0.943	0.824–1.080	0.397	0.450	0.0
Asia	1	–	–	–	–	–

RR relative risk, *CI* confidence interval, *RCT* randomized controlled trial

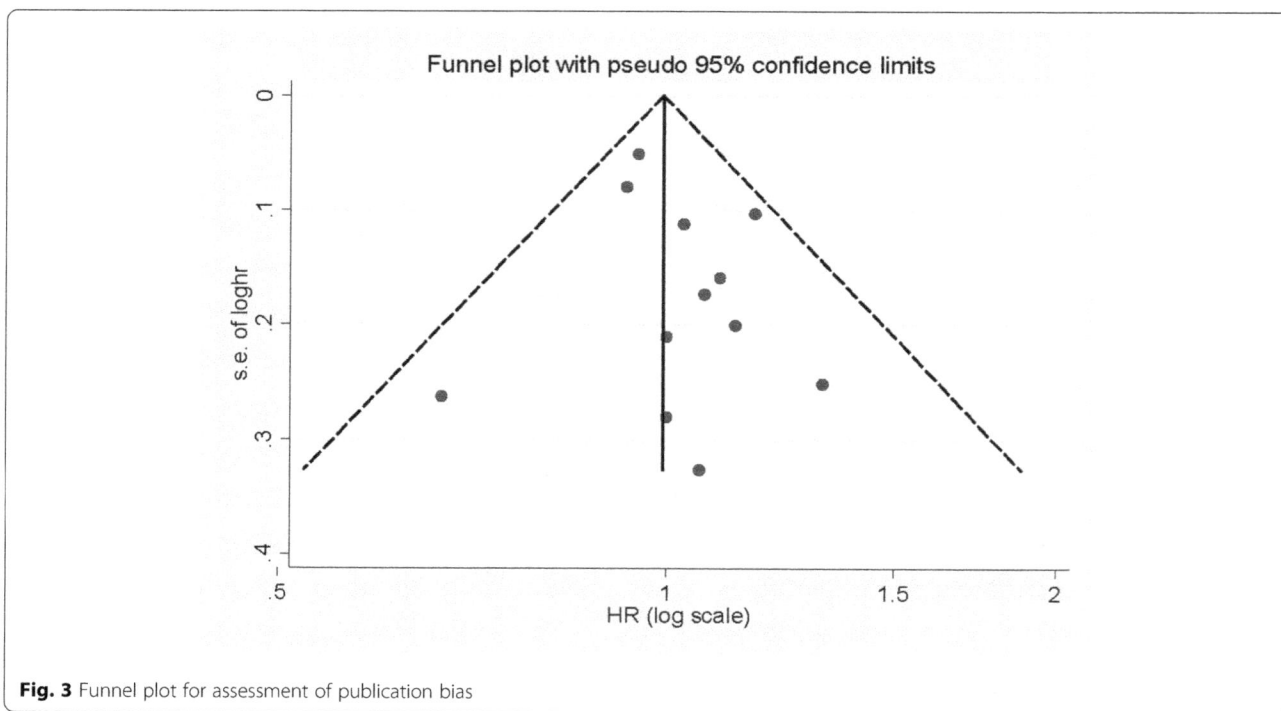

Fig. 3 Funnel plot for assessment of publication bias

Therefore, these mechanisms may support the point that higher category of dietary soy foods intake could reduce the risk of prostate cancer [25]. However, we cannot conclude a reverse relation between vegetable protein and prostate cancer risk. Furthermore, a recent meta-analysis suggested a nonsignificant association on colorectal cancer risk while in high-protein intake [28], as consistent with our results.

The most relevant risk factors on prostate cancer risk had been addressed. Previous study indicated that there was a slight association between metabolic syndrome and prostate cancer (RR = 1.17, 95%CI = 1.00–1.36, $P = 0.04$) [29]. Results from 11 cohort studies found that diabetes

mellitus could significantly increase the incidence of prostate cancer [30]. However, a meta-analysis of 14 prospective studies concluded that cholesterol level in blood was not associated with the risk of prostate cancer [31].

Our study had some strength. Firstly, large numbers of cases and participants were included in this study, yielding a more comprehensive result. Secondly, no between-study heterogeneity was found either in the whole analysis or in the subgroup analyses in this study and this may obtain a stable result. Thirdly, the small study effect was not detected using Begg's funnel plots and Egger's test in our analysis.

To our attention, some potential limitations exited in our report. Firstly, only English or Chinese language publications were searched and all suitable studies were English articles, this may omit some other languages publications. However, no publication bias was found. Secondly, most studies included in this report were European or American populations, and we found significant association neither in European populations nor in American populations. As we know, although the results were consistent in different subgroup analyses by racial, men of African descent showed a high incidence of prostate cancer and it may make some difference [32]. Furthermore, there exists a gap in the knowledge with lower risk populations where dietary or environmental risk may play a disproportionate impact (for example, incidence of prostate cancer is lower in Asians than in Caucasians or African Americans in the USA; however, the incidence of prostate cancer in Asian Americans,

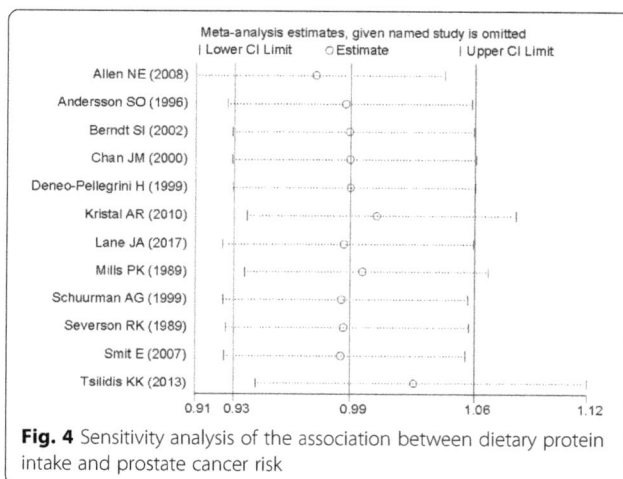

Fig. 4 Sensitivity analysis of the association between dietary protein intake and prostate cancer risk

while lower than that in Caucasians, is nonetheless higher than that in East Asians). Thus, more studies conducted in other countries should be performed to further assess the association on prostate cancer risk with protein intake. Thirdly, three of the included studies followed with case-control design may lead to inherent recall and selection bias of retrospective studies. Although different kinds of studies were included, we did subgroup analysis to exclude the interruption. There is no significant relation between prostate cancer and study design. Fourth, as understanding of prostate cancer growth, genetics, and the natural history of the disease has grown, subsidiary questions are increasingly important. Given the commonality of low-risk disease and evidence of over treatment, a more refined question to be asked is the association with high-grade or intermediate or high-risk disease. Therefore, more refined studies are wanted to answer these questions due to the data from an epidemiological standpoint that does not exist to support such analysis.

Conclusions

In conclusions, findings from this meta-analysis concluded that there is no effect on prostate cancer with high-protein intake. Since some limitations exited in our study, future studies are wanted to confirm the result.

Abbreviations
CI: Confidence intervals; RCTs: Randomized controlled trials; RR: Relative risk

Authors' contributions
YM, YT, and JD are the guarantors of integrity of the entire study who contributed to the definition of intellectual content, data acquisition, data analysis, statistical analysis, and review of the manuscript. JD conceived the concepts of the study. JD and YM contributed to the study design and helped in literature research. YM conducted the clinical and experimental studies and prepared the manuscript. YM and YT edited the manuscript. All authors read and approved the final manuscript.

Competing interests
The authors declare that they have no competing interests.

References
1. Center MM, Jemal A, Lortet-Tieulent J, et al. International variation in prostate cancer incidence and mortality rates. Eur Urol. 2012;61(6):1079–92.
2. Siegel RL, Miller KD, Jemal A. Cancer statistics, 2017. CA Cancer J Clin. 2017; 67(1):7–30.
3. Lopez Fontana CM, Recalde Rincon GM, Messina Lombino D, et al. Body mass index and diet affect prostate cancer development. Actas Urologicas Espanolas. 2009;33(7):741–6.
4. Wu K, Hu FB, Willett WC, et al. Dietary patterns and risk of prostate cancer in U.S. men. Cancer Epidemiol Biomarkers Prev. 2006;15(1):167–71.
5. Montagnese C, Santarpia L, Iavarone F, et al. North and South American countries food-based dietary guidelines: a comparison. Nutrition. 2017; 42:51–63.
6. Aronson WJ, Barnard RJ, Freedland SJ, et al. Growth inhibitory effect of low fat diet on prostate cancer cells: results of a prospective, randomized dietary intervention trial in men with prostate cancer. J Urol. 2010;183(1):345–50.
7. Masko EM, Allott EH, Freedland SJ. The relationship between nutrition and prostate cancer: is more always better? Eur Urol. 2013;63(5):810–20.
8. DerSimonian R, Laird N. Meta-analysis in clinical trials. Control Clin Trials. 1986;7(3):177–88.
9. Higgins JP, Thompson SG, Deeks JJ, et al. Measuring inconsistency in meta-analyses. BMJ. 2003;327(7414):557–60.
10. Higgins JP, Thompson SG. Controlling the risk of spurious findings from meta-regression. Stat Med. 2004;23(11):1663–82.
11. Egger M, Davey Smith G, Schneider M, et al. Bias in meta-analysis detected by a simple, graphical test. BMJ. 1997;315(7109):629–34.
12. Begg CB, Mazumdar M. Operating characteristics of a rank correlation test for publication bias. Biometrics. 1994;50(4):1088–101.
13. Allen NE, Key TJ, Appleby PN, et al. Animal foods, protein, calcium and prostate cancer risk: the European Prospective Investigation into Cancer and Nutrition. Br J Cancer. 2008;98(9):1574–81.
14. Andersson SO, Wolk A, Bergstrom R, et al. Energy, nutrient intake and prostate cancer risk: a population-based case-control study in Sweden. Int J Cancer. 1996;68(6):716–22.
15. Berndt SI, Carter HB, Landis PK, et al. Calcium intake and prostate cancer risk in a long-term aging study: the Baltimore Longitudinal Study of Aging. Urology. 2002;60(6):1118–23.
16. Chan JM, Pietinen P, Virtanen M, et al. Diet and prostate cancer risk in a cohort of smokers, with a specific focus on calcium and phosphorus (Finland). Cancer Causes Control. 2000;11(9):859–67.
17. Deneo-Pellegrini H, De Stefani E, Ronco A, et al. Foods, nutrients and prostate cancer: a case-control study in Uruguay. Br J Cancer. 1999;80(3–4):591–7.
18. Kristal AR, Arnold KB, Neuhouser ML, et al. Diet, supplement use, and prostate cancer risk: results from the prostate cancer prevention trial. Am J Epidemiol. 2010;172(5):566–77.
19. Lane JA, Oliver SE, Appleby PN, et al. Prostate cancer risk related to foods, food groups, macronutrients and micronutrients derived from the UK Dietary Cohort Consortium food diaries. Eur J Clin Nutr. 2017;71(2):274–83.
20. Mills PK, Beeson WL, Phillips RL, et al. Cohort study of diet, lifestyle, and prostate cancer in Adventist men. Cancer. 1989;64(3):598–604.
21. Severson RK, Nomura AM, Grove JS, et al. A prospective study of demographics, diet, and prostate cancer among men of Japanese ancestry in Hawaii. Cancer Res. 1989;49(7):1857–60.
22. Schuurman AG, van den Brandt PA, Dorant E, et al. Animal products, calcium and protein and prostate cancer risk in The Netherlands Cohort Study. Br J Cancer. 1999;80(7):1107–13.
23. Smit E, Garcia-Palmieri MR, Figueroa NR, et al. Protein and legume intake and prostate cancer mortality in Puerto Rican men. Nutr Cancer. 2007;58(2):146–52.
24. Tsilidis KK, Travis RC, Appleby PN, et al. Insulin-like growth factor pathway genes and blood concentrations, dietary protein and risk of prostate cancer in the NCI Breast and Prostate Cancer Cohort Consortium (BPC3). Int J Cancer. 2013;133(2):495–504.
25. Wu J, Zeng R, Huang J, et al. Dietary protein sources and incidence of breast cancer: a dose-response meta-analysis of prospective studies. Nutrients. 2016;8(11).
26. Bylsma LC, Alexander DD. A review and meta-analysis of prospective studies of red and processed meat, meat cooking methods, heme iron, heterocyclic amines and prostate cancer. Nutr J. 2015;14:125.
27. Hwang YW, Kim SY, Jee SH, et al. Soy food consumption and risk of prostate cancer: a meta-analysis of observational studies. Nutr Cancer. 2009; 61(5):598–606.
28. Lai R, Bian Z, Lin H, et al. The association between dietary protein intake and colorectal cancer risk: a meta-analysis. World J Surg Oncol. 2017;15(1):169.
29. Gacci M, Russo GI, De Nunzio C, et al. Meta-analysis of metabolic syndrome and prostate cancer. Prostate Cancer Prostatic Dis. 2017;20(2):146–55.
30. Cai H, Xu Z, Xu T, et al. Diabetes mellitus is associated with elevated risk of mortality amongst patients with prostate cancer: a meta-analysis of 11 cohort studies. Diabetes Metab Res Rev. 2015;31(4):336–43.
31. YuPeng L, YuXue Z, PengFei L, et al. Cholesterol levels in blood and the risk of prostate cancer: a meta-analysis of 14 prospective studies. Cancer Epidemiol Biomarkers Prev. 2015;24(7):1086–93.
32. Ferlay J, Soerjomataram I, Dikshit R, et al. Cancer incidence and mortality worldwide: sources, methods and major patterns in GLOBOCAN 2012. Int J Cancer. 2015;136(5):E359–86.

5

Impact of adjuvant chemotherapy on patients with ypT0–2 ypN0 rectal cancer after neoadjuvant chemoradiation

Christian Galata[1*], Kirsten Merx[2], Sabine Mai[3], Timo Gaiser[4], Frederik Wenz[3], Stefan Post[1], Peter Kienle[6], Ralf-Dieter Hofheinz[2] and Karoline Horisberger[1,5]

Abstract

Background: To investigate the importance of adjuvant chemotherapy in locally advanced rectal cancer ($\geq$ cT3 or N+) staged ypT0–2 ypN0 on final histological work-up after neoadjuvant chemoradiation and radical resection.

Methods: The clinical course of patients with rectal cancer and ypT0–2 ypN0 stages after neoadjuvant chemoradiation and radical resection was analyzed from 1999 to 2012. Patients were divided into two groups depending on whether adjuvant chemotherapy was administered or not. Overall survival, distant metastases, and local recurrence were compared between both groups.

Results: Fifty-four patients with adjuvant (ACT) and 50 patients without adjuvant chemotherapy (NACT) after neoadjuvant chemoradiation followed by radical resection for rectal cancer were included in the analysis. Mean follow-up was 68 ± 33.7 months. One patient without adjuvant chemotherapy and none in the ACT group developed a local recurrence. Five patients in the NACT group and three patients in the ACT group had distant recurrences. Median disease-free survival for all patients was 65.5 ± 34.5 months. Multivariate analysis showed adjuvant chemotherapy to be the most relevant factor for disease-free and overall survival. Patients staged ypT2 ypN0 showed a significantly better disease-free survival after application of adjuvant chemotherapy. Disease-free survival in ypT0–1 ypN0 patients showed no correlation to the administration of adjuvant chemotherapy.

Conclusion: Administration of adjuvant chemotherapy after neoadjuvant chemoradiation and radical resection in rectal cancer improved disease-free and overall survival of patients with ypT0–2 ypN0 tumor stages in our study. In particular, ypT2 ypN0 patients seem to profit from adjuvant treatment.

Keywords: Rectal neoplasms, Neoadjuvant therapy, Chemoradiotherapy, Adjuvant chemotherapy, Disease-free survival

Background

Neoadjuvant chemoradiation is a considered standard treatment for locally advanced rectal cancer [1]. Current guidelines for the treatment of colorectal cancer in Germany recommend the administration of adjuvant chemotherapy for all rectal cancer patients after neoadjuvant chemoradiation and total mesorectal excision (TME),

regardless of the postoperative pathologic staging result [2]. This recommendation is based on the CAO/ARO/AIO-94 and FFCD 9203 studies [1, 3]. However, hard evidence is lacking, especially for patients staged ypT0–2 ypN0. While an exploratory analysis suggested that particular patients with good response (ypT0–2) benefit from adjuvant chemotherapy [4] randomized controlled trials addressing the same question showed no benefit for adjuvant chemotherapy [5, 6]. However, these trials have relevant methodological restrictions. While a recent pooled analysis showed positive effects for adjuvant chemotherapy, another recent meta-analysis failed to do so [7, 8].

---

* Correspondence: christian.galata@umm.de
[1]Department of Surgery, University Hospital Mannheim, Medical Faculty Mannheim, University of Heidelberg, Theodor-Kutzer-Ufer 1-3, 68167 Mannheim, Germany
Full list of author information is available at the end of the article

In adherence to the German national guidelines from before 2008, ypT0–2 ypN0 patients were then not treated with postoperative chemotherapy (NACT) at our institution. After the introduction of the amended guidelines in 2008, adjuvant treatment was routinely administered to the same group of patients (ACT). In the present study, we investigated patients with locally advanced rectal cancer in clinical staging (UICC stages II and III) treated with neoadjuvant chemoradiation and TME and then staged ypT0–2 ypN0. On the basis of a prospectively maintained database, the oncologic outcomes of these patients were analyzed.

Methods

Ethics approval
The institutional review board reviewed and approved the protocol; the study was conducted in accordance with the Declaration of Helsinki.

Patient selection
All surgically treated colorectal carcinomas at the Department of Surgery, University Hospital Mannheim, Germany, between 1999 and 2012 were retrospectively analyzed on the basis of prospective databases. Patients with locally advanced rectal cancer who underwent neoadjuvant chemoradiation and subsequent TME in curative intent were eligible for the study when diagnosed ypT0–2 ypN0 in postoperative pathological staging. Exclusion criteria were postoperative death (in-hospital mortality), UICC stage IV and recurrent disease, or missing information on whether adjuvant chemotherapy was administered. Primary outcome measure was disease-free survival (DFS). Disease was defined as the event of local and/or distant recurrence during follow-up. DFS was defined as absence of local and/or distant recurrence and death by any cause during follow-up after primary hospital stay.

Pre-treatment evaluation
The presence of adenocarcinoma was confirmed by pathological examination in all cases. Clinical staging was performed using rigid rectoscopy, endorectal ultrasound, radiographic imaging of the chest, and abdominal ultrasound. Routine performance of magnetic resonance imaging (MRI) of the pelvis was introduced in 2003. Computed tomography (CT) scans of the thorax and/or abdomen were obtained in the majority of cases.

Preoperative chemoradiation and surgery
Neoadjuvant chemoradiation was administered when locally advanced rectal cancer was diagnosed (uT3-4, uN+). As preoperative chemotherapy regimen, capecitabine, capecitabine + irinotecan (XELIRI), XELIRI + cetuximab, capecitabine + oxaliplatin (XELOX), intravenous 5-FU, or panitumumab were used. Radiation therapy was applied as external-beam radiation with a target dose of 50.4 Gy. TME was scheduled 4 to 5 weeks after completing neoadjuvant chemoradiation before 2008, and 8 to 12 weeks after completion of chemoradiation for patients from 2008 till 2012.

Pathology investigation
Resected specimens were fixated in formalin and pathological work-up was done according to published standards [9]. If no residual tumor was apparent, the initial tumor-bearing area was sliced and embedded. Tumor regression grade was determined based on the classification proposed by the Japanese Society for Cancer of the Colon and Rectum (JSCCR) [10].

Postoperative chemotherapy
According to national colorectal cancer guidelines before the year 2008, patients were not offered postoperative chemotherapy when diagnosed ypT0–2 ypN0 in final pathological staging. After 2008, adjuvant chemotherapy became the treatment of choice for those patients when no contraindications were present. For adjuvant chemotherapy capecitabine, XELOX or intravenous 5-FU was used.

Statistical analysis
Baseline characteristics of all patients together were evaluated with respect to their influence on outcome. The characteristics were then compared between patients who received adjuvant chemotherapy and those who did not. Comparisons of frequencies between the two groups were performed using the Student's t test or the chi-square test. Differences of non-parametric quantitative data were analyzed using the Mann-Whitney U test. Kaplan-Meier estimates were computed for recurrence and survival and were compared between the two treatment groups using the log-rank test. A p value < 0.05 was considered statistically significant. All calculations were made with the SPSS version 22.0 (IBM© SPSS® Statistics).

Results

Patients' characteristics
Initial screening of the database returned 131 patients staged ypT0–2 ypN0 rectal cancer between 1999 and 2012 out of 397 patients who had received neoadjuvant treatment. Twenty-seven patients were excluded due to the above mentioned exclusion criteria. A total of 104 patients met the inclusion criteria, 28 females (26.9%) and 76 males (73.1%) with a mean age of 62.0 ± 10.7 years. Low rectal cancer was present in 48 patients (46.2%); 52 patients (50%) had cancers of the mid rectum, and 4 patients (3.8%) of the upper rectum. Median dose of delivered radiation was 50.4 Gy (range 36 to 50.4 Gy). Sphincter-preserving operation was performed

in 79.8% of the patients ($n = 83$). Postoperative chemotherapy was given to 54 patients (51.9%), while 50 patients (48.1%) did not receive adjuvant treatment. Ten of the patients (18.5%) who had received adjuvant therapy had surgery before 2008. In the group without adjuvant therapy, 41 patients (82%) were operated before 2008.

Data on gender, age, tumor height, preoperative radiation dose, and type of operation did not differ significantly between ACT and NACT (Table 1). A total of 46 patients (44.2%) were diagnosed ypT0 or ypT1 whereas 58 patients (55.8%) were diagnosed ypT2 in the final pathological examination. Distribution of ypT0, T1, and T2 showed a non-significant trend towards a higher rate of ypT0 in the patient group that received no adjuvant treatment (Table 1). Patients with ypT0–1 versus ypT2 showed no difference between the treatment groups. Neither the distribution of tumor regression grading nor the number of retrieved lymph nodes showed differences between both groups.

Oncologic outcomes according to adjuvant chemotherapy
Mean follow-up was 68.0 months ($\pm$ 33.7) for all patients eligible for the study. Follow-up time was significantly longer in the group without adjuvant chemotherapy ($p < 0.005$; Table 2). Mean disease-free survival was 65.5 ± 34.5 months. Overall recurrence of the disease

was seen in nine patients (8.7%). Metachronous metastasis occurred in eight cases (7.7%) and locoregional recurrence in one patient (0.96%).

In the univariate analysis, age, sex, tumor height, and extirpation had no influence on disease-free survival. Log-rank tests showed that adjuvant chemotherapy had no influence on local recurrence ($p = 0.382$), distant metastasis ($p = 0.54$), or overall recurrence ($p = 0.382$) but on disease-free survival ($p = 0.037$) and overall survival ($p = 0.017$) (Fig. 1). The 3-year OS and DFS were 98 and 94% in the ACT group, respectively, and 87 and 86% in the NACT group.

Anastomotic leakage showed a statistical trend towards influencing overall ($p = 0.053$) but not disease-free survival ($p = 0.435$). Adjuvant chemotherapy, after stratification for anastomotic leakage, demonstrated a statistically significant effect on disease-free survival in patients without leakage ($p = 0.016$); however, there was no significant influence of adjuvant chemotherapy on disease-free survival in patients with anastomotic leakage ($p = 0.293$).

ypT stages did not influence disease-free survival ($p = 0.513$), and also ypT stage groups (ypT0–1 versus ypT2) were not correlated to disease-free survival ($p = 0.265$) (Fig. 2). After stratification along these groups, no significant correlation with adjuvant chemotherapy could

Table 1 Patient characteristics of patients without and with adjuvant chemotherapy. In one patient, regression grade could not be determined

	No adjuvant therapy ($n = 50$)	Adjuvant therapy ($n = 54$)	p value
Age	62.9 ± 11.6	61.2 ± 9.8	0.414
Sex (female/male)	36/14	40/14	0.829
Abdominoperineal resection	10/50	11/54	1.0
Anastomotic leakage	9/40	3/43	0.062
T stage			
ypT0	20 (40%)	12 (22%)	0.064
ypT1	6 (12%)	8 (15%)	
ypT2	24 (48%)	34 (63%)	
T stage			
ypT0–1	26	20	0.167
ypT2	24	34	
Lymph nodes retrieved	13.1 ± 0.7	13.5 ± 0.7	0.687
Lymph nodes			
< 12	12 (24%)	12 (22.2%)	1.0
≥ 12	38 (76%)	42(77.8%)	
Regression grade (JSCCR)			
TRG 0	0	1 (2%)	0.384
TRG 1	11 (22%)	9 (17%)	
TRG 2	20 (49%)	32 (60%)	
TRG 3 (pCR)	18 (36%)	12 (22%)	

Table 2 Follow-up, local, and distant recurrence in patients without and with adjuvant chemotherapy

	No adjuvant therapy (n = 50)	Adjuvant therapy (n = 54)	p value
Follow-up (months)	82.2 ± 38.7	54.7 ± 21.4	0.003
Local recurrence	1	0	0.481
Distant recurrence	5	3	0.477

be seen concerning disease-free survival in ypT0–1 (p = 0.556); however, ypT2 patients showed a significantly better disease-free survival after adjuvant chemotherapy (p = 0.014) (Fig. 3). In ypT0 (p = 0.195) and ypT1 (p = 0.386), no correlation between adjuvant chemotherapy and disease-free survival could be detected. After stratification in groups of pCR (pathological complete response) versus ypT1–2, disease-free survival showed no significant correlation to adjuvant treatment in ypT0 patients (p = 0.195), and only marginally in ypT1–2 patients (p = 0.056). The 3-year DFS and OS in the ACT group were both 100% in ypT0, 100 and 88% in ypT1, and 94 and 100% in ypT2, respectively, and in the NACT group both 90% in ypT0, both 100% in ypT1, and 79 and 82% in ypT2.

When patients were classified in groups with more or less than 12 lymph nodes harvested, the number of lymph nodes harvested did not influence the disease-free survival by itself (p = 0.821). The interaction of lymph nodes harvested and adjuvant chemotherapy showed a significantly better disease-free survival in patients with more than 12 lymph nodes (p = 0.009) but no significant

influence of adjuvant chemotherapy in patients with less than 12 lymph nodes (p = 0.809).

Of the patients, 90% had at least half of the indicated chemotherapy cycles, 83% had 5 or 6 chemotherapy cycles, and 7% had 3 or 4 cycles (Table 3). Completeness of chemotherapy had no influence on the outcome.

Discussion

Introduction of neoadjuvant chemoradiation for rectal adenocarcinoma has in combination with TME surgery led to reduce rates of locoregional recurrence [1]. This improvement of local control, however, did not result in prolonged overall survival [11]. Our data show a significant benefit from adjuvant treatment for disease-free and overall survival but no benefits with respect to recurrence.

Adjuvant chemotherapy after neoadjuvant treatment and TME surgery is administered with the intention of reducing the incidence of distant metastasis and thereby improving survival. Although this has been prospectively investigated in several trials, controversy remains [5, 6]. In the just recently published study by Breugom et al.,

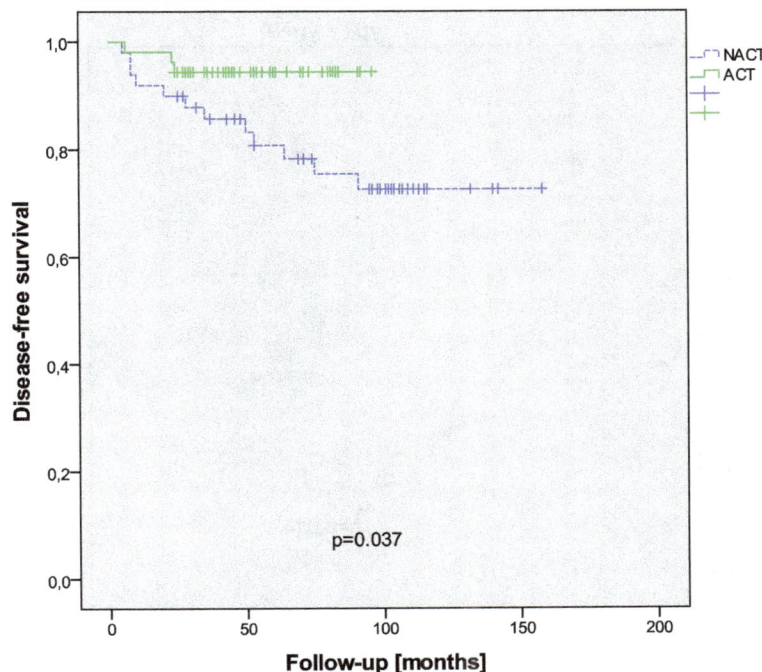

Fig. 1 DFS in all patients with respect to adjuvant chemotherapy

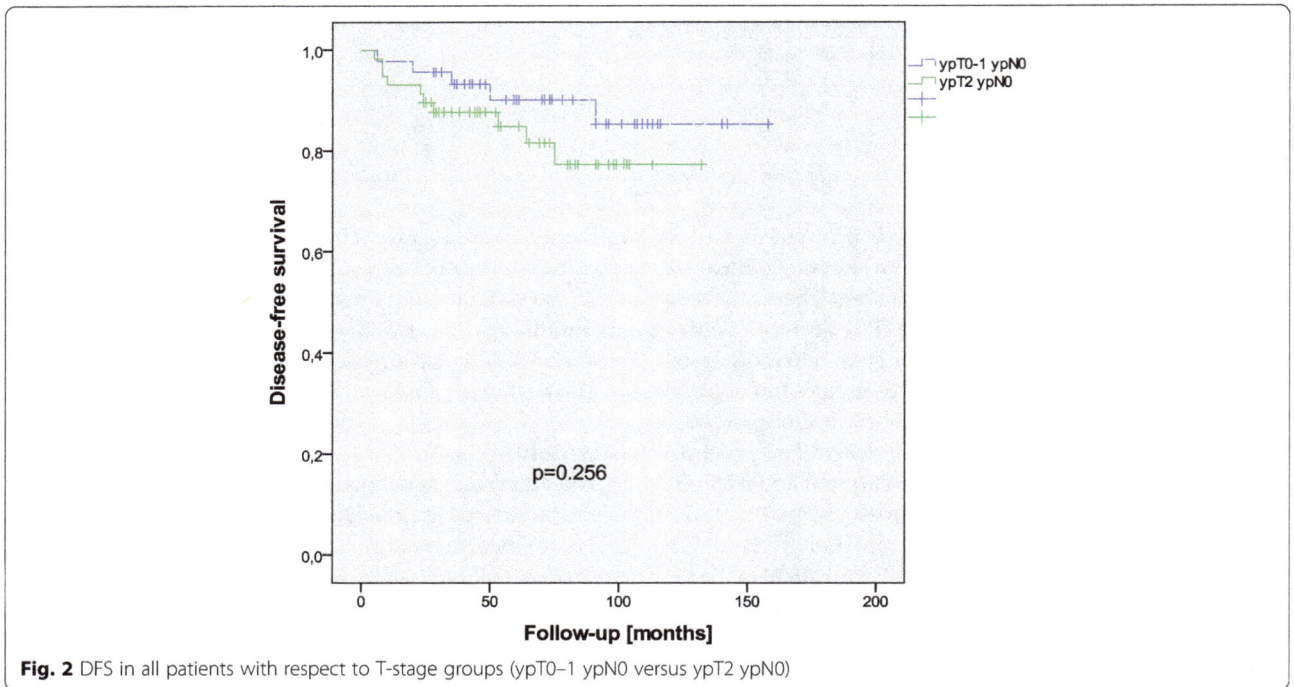

Fig. 2 DFS in all patients with respect to T-stage groups (ypT0–1 ypN0 versus ypT2 ypN0)

patients with ypTNM stage 0 or I were explicitly excluded which was also criticized [8, 12, 13]. A meta-analysis identified this subgroup to profit the most from adjuvant chemotherapy [14]. Maas et al. found the most pronounced effect of adjuvant chemotherapy on disease-free survival in ypT1–2 patients both in comparison to higher stages but also to pCR patients [7]. Our analysis found the most pronounced effect of adjuvant chemotherapy in ypT2 patients. The theoretical consideration that tumors with the combination of

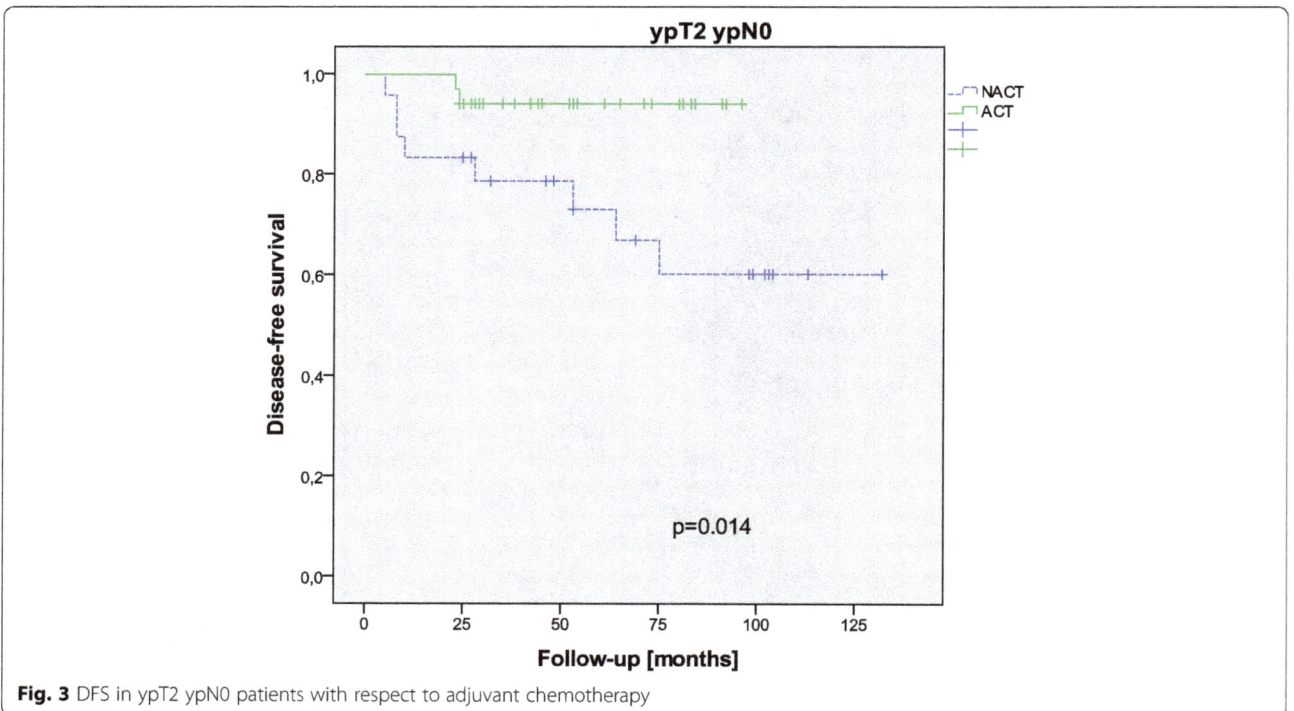

Fig. 3 DFS in ypT2 ypN0 patients with respect to adjuvant chemotherapy

Table 3 Completion of adjuvant chemotherapy (in three patients, the number of cycles could not be clarified anymore)

Completeness of chemotherapy	5–6 cycles	3–4 cycles	1–2 cycles
ACT group (n = 54)	45 (83%)	4 (7%)	2 (4%)

responsiveness (shown by downstaging) and continued considerable risk for local and distant recurrence (> ypT1) would profit from adjuvant treatment might in particular hold true for ypT2 [4].

Another restriction in the analysis of Breugom et al. is that the majority of the patients received bolus 5-FU [8]. However, an explanatory phase III trial showed better disease-free survival after perioperative treatment with capecitabine than with 5-FU [15]. In our analysis, only two patients received 5-FU postoperatively; therefore, a comparison of the effect of the two agents cannot be undertaken.

Our results are in conflict with the EORTC 22921 study that previously reported ypT1–2 patients to benefit from postoperative chemotherapy after 5 years; however, recently published late results after 10 years showed no improvement in disease-free or overall survival [4, 16]. Meta-analyses presented inherently contradictory results with respect to the positive effects of adjuvant chemotherapy on disease-free and overall survival [7, 8, 17, 18]. However, it is difficult to draw conclusions from these meta-analyses as the included studies have relevant shortcomings. As mentioned above, TME was not mandatory in some of the trials; others revealed a questionable quality of surgery with a R1 rate above 10% and finally, but most important, many of the studies showed a high percentage of patients not undergoing any adjuvant chemotherapy or not the initially planned number of cycles [5]. Low adherence to planned postoperative chemotherapy is one of the major problems of the available randomized trials, and it is a serious problem for interpretation of non-significant results as a proof for ineffectiveness of adjuvant chemotherapy [6, 8, 19]. In the EORTC 22921 trial, only 41% of the patients received complete chemotherapy [13, 16].

Anastomotic leakage is a major problem for patients who actually would have been eligible for adjuvant therapy. In our cohort, anastomotic leakage showed a trend towards negatively influencing application of adjuvant chemotherapy ($p = 0.062$). This is well in accord with general clinical experience that anastomotic leakage often prevents application of chemotherapy.

The results of the PROCTOR-SCRIPT trial challenge our study, as this is the first randomized trial on the application of adjuvant chemotherapy in neoadjuvantly treated patients with rectal cancer [6]. In this study, no benefit from adjuvant chemotherapy could be detected. However, again, there are limitations in this study. The

trial had to be closed earlier due to poor patient recruitment and survival was better than expected suggesting that the trial was probably underpowered. In the PROCTOR part of the trial, only 50% of the patients had a CT or MRI scan before treatment, so inaccuracy of staging is probably a major bias. Patients were preoperatively treated either with 5×5 Gy or with long-term chemoradiation; however, the longstanding oncological results of a randomized comparison of these two therapy schedules are still awaited [20]. Furthermore, stagewise analysis was not performed in the PROCTOR-SCRIPT trial and the number of retrieved lymph nodes not reported [6].

The question if the number of lymph nodes retrieved during surgery would influence long-term outcome respectively the application of chemotherapy and thereby the outcome has to be addressed. Most guidelines recommend investigation of at least 12 lymph nodes for determining final pathologic tumor stage [21]. In several studies, the number of detected locoregional lymph nodes was decreased after neoadjuvant chemoradiation [22, 23]. However, when < 12 lymph nodes are investigated, metastasis could be missed and histopathological stage underestimated. As performance of adjuvant treatment is stage-dependent also patients that would need therapy are then excluded. When intensified pathology work-up of the specimens is performed and more lymph nodes are evaluated, the number of metastatic lymph nodes may raise thereby possibly resulting in stage migration ("Will Rogers phenomenon") [24]. While some studies indicate an association between the number of harvested lymph nodes and oncologic outcome [24], the same authors could not reproduce these results when neoadjuvant chemoradiation was administered [25]. Recent studies on this topic continue to give conflicting results; therefore, the significance of retrieving more than 12 lymph nodes remains unclear [26, 27]. In the present study, retrieval of less than 12 lymph nodes showed no influence of adjuvant chemotherapy with respect to disease-free survival, while more than 12 lymph nodes and adjuvant chemotherapy were correlated to a better disease-free survival.

There are several limitations to our study. First, this is a retrospective study. Patients were not prospectively randomized and selection bias cannot be excluded, even though the groups were well matched in size, age, gender, and tumor-specific parameters. As the indication for adjuvant therapy changed in 2008 in Germany, the comparison could be described as historical. Second, follow-up time was significantly longer in the NACT group. The difference is explainable by the consecutive change of guidelines. These two points in turn can be regarded as strength of this study, making it a "quasi-RCT." Furthermore, follow-up in patients who received adjuvant chemotherapy still was 54 months in mean.

Third, a possible sign of selection bias is the higher proportion of ypT0 patients in the group without adjuvant chemotherapy. In fact, clinicians are often averse to the application of adjuvant chemotherapy in pCR patients. Breugom et al. criticized the retrospective character of the study by Maas et al. and the fact that the other study supporting adjuvant chemotherapy was a meta-analysis [7, 14, 28]. However, a meta-analysis usually reduces the risk of confounding.

A more detailed analysis of surgical complications other than anastomotic leakage could not be performed. Even if the database was prospectively performed and updated, the number of parameters documenter increased over time, e.g., the Clavien-Dindo complication grading was only introduced at a later stage. However, anastomotic leakage, which was adequately documented in the database, is one of the most severe complications in rectal surgery and most often the reason why adjuvant chemotherapy is delayed or not started at all. Moreover, leakage has been shown to influence the oncological outcome, and as both groups demonstrated a comparable leakage rate, this factor can be ruled out as a biasing factor.

At last, the sample size is too small to be able to evaluate statistical significant difference in rare incidences such as local recurrence that occurred only once.

Regardless of these limitations, the results support current guideline recommendations that in patients with ypT0−2 tumors adjuvant chemotherapy should continue to be administered, especially in ypT2 stages.

Conclusion

Administration of adjuvant chemotherapy after neoadjuvant chemoradiation and radical resection in rectal cancer improved disease-free and overall survival of patients with ypT0−2 ypN0 tumor stages in our study. In particular, ypT2 ypN0 patients seem to profit from adjuvant treatment.

Acknowledgements
Data from this publication have been previously presented as a poster at the 10th Scientific and Annual Meeting of the European Society of Coloproctology, 23–25 September 2015, Dublin, Ireland [29].

Authors' contributions
CG collected, analyzed, and interpreted the patient data and was a major contributor in writing the manuscript. KM collected the data from the Department of Oncology and was a major contributor in writing and editing the manuscript. SM collected the data from the Department of Radio-Oncology and was a major contributor in writing and editing the manuscript. TG performed the histological examinations and was a major contributor in reviewing and editing the manuscript. FW provided the resources in the Department of Radio-Oncology and was a major contributor in reviewing and editing the manuscript. SP provided the resources in the Department of Surgery and was a major contributor in reviewing and editing the manuscript. PK supervised the project and was a major contributor in writing, reviewing, and editing the manuscript. RDH provided the resources in the Department of Oncology and was a major contributor in writing, reviewing, and editing the manuscript. KH was responsible for the conceptualization, data collection, formal analysis, and writing of the manuscript as well as editing. KH was responsible for the project administration. All authors read and approved the final manuscript.

Competing interests
The authors declare that they have no competing interests.

Author details
[1]Department of Surgery, University Hospital Mannheim, Medical Faculty Mannheim, University of Heidelberg, Theodor-Kutzer-Ufer 1-3, 68167 Mannheim, Germany. [2]Interdisciplinary Tumor Centre, III. Department of Internal Medicine, University Hospital Mannheim, Medical Faculty Mannheim, University of Heidelberg, Mannheim, Germany. [3]Institute for Radiotherapy and Radiooncology, University Hospital Mannheim, Medical Faculty Mannheim, University of Heidelberg, Mannheim, Germany. [4]Institute for Pathology, University Hospital Mannheim, Medical Faculty Mannheim, University of Heidelberg, Mannheim, Germany. [5]Department of Visceral and Transplant Surgery, Universitätsspital Zürich, Zürich, Switzerland. [6]Department of Surgery, Theresienkrankenhaus Mannheim, Mannheim, Germany.

References

1. Sauer R, Becker H, Hohenberger W, Rodel C, Wittekind C, Fietkau R, Martus P, Tschmelitsch J, Hager E, Hess CF, et al. Preoperative versus postoperative chemoradiotherapy for rectal cancer. N Engl J Med. 2004;351(17):1731–40.
2. Leitlinienprogramm Onkologie (Deutsche Krebsgesellschaft DK, AWMF). In: AWMF, editor. S3-Leitlinie Kolorektales Karzinom. vol. Registrierungsnummer: 021-007OL, Langversion 1.1 edn; 2014.
3. Gerard JP, Conroy T, Bonnetain F, Bouche O, Chapet O, Closon-Dejardin MT, Untereiner M, Leduc B, Francois E, Maurel J, et al. Preoperative radiotherapy with or without concurrent fluorouracil and leucovorin in T3-4 rectal cancers: results of FFCD 9203. J Clin Oncol. 2006;24(28):4620–5.
4. Collette L, Bosset JF, den Dulk M, Nguyen F, Mineur L, Maingon P, Radosevic-Jelic L, Pierart M, Calais G. Patients with curative resection of cT3-4 rectal cancer after preoperative radiotherapy or radiochemotherapy: does anybody benefit from adjuvant fluorouracil-based chemotherapy? A trial of the European Organisation for Research and Treatment of Cancer Radiation Oncology Group. J Clin Oncol. 2007;25(28):4379–86.
5. Sainato A, Cernusco Luna Nunzia V, Valentini V, De Paoli A, Maurizi ER, Lupattelli M, Aristei C, Vidali C, Conti M, Galardi A, et al. No benefit of adjuvant fluorouracil leucovorin chemotherapy after neoadjuvant chemoradiotherapy in locally advanced cancer of the rectum (LARC): long term results of a randomized trial (I-CNR-RT). Radiother Oncol. 2014;113(2):223–9.
6. Breugom AJ, van Gijn W, Muller EW, Berglund A, van den Broek CB, Fokstuen T, Gelderblom H, Kapiteijn E, Leer JW, Marijnen CA, et al. Adjuvant chemotherapy for rectal cancer patients treated with preoperative (chemo)radiotherapy and total mesorectal excision: a Dutch Colorectal Cancer Group (DCCG) randomized phase III trialdagger. Ann Oncol. 2015; 26(4):696–701.
7. Maas M, Nelemans PJ, Valentini V, Crane CH, Capirci C, Rodel C, Nash GM, Kuo LJ, Glynne-Jones R, Garcia-Aguilar J, et al. Adjuvant chemotherapy in rectal cancer: defining subgroups who may benefit after neoadjuvant chemoradiation and resection: a pooled analysis of 3,313 patients. Int J Cancer. 2015;137(1):212–20.
8. Breugom AJ, Swets M, Bosset JF, Collette L, Sainato A, Cionini L, Glynne-Jones R, Counsell N, Bastiaannet E, van den Broek CB, et al. Adjuvant chemotherapy after preoperative (chemo)radiotherapy and surgery for patients with rectal cancer: a systematic review and meta-analysis of individual patient data. Lancet Oncol. 2015;16(2):200–7.
9. Nagtegaal ID, van de Velde CJ, van der Worp E, Kapiteijn E, Quirke P, van Krieken JH. Macroscopic evaluation of rectal cancer resection specimen: clinical significance of the pathologist in quality control. J Clin Oncol. 2002; 20(7):1729–34.
10. Rectum JSfCotCa. Japanese classification of colorectal carcinoma, first english edition edn. Tokyo: Kanehara & Co.; 1997.

11. Sauer R, Liersch T, Merkel S, Fietkau R, Hohenberger W, Hess C, Becker H, Raab HR, Villanueva MT, Witzigmann H, et al. Preoperative versus postoperative chemoradiotherapy for locally advanced rectal cancer: results of the German CAO/ARO/AIO-94 randomized phase III trial after a median follow-up of 11 years. J Clin Oncol. 2012;30(16):1926–33.

12. Petrelli F, Coinu A, Barni S. Adjuvant chemotherapy for rectal cancer. Lancet Oncol. 2015;16(4):e152–3.

13. Hofheinz RD, Rodel C, Burkholder I, Kienle P. Adjuvant chemotherapy for rectal cancer. Lancet Oncol. 2015;16(4):e154–5.

14. Petrelli F, Coinu A, Lonati V, Barni S. A systematic review and meta-analysis of adjuvant chemotherapy after neoadjuvant treatment and surgery for rectal cancer. Int J Color Dis. 2015;30(4):447–57.

15. Hofheinz RD, Wenz F, Post S, Matzdorff A, Laechelt S, Hartmann JT, Muller L, Link H, Moehler M, Kettner E, et al. Chemoradiotherapy with capecitabine versus fluorouracil for locally advanced rectal cancer: a randomised, multicentre, non-inferiority, phase 3 trial. Lancet Oncol. 2012;13(6):579–88.

16. Bosset JF, Calais G, Mineur L, Maingon P, Stojanovic-Rundic S, Bensadoun RJ, Bardet E, Beny A, Ollier JC, Bolla M, et al. Fluorouracil-based adjuvant chemotherapy after preoperative chemoradiotherapy in rectal cancer: long-term results of the EORTC 22921 randomised study. Lancet Oncol. 2014; 15(2):184–90.

17. Bujko K, Kolodziejczyk M, Nasierowska-Guttmejer A, Michalski W, Kepka L, Chmielik E, Wojnar A, Chwalinski M. Tumour regression grading in patients with residual rectal cancer after preoperative chemoradiation. Radiother Oncol. 2010;95(3):298–302.

18. Valentini V, van Stiphout RG, Lammering G, Gambacorta MA, Barba MC, Bebenek M, Bonnetain F, Bosset JF, Bujko K, Cionini L, et al. Nomograms for predicting local recurrence, distant metastases, and overall survival for patients with locally advanced rectal cancer on the basis of European randomized clinical trials. J Clin Oncol. 2011;29(23):3163–72.

19. Bosset JF, Collette L, Calais G, Mineur L, Maingon P, Radosevic-Jelic L, Daban A, Bardet E, Beny A, Ollier JC. Chemotherapy with preoperative radiotherapy in rectal cancer. N Engl J Med. 2006;355(11):1114–23.

20. Ngan SY, Burmeister B, Fisher RJ, Solomon M, Goldstein D, Joseph D, Ackland SP, Schache D, McClure B, McLachlan SA, et al. Randomized trial of short-course radiotherapy versus long-course chemoradiation comparing rates of local recurrence in patients with T3 rectal cancer: Trans-Tasman Radiation Oncology Group trial 01.04. J Clin Oncol. 2012;30(31):3827–33.

21. Glimelius B, Pahlman L, Cervantes A, Group EGW. Rectal cancer: ESMO Clinical Practice Guidelines for diagnosis, treatment and follow-up. Ann Oncol. 2010;21(Suppl 5):v82–6.

22. Baxter NN, Morris AM, Rothenberger DA, Tepper JE. Impact of preoperative radiation for rectal cancer on subsequent lymph node evaluation: a population-based analysis. Int J Radiat Oncol Biol Phys. 2005;61(2):426–31.

23. Scabini S, Ferrando V. Number of lymph nodes after neoadjuvant therapy for rectal cancer: how many are needed? World J Gastrointest Surg. 2012; 4(2):32–5.

24. Kim YW, Kim NK, Min BS, Lee KY, Sohn SK, Cho CH. The influence of the number of retrieved lymph nodes on staging and survival in patients with stage II and III rectal cancer undergoing tumor-specific mesorectal excision. Ann Surg. 2009;249(6):965–72.

25. Kim YW, Kim NK, Min BS, Lee KY, Sohn SK, Cho CH, Kim H, Keum KC, Ahn JB. The prognostic impact of the number of lymph nodes retrieved after neoadjuvant chemoradiotherapy with mesorectal excision for rectal cancer. J Surg Oncol. 2009;100(1):1–7.

26. Park IJ, Yu CS, Lim SB, Yoon YS, Kim CW, Kim TW, Kim JH, Kim JC. Prognostic implications of the number of retrieved lymph nodes of patients with rectal cancer treated with preoperative chemoradiotherapy. J Gastrointest Surg. 2014;18(10):1845–51.

27. Blaker H, Hildebrandt B, Riess H, von Winterfeld M, Ingold-Heppner B, Roth W, Kloor M, Schirmacher P, Dietel M, Tao S, et al. Lymph node count and prognosis in colorectal cancer: the influence of examination quality. Int J Cancer. 2015;136(8):1957–66.

28. Breugom AJ, Swets M, van de Velde CJ. Adjuvant chemotherapy for rectal cancer – authors' reply. Lancet Oncol. 2015;16(4):e155.

29. Galata C, Merx K, Mai S, Gaiser T, Kienle P, Post S, Hofheinz RD, Horisberger K. Impact of adjuvant chemotherapy in ypT0-2 ypN0 rectal cancer patients. Poster Abstracts (P177). Color Dis. 2015;17:38–101. https://doi.org/10.1111/codi.13053.

6

Survival benefit of pure dose-dense chemotherapy in breast cancer

Wenqi Zhou[1], Shizhe Chen[2], Faliang Xu[1] and Xiaohua Zeng[1]* ⓘ

Abstract

Background: Dose-dense chemotherapy is a widely accepted regimen for high-risk breast cancer patients. However, conflicting survival benefits of pure dose-dense chemotherapy have been reported in different randomized controlled trials (RCTs). This meta-analysis aimed to further assess the efficacy and safety of pure dose-dense chemotherapy in breast cancer.

Methods: A literature search of electronic databases and websites was performed to identify phase III RCTs reporting the efficacy and toxicity of pure dose-dense chemotherapy. The endpoints of interest were overall survival (OS), disease-free survival (DFS), and toxicities. The hazard ratios (HRs) of death and recurrence and the odds ratios (ORs) of adverse events were estimated and pooled.

Results: Seven studies (five trials) were eligible, encompassing a total of 9851 patients. Patients treated with dose-dense chemotherapy obtained better DFS (HR = 0.83; 95% CI 0.75–0.91; p = 0.0001) than those treated with the conventional schedule, while OS benefit of dose-dense chemotherapy was less impressive (HR = 0.86; 95% CI 0.73–1.02; p = 0.08). However, significant OS benefit was observed in node-positive patients (HR = 0.77; 95% CI 0.66–0.90; p = 0.001). The incidence of anemia, pain, and transaminase elevation was higher in the dose-dense chemotherapy arm.

Conclusions: Dose-dense chemotherapy leads to better prognosis; these findings suggest that it may be a potentially preferred treatment for breast cancer patients, particularly for women with lymph node involvement. However, more RCTs are warranted to better define the best candidates for dose-dense chemotherapy.

Keywords: Dose-dense, Chemotherapy, Breast cancer, Overall survival, Meta-analysis

Background

Breast cancer is the most commonly diagnosed cancer and the second leading cause of cancer death among women in the USA [1]. Although adjuvant chemotherapy confers about a one-third reduction for 10-year risk of death from breast cancer [2], a large number of patients will suffer from recurrence and breast cancer-related death. Thus, to further optimize prognoses of breast cancer patients with elevated recurrence risk, different approaches have been taken to improve the efficacy of chemotherapy, including the addition of new drugs or modifications of drug delivery.

According to the Norton-Simon hypothesis [3] and the Gomepertzian growth pattern [4], delivering drugs at shorter intervals may maximize the possibility of eradicating tumor cells by shortening the time for tumor regression between treatments. Dose-dense chemotherapy, in which drugs are delivered with shorter interval between treatments, is a widely accepted regimen for high-risk breast cancer patients [5]. Even so, treatment guidelines vary from Europe [6] to America [5]. According to the St. Gallen International Breast Cancer Consensus in 2017 [6], there were no clear recommendations for dose-dense chemotherapy, and less than half of the attendees thought that dose-dense regimens should be preferred in triple-negative patients. Furthermore, the few existing studies based on pure dose-dense chemotherapy, in which

* Correspondence: qq-zxh@126.com; 691155466@qq.com
[1]Breast Center, Chongqing University Cancer Hospital & Chongqing Cancer Institute & Chongqing Cancer Hospital, Chongqing 400030, People's Republic of China
Full list of author information is available at the end of the article

drugs were administered at shorter intervals with the same cycles and doses of conventional regimen, have reported conflicting results. The CALGB 9741 [7] and GIM2 [8] trials demonstrated that dose-dense chemotherapy significantly improved disease-free survival (DFS) and overall survival (OS), while no survival benefit of dose-dense chemotherapy was observed in the MIG-1 [9] and TACT2 [10] trials. Meta-analyses have shown that dose-dense chemotherapy produces a significant improvement in DFS, especially in patients with negative hormone receptor, while the results of OS were controversial [11–13]. However, few of them were based on pure dose-dense trials, and thus, the real benefit of the increase in dose density cannot be assessed appropriately due to the introduction of confounding factors. Furthermore, none of the previous meta-analyses included the new results of the TACT2 trial. Therefore, this updated meta-analysis was performed to further investigate the efficacy and toxicity of pure dose-dense chemotherapy.

Methods

This meta-analysis was performed in accordance with the recommendation outlined in the Preferred Reporting Items for Systematic Reviews and Meta-Analyses (PRISMA) statement [14]. A literature search was performed using the databases of PubMed/MEDLINE, Cochrane library, EMBASE through 1 September 2017. In addition, the ASCO, SABCS, and ESMO Meeting websites were scrutinized. The search strategy was developed using the following terms: (breast cancer OR breast tumor OR breast neoplasms OR breast carcinoma) and (drug therapy OR chemotherapy) and ((dose dense) OR accelerat* OR (14 days) OR (2 weeks) OR biweekly OR weekly OR (2 weekly)) and (random* OR prospective*).

Selection criteria

This meta-analysis was based on phase III RCTs in which the dose-dense regimen of the experimental arm was narrowly defined as delivering drugs over a shorter interval with the same cycle and dosage of the conventional schedule in the control arm. Full papers and conference abstracts providing sufficient data were eligible. Studies that included metastatic breast cancer patients and studies based on impure dose-dense regimens (with different type or dosage of drugs) were ineligible. In addition, studies without outcomes of interest were excluded.

Quality assessment

The methodological quality of the eligible studies was independently assessed by two reviewers using the Cochrane risk-of-bias tool, which consists of the following domains of bias: selection bias, performance bias, detection bias, attrition bias, and reporting bias [15, 16]. Disagreements were resolved through discussion and consensus.

Data extraction

A standardized Excel form was used to extract data from eligible studies, including first author, year of publication, sample size, inclusion criteria, chemotherapy regimen, and median follow-up. The primary endpoint was OS (measured from randomization until death from any cause); other outcomes of interest were DFS (measured from randomization until local recurrence, distant relapse, or death without relapse, whichever occurred first) and incidence of grade 3 to 5 toxicities. The hazard ratios (HRs) and variances of time-to-event data were extracted from the original studies or were estimated as described by Parmar et al. [17] and Tierney et al. [18].

Statistical analysis

Hazard ratios (HRs) and odds ratios (ORs) were calculated to compare time to event outcomes and dichotomous data, respectively. An HR or OR less than one favored the dose-dense chemotherapy arm. The meta-analyses of outcomes were based on a fixed-effect model, except the outcomes with significant heterogeneity, for which a random-effect model was used.

Heterogeneity was quantified using the inconsistency index (I^2) and the p value of the χ^2 test. Significant heterogeneity was considered to exist for p values less than 0.1 or I^2 greater than 50%. Subgroup analyses were conducted according to hormone receptor status of the tumors and the inclusion criteria of the studies to assess potential contributions to outcomes. Publication bias was evaluated by funnel plots and Egger's test [19]. The meta-analysis was performed using RevMan version 5.3.

Results

Study selection

According to the research strategy, a total of 4079 studies were retrieved, of which 3081 studies were removed owing to duplication or overlap using Endnote software. Another 917 studies were excluded by screening the titles and abstracts. After reading the remaining 81 full-text articles, 74 studies were excluded. Ultimately, 7 studies [7–10, 20–22] based on 5 phase III RCTs that compared pure dose-dense chemotherapy with conventional chemotherapy were included. Figure 1 shows the details of the study selection process and the exclusion criteria.

Characteristics of eligible studies

The characteristics of the included studies are listed in Table 1. A total of 9851 node-positive or high-risk

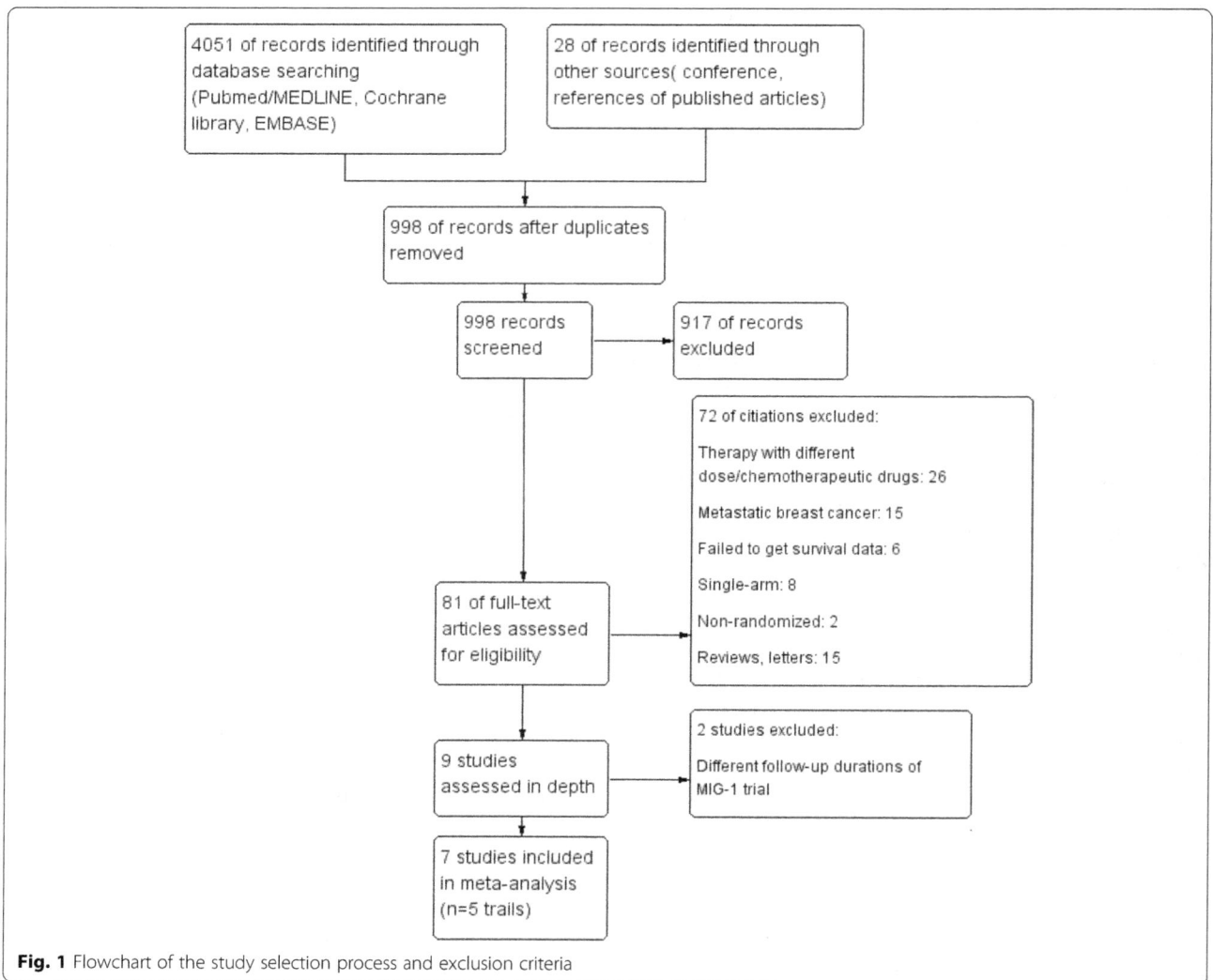

Fig. 1 Flowchart of the study selection process and exclusion criteria

node-negative patients were included in this meta-analysis. Four studies (three trials) [9, 10, 20, 21] were based on anthracycline, while the other three studies (two trials) [7, 8, 22] were based on anthracycline and taxane. Among the five included trials, survival data of the CALGB 9741 trial and MIG-1 trial were updated in abstract forms at the San Antonio Breast Cancer Symposium in 2005 [22] and the European Society for Medical Oncology in 2016 [21], respectively. The risk of bias for each study is reported in Table 2. TACT2 trial [10] was judged as high risk for reporting bias due to incomplete reporting of the DFS outcome.

Overall survival

A total of 9731 patients were included in the OS meta-analysis. Updated abstracts [21, 22] of two eligible trials [7, 9] were included in this meta-analysis. Patients in the dose-dense arm failed to obtain a significant OS

benefit compared with those in the conventional arm (HR = 0.86; 95%CI 0.73–1.02; p = 0.08). A random effect model was used due to the high heterogeneity among studies (I^2 = 59%) (Fig. 2). According to the subgroup analysis based on hormone receptor status, dose-dense chemotherapy produced significant OS benefit in patients with negative hormone receptor status (HR = 0.73; 95%CI 0.59–0.90; p = 0.003; I^2 = 0%), but not in hormone receptor-positive patients (HR = 0.83; 95% CI 0.69–1.00; p = 0.05; I^2 = 0%). However, there was no sign of interaction between survival benefit of the dose-dense regimen and hormone receptor status (interaction test, p = 0.36). Figure 3 illustrates the analysis according to hormone receptor status.

Disease-free survival

The meta-analysis of DFS covered 5340 patients. According to the result, DFS was significantly improved in the dose-dense arm (HR = 0.83; 95% CI 0.75–0.91; p = 0.0001),

Table 1 Characteristics of included studies

Study	N	Patients	Treatment	MF	DFS HR(95%CI) DD vs Con	OS HR(95%CI) DD vs Con
Baldini 2003	150	IIIA/B	dd(CEF → CMF/CEF) CEF → CMF/CEF	5 years	0.77(0.47–1.26)	0.87(0.49–1.53)
CALGB 9741						
(1)Citron 2003	2005	T0–3, N1–2, M0	dd(A → P → C) A → P → C	36 months	0.74(0.59–0.93)	0.69(050–0.93)
(2)Hudis 2005			dd(AC → P) AC → P	69 months	0.80(0.67–0.96)	0.85(0.68–1.05)
MIG-1						
(1)Venturini 2005	1214	pN+(≤ 10); pN– and high risk	ddFEC FEC	10.4 years	0.88(0.71–1.08)	0.87(0.67–1.13)
(2)Giraudi 2016				15.8 years	0.90(0.77–1.05)	0.89(0.72–1.09)
GIM2 Mastro 2015	2091	pN+(≥ 1)	dd(EC → P) EC → P dd(FEC → P) FEC → P	7 years	0.77(0.65–0.92)	0.65(0.51–0.84)
TACT2 Cameron 2017	4391	≥ 18 years; pN+; pN– and high risk (T0–3,N0–2,M0)	ddE → CMF E → CMF ddE → X E → X	85.6 months	NA	1.04(0.88–1.21)

N number of patients, MF median follow-up, DFS disease-free survival, OS overall survival, HR hazard ratio, CI confidence interval, DD dose-dense chemotherapy, Con conventional chemotherapy, NA not available, CEF cyclophosphamide + epirubicin + 5-fluorouracil; CMF, cyclophosphamide + methotrexate + 5-fluorouracil, A doxorubicin, P paclitaxel, C cyclophosphamide, AC doxorubicin + cyclophosphamide, FEC 5-fluorouracil + epirubicin + cyclophosphamide, X capecitabine

with no heterogeneity (I^2 = 0%) (Fig. 4). Considering the different hormone receptor status, dose-dense chemotherapy conferred a significant improvement in DFS in patients with hormone receptor-negative tumor (HR = 0.74; 95%CI 0.62–0.89; p = 0.001; I^2 = 0%), while patients with hormone receptor-positive tumor obtained no significant DFS benefit (p = 0.53) (interaction test, p = 0.20).

Toxicities

The incidences of grade 3 to 5 neutropenia (OR = 0.14; 95% CI 0.09–0.24; p < 0.0001), leukopenia (OR = 0.39; 95% CI 0.28–0.55; p < 0.0001), and neuropathy (OR = 0.72; 95% CI 0.54–0.97; p = 0.03) were significantly lower in the dose-dense arm than those in the conventional arm. However, pooled analyses demonstrated that dose-dense chemotherapy significantly increased the incidences of grade 3 to 5 anemia (OR = 4.08; 95% CI 0.67–9.99; p = 0.002), pain

(OR = 1.67; 95% CI 1.24–2.55; p = 0.0007), and transaminase elevation (OR = 3.71; 95% CI 1.50–9.17; p = 0.005) compared with the conventional regimen. There was no difference between dose-dense and conventional chemotherapy in terms of thrombocytopenia, asthenia, diarrhea, stomatitis, nausea/vomiting, and infection. The details are shown in Table 3.

Heterogeneity

As previously mentioned, there was high heterogeneity in the pooled analysis of OS (I^2 = 59%). Neither the funnel plot (Fig. 5) nor Egger's test (p = 0.729) indicated significant publication bias. To explore the between-study heterogeneity, a subgroup analysis was performed based on the characteristics of the included patients. The pooled analysis of three studies in which eligible patients all had nodal involvement demonstrated significantly better OS in the dose-dense arm (HR = 0.77; 95% CI

Table 2 Risk of bias summary for each included study

Study	Selection bias	Performance bias	Detection bias	Attrition bias	Reporting bias	Other bias
Cameron 2017 (TACT2)	Low	Low	Low	Low	High	Low
Baldini 2003	Low	Low	Low	Low	Low	Low
Citron 2003/Hudis 2005 (CALGB 9741)	Unclear	Low	Low	Low	Low	Low
Venturini 2005/Giraudi 2016 (MIG-1)	Low	Low	Low	Low	Low	Low
Mastro 2015 (GIM2)	Low	Low	Low	Low	Low	low

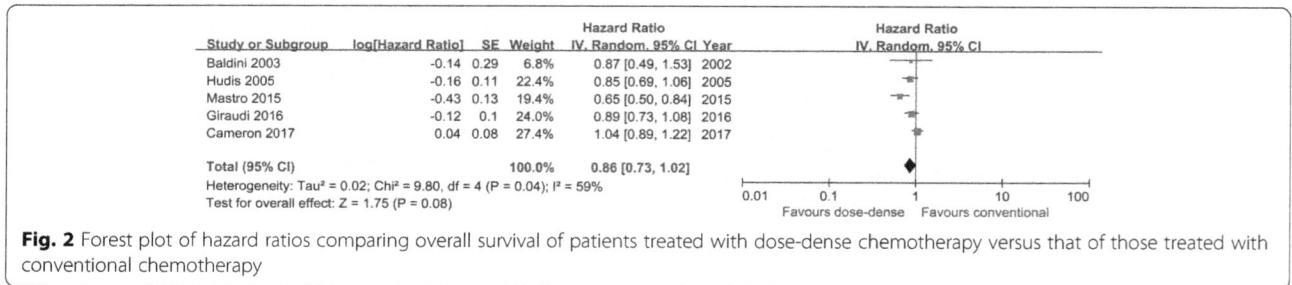

Fig. 2 Forest plot of hazard ratios comparing overall survival of patients treated with dose-dense chemotherapy versus that of those treated with conventional chemotherapy

0.66–0.90; $p = 0.001$; $I^2 = 26\%$). While the pooled results from the other two studies, which included both node-positive and high-risk node-negative patients, failed to show significant benefit (HR = 0.98; 95% CI 0.87–1.11; $p = 0.72$; $I^2 = 36\%$). In addition, there was a significant interaction between OS benefit of dose-dense chemotherapy and patient characteristics ($p = 0.02$; see Fig. 6).

Discussion

As a newly updated meta-analysis based on phase III RCTs regarding the efficacy and safety of pure dose-dense chemotherapy, the pooled results demonstrated a 17% reduction in risk of recurrence and a 14% reduction in risk of death, though the OS benefit was less obvious. A possible explanation for the lack of significant OS benefit may be the insufficient follow-up duration, which prevents the real impact of the dose-dense regimen to be verified. Additionally, the specific agents and total dose in eligible studies may vary from state-of-the-art regimens, especially those conducted in early years. According to the subgroup analysis by inclusion criterion, the pooled analysis of studies based on patients with lymph node involvement showed a significant OS benefit in the dose-dense arm, while

studies including patients without lymph node involvement did not. Furthermore, the interaction test showed significant evidence of interaction between dose-dense benefit and patient selection (interaction test, $p = 0.02$). Therefore, the heterogeneity may largely be driven by the different inclusion criteria, especially the nodal status of patients. This was supported by the AGO trial [23], which demonstrated a more pronounced benefit of intense dose-dense chemotherapy among patients with 10 or more involved lymph nodes (HR = 0.64; $p = 0.0012$). A similar effect was also observed in the MIG-1 trial [9]. In this study, the OS benefit of dose-dense chemotherapy seemed to be restricted to patients with lymph node involvement, but there were insufficient primary studies to further assess the survival benefit of dose-dense chemotherapy in patients with different nodal status.

With the support of pegfilgrastim, the incidence of neutropenia was significantly reduced in the dose-dense arm. The high heterogeneity ($I^2 = 87\%$) may be due to higher incidence of neutropenia resulting from FEC-P (fluorouracil, epirubicin, cyclophosphamide followed by paclitaxel) in the GIM2 trial [8]. However, dose-dense schedules inevitably increased the risk of anemia, pain, and transaminase elevation. There was insufficient data for this meta-analysis to assess treatment-induced amenorrhea. The TACT2 trial

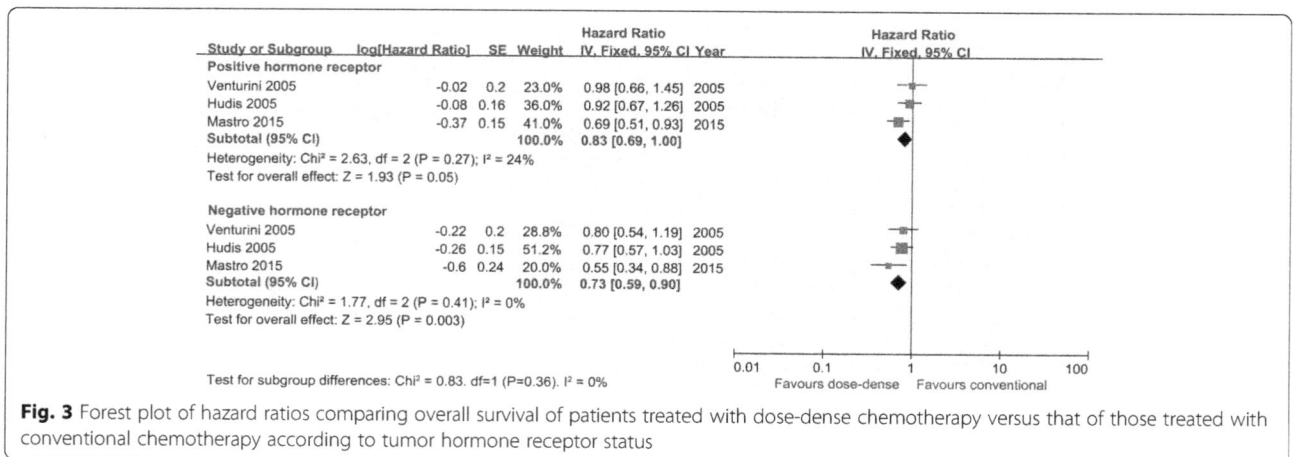

Fig. 3 Forest plot of hazard ratios comparing overall survival of patients treated with dose-dense chemotherapy versus that of those treated with conventional chemotherapy according to tumor hormone receptor status

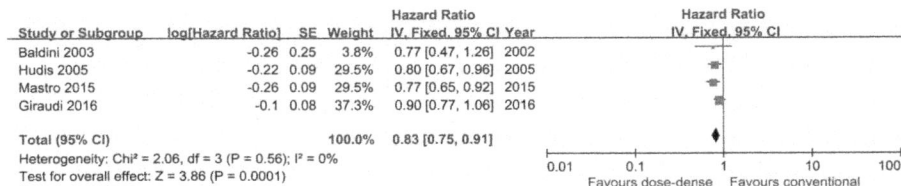

Study or Subgroup	log[Hazard Ratio]	SE	Weight	Hazard Ratio IV, Fixed, 95% CI	Year	Hazard Ratio IV, Fixed, 95% CI
Baldini 2003	-0.26	0.25	3.8%	0.77 [0.47, 1.26]	2002	
Hudis 2005	-0.22	0.09	29.5%	0.80 [0.67, 0.96]	2005	
Mastro 2015	-0.26	0.09	29.5%	0.77 [0.65, 0.92]	2015	
Giraudi 2016	-0.1	0.08	37.3%	0.90 [0.77, 1.06]	2016	
Total (95% CI)			100.0%	0.83 [0.75, 0.91]		

Heterogeneity: Chi² = 2.06, df = 3 (P = 0.56); I² = 0%
Test for overall effect: Z = 3.86 (P = 0.0001)

Favours dose-dense   Favours conventional

Fig. 4 Forest plot of hazard ratios comparing disease-free survival of patients treated with dose-dense chemotherapy versus that of those treated with conventional chemotherapy

[10] demonstrated that the risk of permanently discontinued menstruation did not differ between dose-dense and conventional chemotherapy. In addition, a pooled analysis focusing on premenopausal patients also confirmed no increased risk of amenorrhea with dose-dense chemotherapy [24]. Hence, dose-dense chemotherapy seems to be an effective and tolerable treatment choice for breast cancer patients.

Similar meta-analyses performed by Bonilla et al. [11] and Petrelli et al. [13] both suggested that dose-dense chemotherapy was associated with improved OS and DFS, especially in hormone receptor-negative patients. However, it should be noted that both of these meta-analyses included trials with impure study design. Therefore, the interpretability of these results was confounded by the variety of dose intensity, type of drug, and cycle number of chemotherapy between dose-dense and control groups. To conduct a true test of the dose-dense concept without confounders, we narrowly defined the dose-dense schedule. Thus, metronomic chemotherapy, which is a variation of the dose-dense schedule whereby drugs are administered at lower doses and shorter intervals [25], is ineligible for this meta-analysis. As evaluated in the E1199 [26] and S0221 [27] trials, metronomic chemotherapy always represents

an intense dose-dense schedule. Unlike these studies, Duarte et al. [12] performed a meta-analysis based on pure dose-dense regimens and reported a similar finding as our study, although they did not include the results of the GIM2 trial [8], the TACT2 trial [10], or the updated result of the MIG1 trial [21].

Therefore, this newest updated meta-analysis further confirms that pure dose-dense chemotherapy leads to prolonged DFS and highlights a significant OS benefit in node-positive patients. Despite the significant improvement in OS among hormone receptor-negative patients treated with dose-dense chemotherapy, there was no sign of interaction between dose-dense benefit and hormone receptor status (interaction test, $p = 0.36$). Thus, the subgroup analysis should be interpreted cautiously, and the greater efficacy of dose-dense chemotherapy in hormone receptor-negative patients elucidated in previous studies may need further investigation. To our knowledge, an EBCTCG meta-analysis reported at the 40th San Antonio Breast Cancer Symposium at an oral session revealed significant reductions in DFS and 10-year breast cancer mortality with dose-dense chemotherapy, which, together with our results, provides further evidence of the efficacy and safety of dose-dense chemotherapy [28].

There are some limitations of this meta-analysis that need to be addressed. First, the limited number of eligible studies may contribute to unstable results, which

Table 3 Meta-analysis of toxicities comparing dose-dense chemotherapy versus conventional chemotherapy

Toxicity (grade 3 to 5)	N	OR (95%CI)	I^2 (%)	p value
Anemia	7379	4.08 [1.67, 9.99]	0	0.002
Neutropenia	6049	0.14 [0.09, 0.24]	87	< 0.0001
Leukopenia	5407	0.39 [0.28, 0.55]	26	< 0.0001
Thrombocytopenia	7379	1.10 [0.47, 2.54]	0	0.83
Asthenia	5271	1.28 [0.93, 1.75]	0	0.13
Diarrhea	7233	1.16 [0.73, 1.86]	0	0.53
Pain	7379	1.67 [1.24, 2.25]	0	0.0007
Stomatitis	7379	1.37 [0.88, 2.15]	0	0.17
Nausea/vomiting	7379	1.18 [0.97, 1.42]	0	0.09
Neuropathy	7233	0.72 [0.54, 0.97]	0	0.03
Transaminase elevation	5271	3.71 [1.50, 9.17]	0	0.005
Infection	5271	0.86 [0.62, 1.19]	0	0.35

N number of patients, OR odds ratio, CI confidence interval

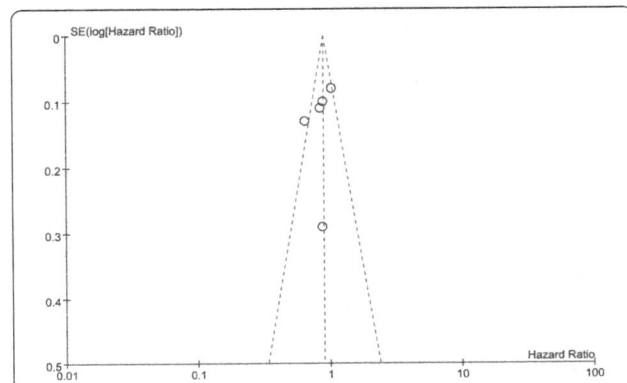

Fig. 5 Funnel plot of overall survival in all eligible trials for the visual detection of systematic publication bias and small study effects

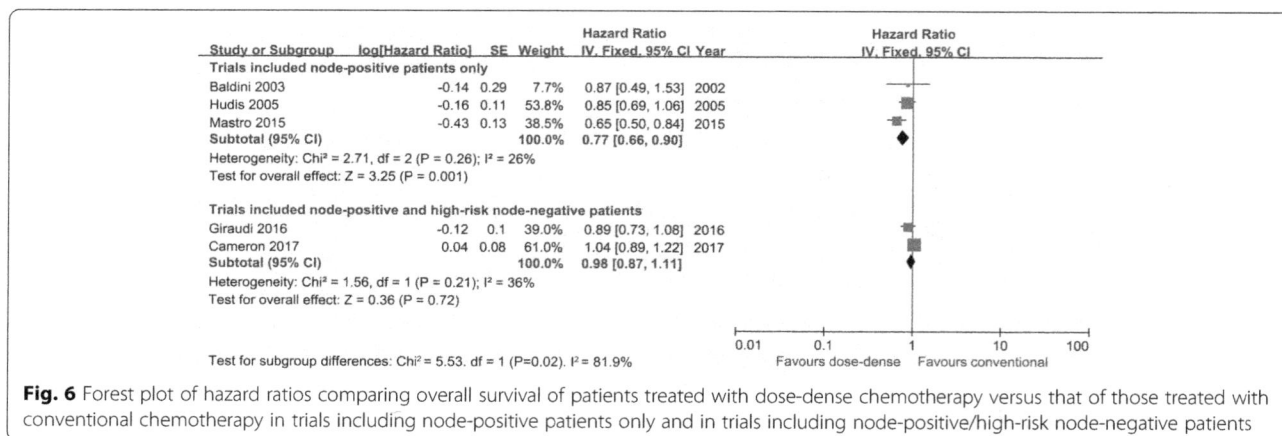

Fig. 6 Forest plot of hazard ratios comparing overall survival of patients treated with dose-dense chemotherapy versus that of those treated with conventional chemotherapy in trials including node-positive patients only and in trials including node-positive/high-risk node-negative patients

may be influenced by unpublished data and further studies, even though there was no sign of significant publication bias according to the funnel plot and Egger's test. Second, this is a meta-analysis based on published literature instead of individual patients, inevitable bias resulting from different study designs may lead to a less reliable result. Third, the chemotherapy regimens of the studies were different, and therefore, it is unclear whether the benefit of dose-dense chemotherapy was derived from taxane or anthracycline. Therefore, to gain further understanding of the survival benefit of dose-dense chemotherapy and to identify subgroups of patients who could gain significant benefit from a dose-dense schedule, more RCTs with pure dose-dense designs and longer follow-ups are warranted.

Conclusion

This study demonstrates that dose-dense chemotherapy leads to improved DFS and highlights a significant OS benefit in node-positive patients. Although limitations exist, this meta-analysis provides further evidence of the dominance and manageable toxicities of dose-dense chemotherapy. It may be a potential preferred treatment for breast cancer patients, particularly for women with lymph node involvement. However, further investigations are needed to better define specific groups of patients who may derive greater benefit from dose-dense chemotherapy.

Authors' contributions
WQZ and XHZ designed the concept. WQZ and SZC acquired the data and performed the analysis and interpretation of the data. WQZ drafted the manuscript. SZC, FLX, and XHZ provided a critical revision of the manuscript. All authors read and approved the final manuscript.

Competing interests
The authors declare that they have no competing interests.

Author details
[1]Breast Center, Chongqing University Cancer Hospital & Chongqing Cancer Institute & Chongqing Cancer Hospital, Chongqing 400030, People's Republic of China. [2]Xiehe Affiliated Hospital of Fujian Medical University, Fuzhou 350000, Fujian, People's Republic of China.

References
1. Siegel RL, Miller KD, Jemal A. Cancer statistics, 2017. CA Cancer J Clin. 2017; 67(1):7–30. https://doi.org/10.3322/caac.21387.
2. Cameron D. Comparisons between different polychemotherapy regimens for early breast cancer: meta-analyses of long-term outcome among 100 000 women in 123 randomised trials. Lancet. 2012;379(9814):432–44.
3. Simon R, Norton L. The Norton-Simon hypothesis: designing more effective and less toxic chemotherapeutic regimens. Nat Clin Pract Oncol. 2006;3(8):406–15.
4. Norton LA. Gompertzian model of human breast cancer growth. Cancer Res. 1988;48(1):7067–71.
5. Denduluri N, Somerfield MR, Eisen A, Holloway JN, Hurria A, King TA, et al. Selection of optimal adjuvant chemotherapy regimens for human epidermal growth factor receptor 2 (HER2)–negative and adjuvant targeted therapy for HER2-positive breast cancers: an American Society of Clinical Oncology Guideline adaptation of the Cancer Care Ontario Clinical Practice Guideline. J Clin Oncol. 2016;34(20):2416–27. https://doi.org/10.1200/jco.2016.67.0182.
6. Gnant M, Harbeck N, Thomssen C. St. Gallen/Vienna 2017: a brief summary of the consensus discussion about escalation and de-escalation of primary breast cancer treatment. Breast Care. 2017;12(2):102.
7. Citron ML, Berry DA, Cirrincione C, Hudis C, Winer EP, Gradishar WJ, et al. Randomized trial of dose-dense versus conventionally scheduled and sequential versus concurrent combination chemotherapy as postoperative adjuvant treatment of node-positive primary breast cancer: first report of intergroup trial C9741/cancer and leukemia group B trial 9741. J Clin Oncol. 2003;21(8):1431–9. https://doi.org/10.1200/jco.2003.09.081.
8. Mastro LD, Placido SD, Bruzzi P, Laurentiis MD, Boni C, Cavazzini G, et al. Fluorouracil and dose-dense chemotherapy in adjuvant treatment of patients with early-stage breast cancer: an open-label, 2×2 factorial, randomised phase 3 trial. Lancet. 2015;385(9980):1863.
9. Venturini M, Mastro LD, Aitini E, Baldini E, Caroti C, Contu A, et al. Dose-dense adjuvant chemotherapy in early breast cancer patients: results from a randomized trial. J Natl Cancer Inst. 2005;97(23):1724–33.
10. Cameron D, Morden JP, Canney P, Velikova G, Coleman R, Bartlett J, et al. Accelerated versus standard epirubicin followed by cyclophosphamide, methotrexate, and fluorouracil or capecitabine as adjuvant therapy for breast cancer in the randomised UK TACT2 trial (CRUK/05/19): a multicentre, phase 3, open-label, randomised, controlled trial. Lancet Oncol. 2017;18(7): 929–45. https://doi.org/10.1016/s1470-2045(17)30404-7.

11. Bonilla L, Benaharon I, Vidal L, Gaftergvili A, Leibovici L, Stemmer SM. Dose-dense chemotherapy in nonmetastatic breast cancer: a systematic review and meta-analysis of randomized controlled trials. J Natl Cancer Inst. 2010; 102(24):1845–54.

12. Duarte IL, Lima CSP, Sasse AD. Dose-dense chemotherapy versus conventional chemotherapy for early breast cancer: a systematic review with meta-analysis. Breast. 2012;21(3):343–9.

13. Petrelli F, Cabiddu M, Coinu A, Borgonovo K, Ghilardi M, Lonati V, et al. Adjuvant dose-dense chemotherapy in breast cancer: a systematic review and meta-analysis of randomized trials. Breast Cancer Res Treat. 2015;151(2):1–9.

14. Knobloch K, Yoon U, Vogt PM. Preferred reporting items for systematic reviews and meta-analyses (PRISMA) statement and publication bias. J Craniomaxillofac Surg. 2011;39(2):91–2. https://doi.org/10.1016/j.jcms.2010.11.001.

15. Higgins JPT, Green S. Cochrane Handbook for Systematic Reviews of Interventions Version 5.0. The Cochrane Collaboration; 2008. www.cochrane-handbook.org. Accessed 30 Sept 2008.

16. Higgins JPT, Altman DG, Gøtzsche PC, Jüni P, Moher D, Oxman AD et al. The Cochrane Collaboration's tool for assessing risk of bias in randomised trials. Bmj British Medical Journal. 2011;343(7829):889–93.

17. Parmar MK, Torri V, Stewart L. Extracting summary statistics to perform meta-analyses of the published literature for survival endpoints. Stat Med. 1998;17(24):2815–34.

18. Tierney JF, Stewart LA, Ghersi D, Burdett S, Sydes MR. Practical methods for incorporating summary time-to-event data into meta-analysis. Trials. 2007;8(1):16.

19. Egger M, Smith GD, Schneider M, Minder C. Bias in meta-analysis detected by a simple, graphical test. BMJ. 1997;315(7109):629–34. https://doi.org/10.1136/bmj.315.7109.629.

20. Baldini E, Gardin G, Giannessi PG, Evangelista G, Roncella M, Prochilo T, et al. Accelerated versus standard cyclophosphamide, epirubicin and 5-fluorouracil or cyclophosphamide, methotrexate and 5-fluorouracil: a randomized phase III trial in locally advanced breast cancer. Annals of Oncology Official Journal of the European Society for. Med Oncol. 2003;14(2):227.

21. Giraudi S, Cavazzini MG, Michelotti A, Censi AD, Testore F, Benasso M, et al. F08Dose-dence adjuvant chemotherapy in early breast cancer: the results of 15 years of follow-up. Ann Oncol. 2016;27(suppl_4):iv61–iv.

22. Hudis C, Citron M, Berry D, Cirrincione C, Gradishar W, Davidson N et al., editors. Five year follow-up of INT C9741: dose-dense (DD) chemotherapy (CRx) is safe and effective. San Antonio Breast Cancer Symposium; 2005.

23. Moebus V, Jackisch C, Lueck HJ, Du BA, Thomssen C, Kurbacher C, et al. Intense dose-dense sequential chemotherapy with epirubicin, paclitaxel, and cyclophosphamide compared with conventionally scheduled chemotherapy in high-risk primary breast cancer: mature results of an AGO phase III study. Journal of Clinical Oncology Official Journal of the American Society of Clinical Oncology. 2010;28(17):2874.

24. Lambertini M, Ceppi M, Cognetti F, Cavazzini G, Laurentiis MD, Placido SD, et al. Dose-dense adjuvant chemotherapy in premenopausal breast cancer patients: a pooled analysis of the MIG1 and GIM2 phase III studies. Eur J Cancer. 2017;71:34–42.

25. Mcarthur HL, Hudis CA. Dose-dense therapy in the treatment of early-stage breast cancer: an overview of the data. Clin Breast Cancer. 2007; 8(suppl 1):S6–S10.

26. Sparano JA, Zhao F, Martino S, Ligibel JA, Perez EA, Saphner T, et al. Long-term follow-up of the E1199 phase III trial evaluating the role of taxane and schedule in operable breast cancer. J Clin Oncol. 2015;33(21):2353–60.

27. Budd GT, Barlow WE, Moore HCF, Hobday TJ, Stewart JA, Isaacs C, et al. SWOG S0221: a phase III trial comparing chemotherapy schedules in high-risk early-stage breast cancer. Journal of Clinical Oncology Official Journal of the American Society of Clinical Oncology. 2015;33(1):58.

28. Gray R, Bradley R, Braybrooke J, Davies C, Pan H, Peto R et al. Increasing the dose density of adjuvant chemotherapy by shortening intervals between courses or by sequential drug administration significantly reduces both disease recurrence and breast cancer mortality: an EBCTCG meta-analysis of 21,000 women in 16 randomised trials. San Antonio Breast Cancer Symposium, 2017 Oral Session: General Session 1. 2017.

7

Prognostic and clinicopathological value of Beclin-1 expression in hepatocellular carcinoma

Zhiqiang Qin[1], Xinjuan Yu[2], Mei Lin[1*], Jinkun Wu[1], Shupei Ma[3] and Ning Wang[1]

Abstract

Background: The abnormal expression of Beclin-1 has recently been investigated in a variety of tumors. However, previous studies have obtained contradicting results regarding the clinical and prognostic value of Beclin-1 in hepatocellular carcinoma (HCC). We performed a meta-analysis to clarify the prognostic value of Beclin-1 and its correlations with clinical pathological parameters in HCC.

Methods: Relevant studies were systematically retrieved from PubMed, EMBASE, China National Knowledge Infrastructure (CNKI), Wan Fang and Chinese VIP databases. We used the Newcastle-Ottawa scale (NOS) to estimate the quality of the involved studies.

Results: Ten eligible studies with 1086 HCC patients were included in this study. Our results showed that decreased Beclin-1 expression in HCC related to histological grade [poor-undifferentiated vs. well-moderate: odds ratio (OR) = 2.34, 95% confidence interval (CI) = 1.65–3.32, $P < 0.00001$]. The pooled hazard ratio (HR) (HR = 1.43, 95% CI = 1.17–1.75, $P = 0.0004$) indicated that decreased Beclin-1 expression correlated with poor overall survival (OS).

Conclusions: This meta-analysis indicated that decreased Beclin-1 expression might relate to poor differentiation and unfavorable outcome in HCC.

Keywords: Beclin-1, Hepatocellular carcinoma (HCC), Clinicopathological factors, Prognosis, Meta-analysis

Background

Hepatocellular carcinoma (HCC) is a principal cause of human cancer death worldwide [1]. Thus far, surgical excision is one of the most effective treatments for HCC [2]. Most early diagnosed HCC patients are treated by surgical excision. However, the post-operative recurrence remains high [3], and the 5-year overall survival (OS) is currently only approximately 18% [4]. Therefore, it is essential to identify an effective biomarker to predict the prognosis of HCC.

Autophagy is an intracellular catabolic process by which cytoplasmic proteins and organelles are delivered to lysosomes and subsequently degraded and recycled [5]. An increasing number of publications have shown

that autophagy is closely related to the occurrence and progression of tumors [6]. However, the roles of autophagy in these processes are still controversial. Previous research reported that autophagy might mitigate metabolic stress and increase genomic stability to inhibit tumor development [7]. However, Ma et al. [8] showed that autophagy enhanced the resistance of glioblastoma to chemotherapy. At present, the impact of autophagy in HCC is also a subject of debate [9].

In 1998, Liang et al. [10] identified and cloned the mammalian homolog of yeast Atg6/Vps30 gene, namely, Beclin-1, which is located on human chromosome 17q21. It is a key regulator of autophagy. It induces autophagy by participating in autophagosome formation and endosome maturation, which are major steps of autophagy [11]. Abnormal expression of Beclin-1 was shown to relate to the occurrence and prognosis of breast cancer, gastric cancer, and lymphoma [12]. However, controversial results have

* Correspondence: linmei70@hotmail.com
[1]Department of Pathology, School of Basic Medicine, Medical College, Qingdao University, No. 308 Ningxia Road, Qingdao 266071, Shandong, People's Republic of China
Full list of author information is available at the end of the article

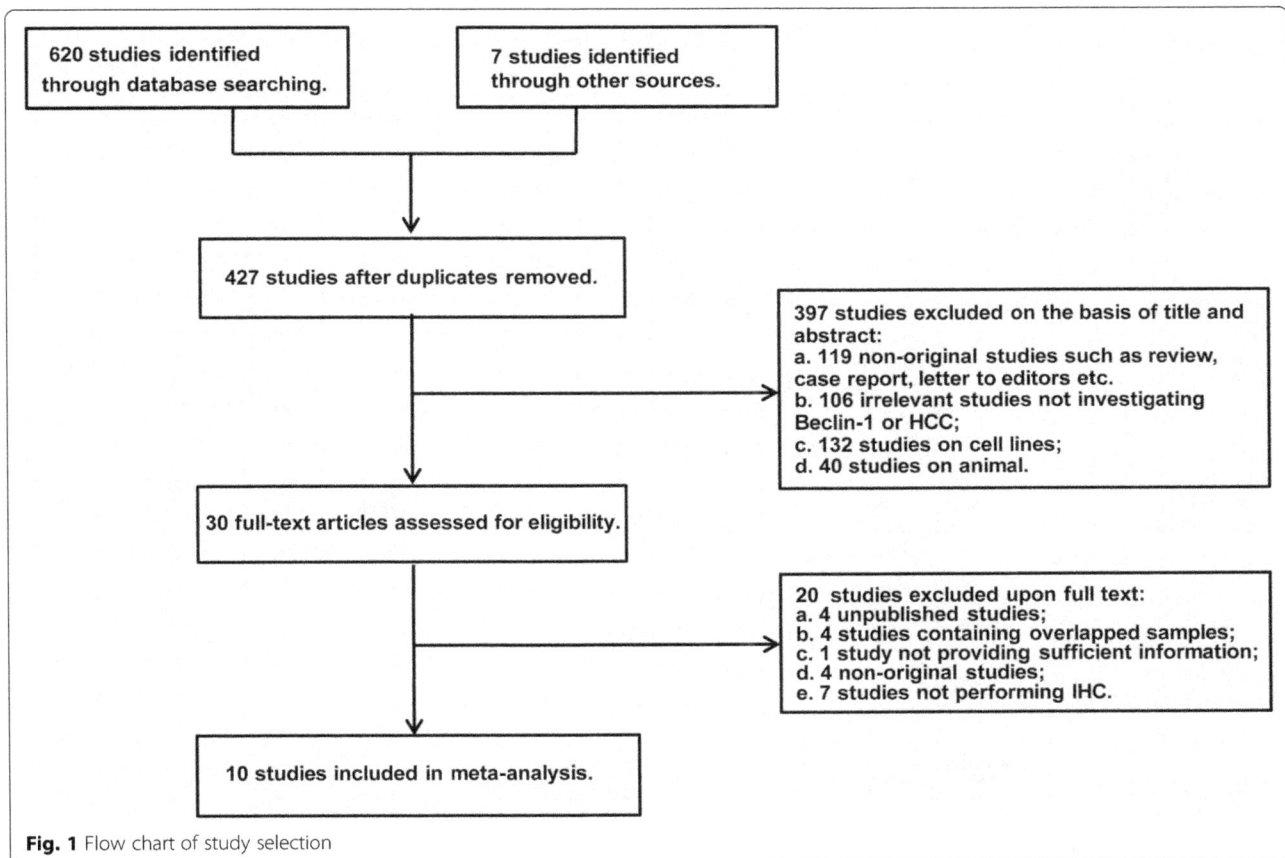

Fig. 1 Flow chart of study selection

been obtained in HCC. Yue et al. [13] found that Beclin-1 +/− mice were more prone to develop malignant tumors, including HCC, than wild-type mice. Qiu et al. [14] showed that Beclin-1 expression was correlated with liver cirrhosis, Edmondson grades and vascular invasion. Ding et al. [15] showed that positive Beclin-1 expression was related to

favorable outcome in HCC patients, while Wu et al. [16] demonstrated that Beclin-1 expression was not related to prognosis and any clinicopathological factors investigated in HCC. Hence, we conducted a meta-analysis to evaluate the clinical and prognostic value of Beclin-1 in HCC.

Table 1 Characteristics of the included studies

References	Year	Country	No. of patients	Gender (M/F, n)	Age range (years)	Method	Antibody dilution	Counting method	Cut-off staining	Reduced Beclin-1 expression (%)	OS data provided
Ding [15]	2008	China	300	252/48	NR	IHC	1:50	IRS*	10%	205/300 (68.33)	Yes
Kang [21]	2013	China	50	47/3	28–71	IHC	NR	IRS	4	11/50 (22.00)	No
Lee [22]	2013	Korea	190	158/32	29–76	IHC	NR	IRS	6	179/190 (94.21)	Yes
Guo [26]	2013	China	54	39/15	33–75	IHC	1:150	IRS	3	10/54 (18.52)	No
Qiu [14]	2014	China	103	85/18	21–79	IHC	1:100	IRS	8	81/103 (78.64)	Yes
Wu [16]	2014	China	156	143/13	NR	IHC	1:100	IRS	6	83/156 (53.21)	Yes
Osman [23]	2015	Egypt	65	51/14	40–74	IHC	1:100	IRS*	10%	32/65 (49.23)	No
Yang [27]	2015	China	50	39/11	26–74	IHC	NR	IRS	3	11/50 (22.00)	No
Al-Shenawy [24]	2016	Egypt	35	20/15	23–75	IHC	1:350	IRS	1	18/35 (51.43)	No
Zhou [25]	2016	China	83	69/14	NR	IHC	1:100	NR	NR	45/83 (54.22)	Yes

M male, *F* female, *NR* not reported, *IHC* immunohistochemistry, *IRS* immunoreactive score, IHC expression was evaluated integrating proportion and intensity of positive staining, *IRS** IHC expression was evaluated by percent positivity, *OS* overall survival

Table 2 Newcastle-Ottawa scale for quality assessment

Study	Selection				Comparability	Outcome			Total
	Exposed cohort	Non-exposed cohort	Ascertainment of exposure	Outcome of interest	Control for factor	Assessment of outcome	Follow-up long enough	Adequacy of follow-up	score
Ding [15]	*	*	*	*	**	*	*	*	9
Kang [21]	*	*	*	*	*	*	*	*	8
Lee [22]	*	*	*	*	**	*	*		8
Guo [26]	*	*	*	*	**	*	*	*	9
Qiu [14]	*	*	*	*	**	*	*	*	9
Wu [16]	*	*	*	*	**	*	*	*	9
Osman [23]	*	*	*	*	*	*	*	*	8
Yang [27]	*	*	*	*	**	*	*	*	9
Al-Shenawy [24]	*	*	*	*	**	*	*	*	9
Zhou [25]	*	*		*	*	*	*		6

*A study can be awarded a maximum of one star for each numbered item within the selection and outcome categories. A maximum of two stars can be given for comparability. http://www.ohri.ca/programs/clinical_epidemiology/oxford.asp

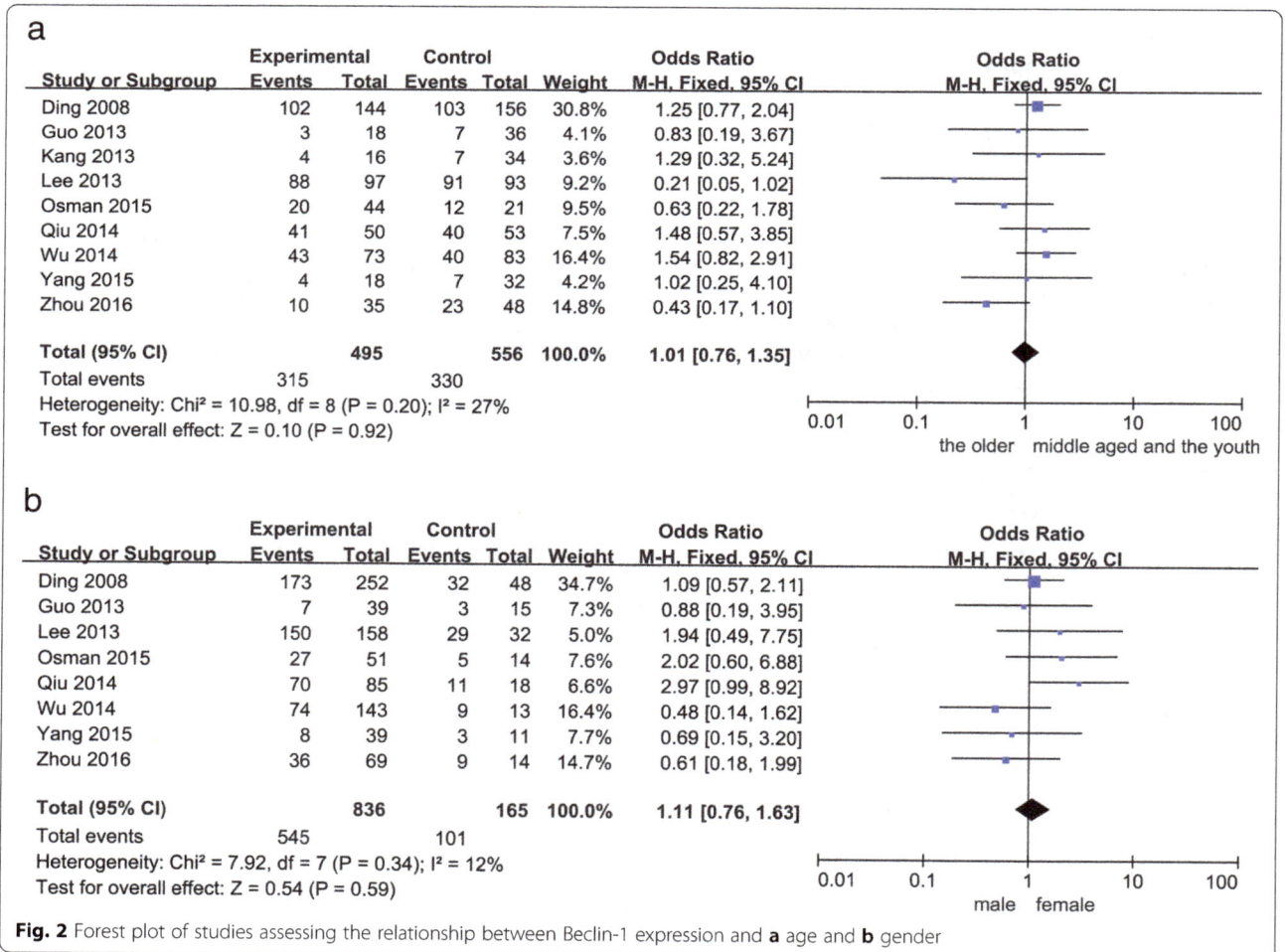

Fig. 2 Forest plot of studies assessing the relationship between Beclin-1 expression and **a** age and **b** gender

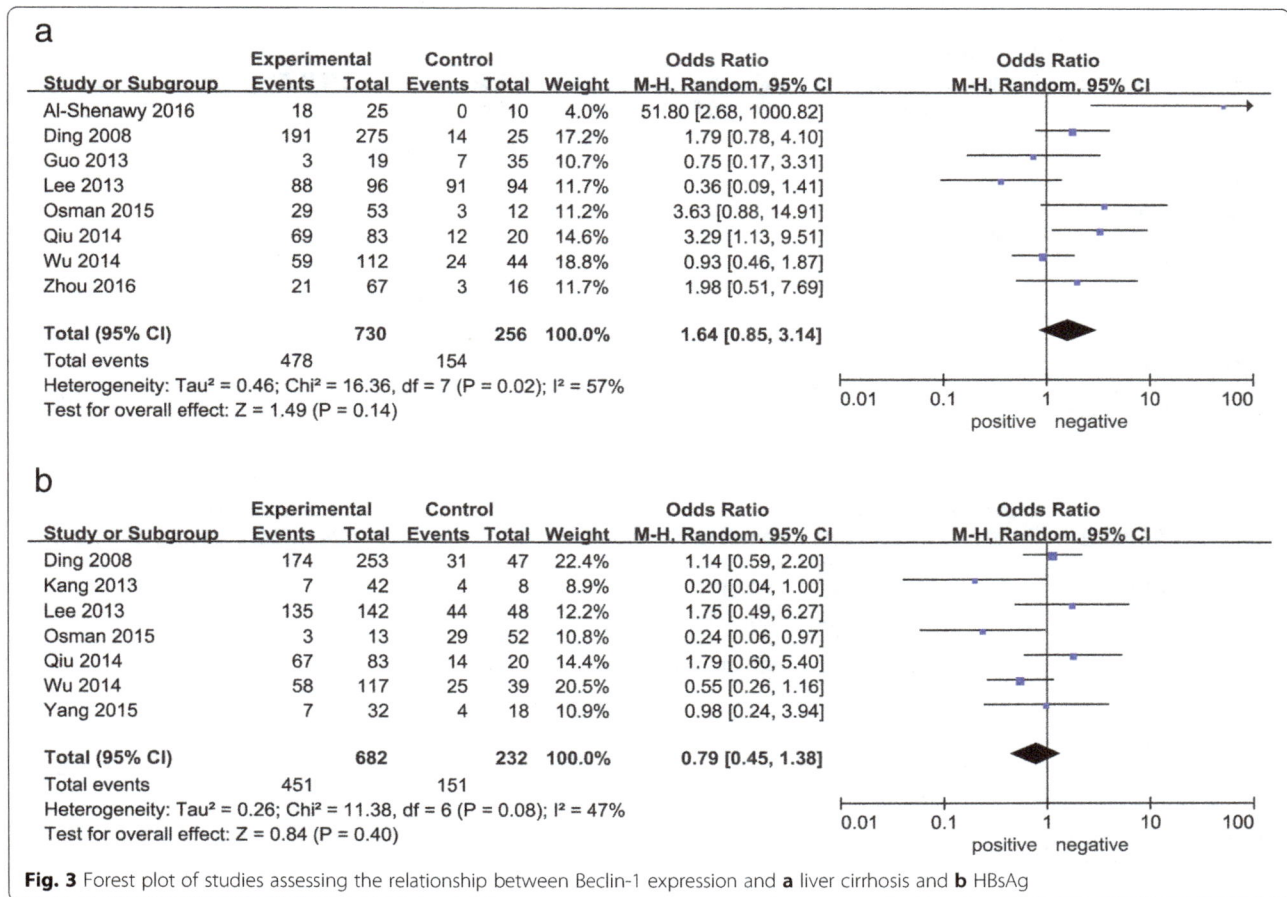

a

Study or Subgroup	Experimental Events	Total	Control Events	Total	Weight	Odds Ratio M-H, Random, 95% CI
Al-Shenawy 2016	18	25	0	10	4.0%	51.80 [2.68, 1000.82]
Ding 2008	191	275	14	25	17.2%	1.79 [0.78, 4.10]
Guo 2013	3	19	7	35	10.7%	0.75 [0.17, 3.31]
Lee 2013	88	96	91	94	11.7%	0.36 [0.09, 1.41]
Osman 2015	29	53	3	12	11.2%	3.63 [0.88, 14.91]
Qiu 2014	69	83	12	20	14.6%	3.29 [1.13, 9.51]
Wu 2014	59	112	24	44	18.8%	0.93 [0.46, 1.87]
Zhou 2016	21	67	3	16	11.7%	1.98 [0.51, 7.69]
Total (95% CI)		**730**		**256**	**100.0%**	**1.64 [0.85, 3.14]**
Total events	478		154			

Heterogeneity: Tau² = 0.46; Chi² = 16.36, df = 7 (P = 0.02); I² = 57%
Test for overall effect: Z = 1.49 (P = 0.14)

b

Study or Subgroup	Experimental Events	Total	Control Events	Total	Weight	Odds Ratio M-H, Random, 95% CI
Ding 2008	174	253	31	47	22.4%	1.14 [0.59, 2.20]
Kang 2013	7	42	4	8	8.9%	0.20 [0.04, 1.00]
Lee 2013	135	142	44	48	12.2%	1.75 [0.49, 6.27]
Osman 2015	3	13	29	52	10.8%	0.24 [0.06, 0.97]
Qiu 2014	67	83	14	20	14.4%	1.79 [0.60, 5.40]
Wu 2014	58	117	25	39	20.5%	0.55 [0.26, 1.16]
Yang 2015	7	32	4	18	10.9%	0.98 [0.24, 3.94]
Total (95% CI)		**682**		**232**	**100.0%**	**0.79 [0.45, 1.38]**
Total events	451		151			

Heterogeneity: Tau² = 0.26; Chi² = 11.38, df = 6 (P = 0.08); I² = 47%
Test for overall effect: Z = 0.84 (P = 0.40)

Fig. 3 Forest plot of studies assessing the relationship between Beclin-1 expression and **a** liver cirrhosis and **b** HBsAg

Methods

Literature search

A systematic literature search was carried out separately by two investigators (Zhiqiang Qin and Xinjuan Yu) in the English databases PubMed and EMBASE and the Chinese databases China National Knowledge Infrastructure (CNKI), Wan Fang and Chinese VIP, with an end date of 30 September 2017. Search terms were "Beclin-1" OR "beclin 1" OR "BECN1" OR "ATG6" AND "hepatocellular" OR "liver" OR "hepatic" AND "carcinoma" OR "tumor" OR "neoplasm" OR "cancer." In addition, we manually retrieved the references of relevant reviews and the included literatures.

Criteria for inclusion and exclusion

The following inclusion criteria were required for studies to be eligible: (1) were published in English or Chinese, and full-text articles can be retrieved; (2) were retrospective cohort studies; (3) had proven diagnosis of HCC in humans; (4) detected Beclin-1 protein expression by immunohistochemistry (IHC); (5) odds ratio (OR) or hazard ratio (HR) and 95% confidence interval (CI) on Beclin-1 expression and clinicopathological

factors or OS could be obtained. Any study that met the following exclusion criteria was excluded: (1) non-original studies, such as review, case reports, letter to editors, or conference abstracts; (2) laboratory studies, such as studies on animal or cancer cell lines; (3) duplication of previous publications.

Quality assessment

Newcastle-Ottawa scale (NOS), a recommended methodological quality assessment tool, was used to estimate the quality of the eligible literature [17]. Two investigators (Zhiqiang Qin and Xinjuan Yu) conducted the assessment independently. When disagreement occurred, the two investigators had a discussion or the third reviewer (Mei Lin) was recruited until consensus was reached. A study with a score ≥ 6 was graded as a high-quality study and others were graded as low quality [18].

Data extraction

Two investigators (Zhiqiang Qin and Xinjuan Yu) independently extracted data from the included studies. Disagreements regarding data extraction were crosschecked

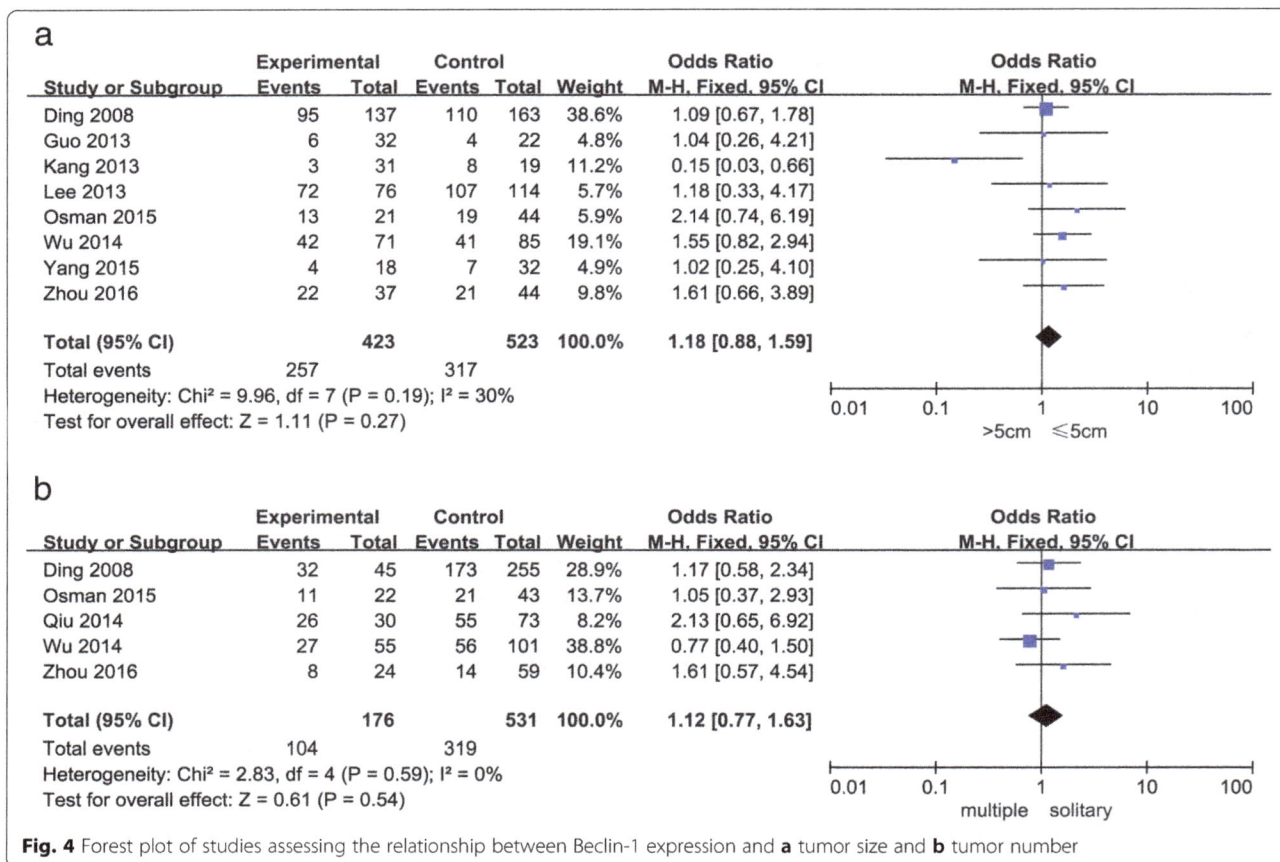

Fig. 4 Forest plot of studies assessing the relationship between Beclin-1 expression and **a** tumor size and **b** tumor number

until achieving consensus. The following information were extracted: surname of the first author, publication year, country, number of patients, gender, age range, antibody dilution, evaluation methods, cut-off value, percentage of decreased Beclin-1 expression, histopathological parameters, and HR and 95% CI of Beclin-1 expression for OS. When HR and its 95% CI were not explicitly given in the article, we performed the calculation using data provided by the literature according to the methods reported by Tierney et al. [19].

Statistical analysis

The current study was conducted based on the Preferred Reporting Items for Systematic Reviews and Meta-Analyses (PRISMA) guidelines [20] (Additional file 1). Pooled ORs and 95% CIs were used to evaluate the associations between Beclin-1 expression and clinicopathological factors. Pooled HR and 95% CI were applied to estimate the effect of Beclin-1 expression on OS. Interstudy heterogeneity was assessed by chi-squared test (Q test) and I^2 test (range from 0-100%). A P value (Q test) > 0.10 and $I^2 \leq 50\%$ indicated no significant heterogeneity. In this case, we used the fixed effect model. When heterogeneity was evident (P value ≤ 0.10 or $I^2 > 50\%$), we used the

random effect model. Subgroup analysis and sensitivity analysis were performed to explore sources of heterogeneity. Publication bias was evaluated by funnel plots. All analyses were carried out using Review Manager (version: 5.3, Cochrane Informatics and Knowledge Management Department, http://tech.cochrane.org/revman/download). $P < 0.05$ was considered statistically significant.

Results
Selection of included articles

Six hundred and twenty potential articles were initially retrieved from relevant electronic databases, and 7 articles were obtained from a manual search of references. A total of 200 repeated documents were excluded. After reviewing the titles and abstracts, 119 non-original articles, 106 irrelevant articles, and 172 laboratory studies on animals or cell lines were removed. The remaining 30 articles were further investigated by attentively reading the full text. Twenty articles were then excluded due to not fulfilling the inclusion criteria or fulfilling the exclusion criteria. Ultimately, 10 articles with a total of 1086 HCC patients were eligible for further analysis.

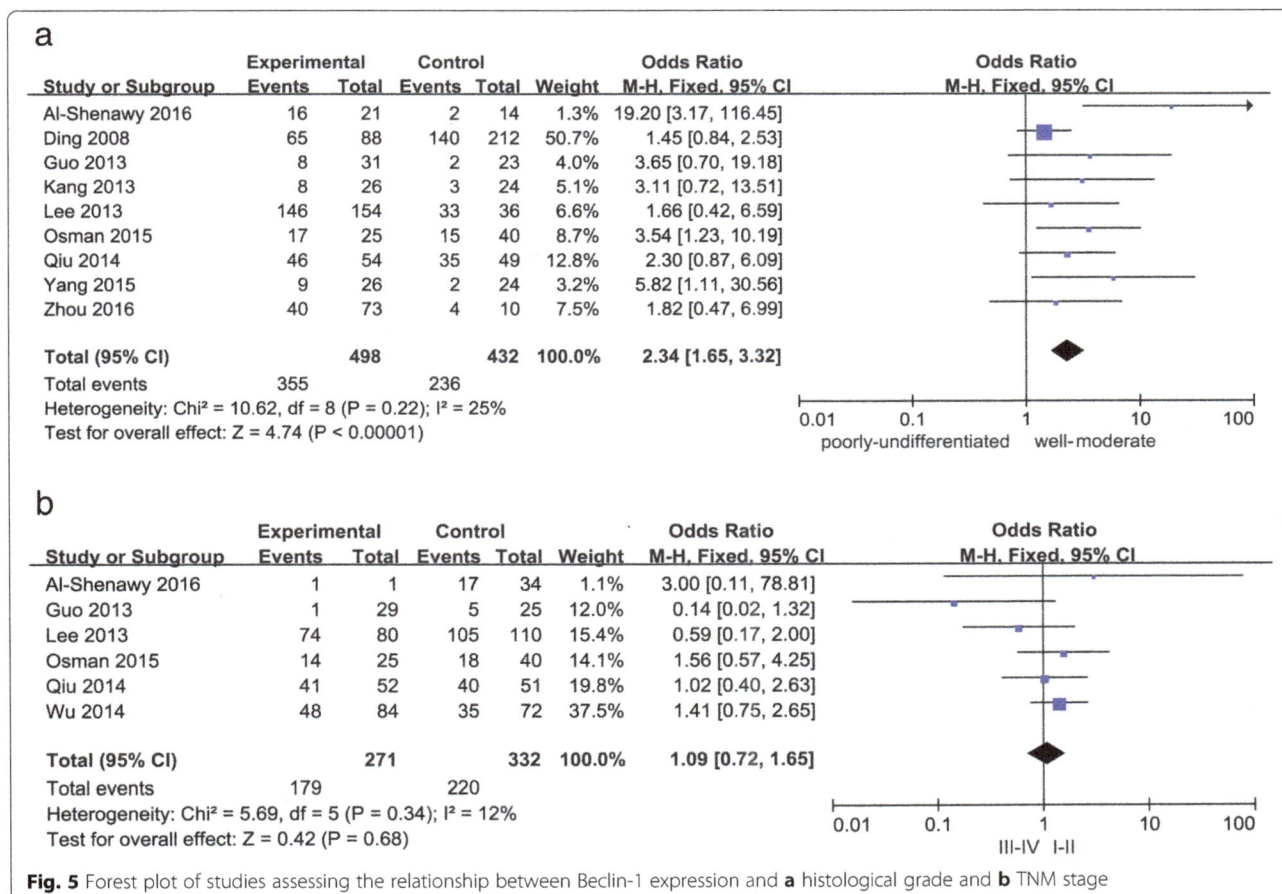

a

Study or Subgroup	Experimental Events	Total	Control Events	Total	Weight	Odds Ratio M-H, Fixed, 95% CI
Al-Shenawy 2016	16	21	2	14	1.3%	19.20 [3.17, 116.45]
Ding 2008	65	88	140	212	50.7%	1.45 [0.84, 2.53]
Guo 2013	8	31	2	23	4.0%	3.65 [0.70, 19.18]
Kang 2013	8	26	3	24	5.1%	3.11 [0.72, 13.51]
Lee 2013	146	154	33	36	6.6%	1.66 [0.42, 6.59]
Osman 2015	17	25	15	40	8.7%	3.54 [1.23, 10.19]
Qiu 2014	46	54	35	49	12.8%	2.30 [0.87, 6.09]
Yang 2015	9	26	2	24	3.2%	5.82 [1.11, 30.56]
Zhou 2016	40	73	4	10	7.5%	1.82 [0.47, 6.99]
Total (95% CI)		**498**		**432**	**100.0%**	**2.34 [1.65, 3.32]**
Total events	355		236			

Heterogeneity: Chi² = 10.62, df = 8 (P = 0.22); I² = 25%
Test for overall effect: Z = 4.74 (P < 0.00001)

b

Study or Subgroup	Experimental Events	Total	Control Events	Total	Weight	Odds Ratio M-H, Fixed, 95% CI
Al-Shenawy 2016	1	1	17	34	1.1%	3.00 [0.11, 78.81]
Guo 2013	1	29	5	25	12.0%	0.14 [0.02, 1.32]
Lee 2013	74	80	105	110	15.4%	0.59 [0.17, 2.00]
Osman 2015	14	25	18	40	14.1%	1.56 [0.57, 4.25]
Qiu 2014	41	52	40	51	19.8%	1.02 [0.40, 2.63]
Wu 2014	48	84	35	72	37.5%	1.41 [0.75, 2.65]
Total (95% CI)		**271**		**332**	**100.0%**	**1.09 [0.72, 1.65]**
Total events	179		220			

Heterogeneity: Chi² = 5.69, df = 5 (P = 0.34); I² = 12%
Test for overall effect: Z = 0.42 (P = 0.68)

Fig. 5 Forest plot of studies assessing the relationship between Beclin-1 expression and **a** histological grade and **b** TNM stage

The selection steps and the reasons for exclusion are summarized in Fig. 1.

Characteristics and quality assessment of studies

The basic characteristics of the 10 included articles are listed in Table 1. In all, the involved studies consisted of 8 English studies [14–16, 21–25] and 2 Chinese studies [26, 27]. These studies were published between 2008 and 2016, and the number of participants ranged from 35 to 300. Of the 10 studies, 7 were from China, 2 from Egypt, and 1 from Korea. All the patients included had proven pathological diagnosis of HCC. IHC staining was used to investigate Beclin-1 expression, and immunoreactive score (IRS) was used to assess Beclin-1 expression. The percentage of decreased Beclin-1 expression ranged from 18.52 to 94.21%. Five studies provided information on OS. However, HR and 95% CI could only be obtained in four studies.

The quality of the 10 eligible studies was evaluated by NOS. The scores were all ≥ 6 points (Table 2). This indicated that all the included studies were high-quality studies.

Beclin-1 expression and clinicopathological parameters

As shown in Figs. 2, 3, 4 and 5, decreased Beclin-1 expression was significantly correlated with histological grade (poorly undifferentiated vs. well-moderated: OR = 2.34, 95% CI = 1.65–3.32, $P < 0.00001$), with slight heterogeneity ($P = 0.22$, $I^2 = 25\%$). However, decreased Beclin-1 expression was not related to age (older vs. middle aged and youth: OR = 1.01, 95% CI = 0.76–1.35, $P = 0.92$), gender (male vs. female: OR = 1.11, 95% CI = 0.76–1.63, $P = 0.59$), liver cirrhosis (positive vs. negative: OR = 1.64, 95% CI = 0.85–3.14, $P = 0.14$), HBsAg (positive vs. negative: OR = 0.79, 95% CI = 0.45–1.38, $P = 0.40$), tumor size (> 5 cm vs. ≤ 5 cm: OR = 1.18, 95% CI = 0.88–1.59, $P = 0.27$), tumor number (multiple vs. solitary: OR = 1.12, 95% CI = 0.77–1.63, $P = 0.54$), or TNM stage (III–IV vs. I–II: OR = 1.09, 95% CI = 0.72–1.65, $P = 0.68$). Considerable interstudy heterogeneity was observed in the analyses of the correlation between Beclin-1 expression and liver cirrhosis ($P = 0.02$, $I^2 = 57\%$) or HBsAg ($P = 0.08$, $I^2 = 47\%$). The analyses of Beclin-1 expression and other clinicopathological factors exhibited slight or no heterogeneity.

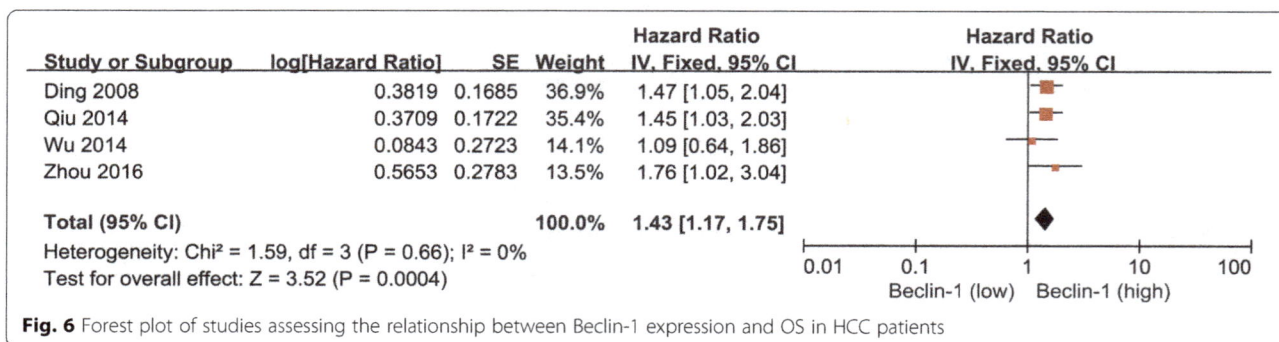

Fig. 6 Forest plot of studies assessing the relationship between Beclin-1 expression and OS in HCC patients

Beclin-1 expression and OS

Four reports that included 642 HCC patients were eligible to investigate the correlation between reduced Beclin-1 expression and OS. As shown in Fig. 6, decreased Beclin-1 expression in HCC was related to poor OS (Beclin-1 low vs. Beclin-1 high: HR = 1.43, 95% CI = 1.17–1.75, $P = 0.0004$). There was no heterogeneity in this analysis ($P = 0.66$, $I^2 = 0$%).

Sensitivity analysis

We conduct a sensitivity analysis by excluding one study in turn. In the study of the correlation between Beclin-1 expression and liver cirrhosis, Beclin-1 expression was lower in patients with cirrhosis than in those without cirrhosis (OR = 1.95, 95% CI = 1.04–3.66, $P = 0.04$) after removing Lee et al.'s study [22], and heterogeneity was still obvious ($P = 0.06$, $I^2 = 50$%). Except Lee et al.'s study, none of the individual studies evidently impacted the outcomes of the current study.

Subgroup analysis

Remarkable heterogeneity was observed in the meta-analysis of the correlation between Beclin-1 expression and liver cirrhosis or HBsAg. To explore the sources of the heterogeneities, we performed subgroup analysis based on geographic region (Table 3). Beclin-1 was irrelevant to liver cirrhosis of HCC patients from both Asia (OR = 1.27, 95% CI = 0.72–2.25, $P = 0.42$) and Egypt (OR = 10.03, 95% CI = 0.74–136.23, $P = 0.08$).

Table 3 Subgroup analysis of liver cirrhosis and HBsAg

Subgroups	No. of studies	Pooled OR (95% CI)	P value	Heterogeneity I^2	P value
Liver cirrhosis					
Asia	6	1.27 (0.72–2.25)	0.42	42%	0.12
Egypt	2	10.03 (0.74–136.23)	0.08	63%	0.10
HBsAg					
Asia	6	0.91 (0.61–1.34)	0.62	38%	0.15
Egypt	1	0.24 (0.06–0.97)	0.04	–	–

HBsAg hepatitis B surface antigen, *OR* odds ratio, *CI* confidence interval

Evident heterogeneity existed in Egyptian HCC patients ($P = 0.10$, $I^2 = 63$%), but not in Asian HCC patients ($P = 0.12$, $I^2 = 42$%). Beclin-1 was not related to the status of HBsAg in Asian HCC patients (OR = 0.91, 95% CI = 0.61–1.34, $P = 0.62$) with no evident heterogeneity ($P = 0.15$, $I^2 = 38$%). However, Beclin-1 expression was significantly decreased in Egyptian HBsAg negative HCC patients (OR = 0.24, 95% CI = 0.06–0.97, $P = 0.04$).

Publication bias

Funnel plots of all included studies were symmetrical (Figs. 7 and 8), indicating that there was no significant publication bias present in the current study.

Discussion

In this meta-analysis, the electronic databases PubMed, EMBASE, CNKI, Wan Fang, and Chinese VIP were systematically searched, and 10 studies with 1086 HCC patients matched the inclusion criterion. The current study demonstrated that decreased Beclin-1 expression related to poor differentiation in HCC. This was in accordance with Xia et al.'s meta-analysis [28], which showed that reduced Beclin-1 expression was related to poor differentiation in gastric cancer. Consistent with the results obtained in cholangiocarcinoma, bladder, and ovarian cancers [29–31], we demonstrated that decreased Beclin-1 expression was associated with unfavorable outcome in HCC patients. These suggested that decreased Beclin-1 might have tumor suppressor function in HCC and indicated that decreased Beclin-1 expression may signify the poor prognosis of HCC. Hence, activation of autophagy may improve the prognosis of HCC patients. Previous studies demonstrated that Beclin-1 downregulated angiogenesis and proliferation of malignant cells [32] and postponed cell cycle progression [33]. In addition, Mathew et al. [34] demonstrated that Beclin-1 could limit genome instability. These may contribute to the tumor suppressor function of Beclin-1. In contrast, other groups discovered that increased Beclin-1 expression was correlated with unfavorable outcome in oral squamous cell carcinoma

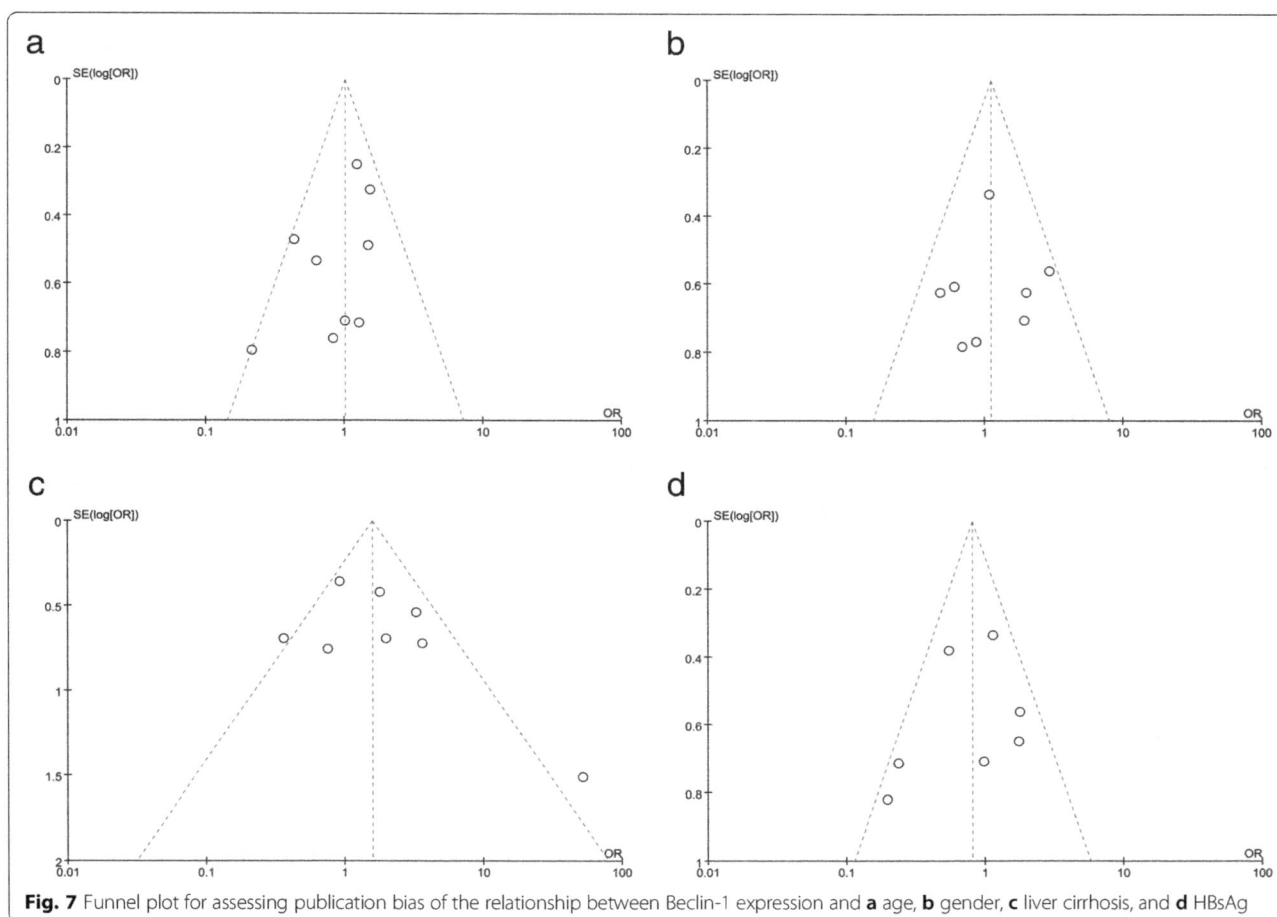

Fig. 7 Funnel plot for assessing publication bias of the relationship between Beclin-1 expression and **a** age, **b** gender, **c** liver cirrhosis, and **d** HBsAg

[35], nasopharyngeal carcinoma [36], and pancreatic ductal adenocarcinoma [37]. This discrepancy might be because the role of autophagy on tumor progression was tissue specific.

Significant heterogeneity existed in the analysis of the correlation of Beclin-1 expression and liver cirrhosis or HBsAg. Thus, we performed sensitivity analysis and subgroup analysis to discover the sources of the heterogeneities. In sensitivity analysis, Beclin-1 expression was significantly decreased in HCC patients with liver cirrhosis compared to those without liver cirrhosis, but heterogeneity was still obvious after excluding Lee et al.'s study [22]. The rate of decreased Beclin-1 expression was 94.21% in Lee et al.'s study [22], which was higher than the other 7 studies (18.52–78.64%). We hypothesized that the high rate of decreased Beclin-1 expression in Lee et al.'s study might alter the result of analysis. Subgroup analysis based on geographic region showed that Beclin-1 expression was irrelevant to liver cirrhosis of HCC patients from both Asia and Egypt. This suggested that regional difference did not influence the association between Beclin-1 expression and liver cirrhosis in this study. The heterogeneity mainly existed in Egyptian study. The heterogeneity mainly existed in Egyptian

HCC patients. This may be because only two studies from Egypt were involved in this study.

Until now, this study has been the first comprehensive and systematic meta-analysis investigating the clinical and prognostic value of autophagic-related protein Beclin-1 in HCC. This study solved the debate regarding whether Beclin-1 was correlated with clinicopathological factors and prognosis of HCC patients. However, several limitations in this study should be acknowledged. First, although Beclin-1 expression in all of the included reports was detected by IHC, the evaluation methods and cut-off values were diverse. This may be a potential source of heterogeneity. Second, in addition to Beclin-1, other autophagy-related proteins, such as LC3 or Atg-9, can also be investigated to clarify the role of autophagy in HCC. Third, of the 10 included studies, 8 were from Asia and 2 were from Egypt. Studies from other areas were not available. This may cause publication bias and make it difficult to indicate the correlation of Beclin-1 and clinicopathological factors or prognosis among HCC patients from Europe and America. Fourth, studies with positive results are more likely to be published

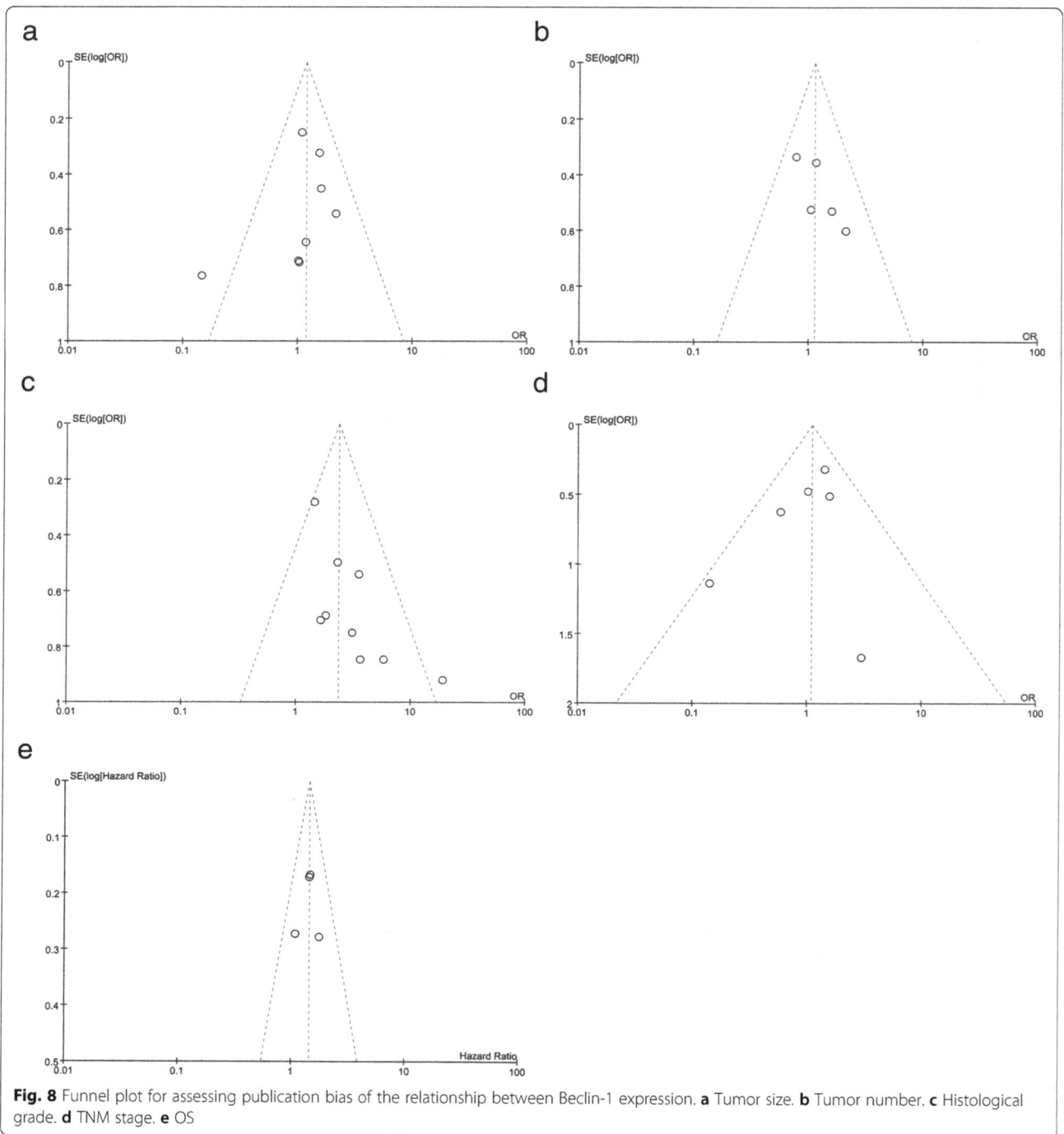

Fig. 8 Funnel plot for assessing publication bias of the relationship between Beclin-1 expression. **a** Tumor size. **b** Tumor number. **c** Histological grade. **d** TNM stage. **e** OS

than those reporting negative results. This may also cause publication bias and might potentially contribute to the limited geographical regions involved in the current study. Finally, only four studies were eligible for analyzing the prognostic role of Beclin-1 in the current study. Therefore, more studies are needed to verify the results obtained by the current study.

Conclusion

In conclusion, this study demonstrated that decreased Beclin-1 expression might relate to poor differentiation and unfavorable outcome in HCC. With regard to the shortcomings of this meta-analysis, we expect studies with larger sample sizes to verify our results.

Abbreviations
CI: Confidence interval; CNKI: Chinese databases China National Knowledge Infrastructure; HCC: Hepatocellular carcinoma; HR: Hazard ratio; IHC: Immunohistochemistry; IRS: Immunoreactive score; NOS: Newcastle-Ottawa scale; OR: Odds ratio; OS: Overall survival; PRISMA: Preferred Reporting Items for Systematic Reviews and Meta-Analyses

Funding
The study was funded by Shandong Provincial Health Department, China (no. 2016WS0318), Shandong Provincial Natural Science Foundation, China (no. ZR2016HM39), and National Natural Science Foundation of China (no. 81702677).

Authors' contributions
ML designed the study. ZQQ and JKW retrieved relevant literatures. ZQQ, XJY, and ML extracted data from included studies. JKW, SPM, and NW performed the statistical analysis. ZQQ drafted the manuscript. ML and XJY revised the manuscript. All authors read and approved the final manuscript.

Competing interests
The authors declare that they have no competing interests.

Author details
[1]Department of Pathology, School of Basic Medicine, Medical College, Qingdao University, No. 308 Ningxia Road, Qingdao 266071, Shandong, People's Republic of China. [2]Central Laboratories, Qingdao Municipal Hospital, Qingdao 266071, Shandong, People's Republic of China. [3]Department of Hematology, Qingdao Municipal Hospital, Qingdao 266011, Shandong, People's Republic of China.

References
1. Shiraha H, Yamamoto K, Namba M. Human hepatocyte carcinogenesis. Int J Oncol. 2013;42:1133–8.
2. Hanazaki K, Kajikawa S, Shimozawa N, Mihara M, Shimada K, Hiraguri M, et al. Survival and recurrence after hepatic resection of 386 consecutive patients with hepatocellular carcinoma. J Am Coll Surg. 2000;191:381–8.
3. Schlachterman A, Craft WW Jr, Hilgenfeldt E, Mitra A, Cabrera R. Current and future treatments for hepatocellular carcinoma. World J Gastroenterol. 2015; 21:8478–91.
4. Kulik LM, Chokechanachaisakul A. Evaluation and management of hepatocellular carcinoma. Clin Liver Dis. 2015;19:23–43.
5. Klionsky DJ, Emr SD. Autophagy as a regulated pathway of cellular degradation. Science. 2000;290:1717–21.
6. Chen P, Cescon M, Bonaldo P. Autophagy-mediated regulation of macrophages and its applications for cancer. Autophagy. 2014;10:192–200.
7. Karantza-Wadsworth V, Patel S, Kravchuk O, Chen G, Mathew R, Jin S, et al. Autophagy mitigates metabolic stress and genome damage in mammary tumorigenesis. Genes Dev. 2007;21:1621–35.
8. Ma B, Yuan Z, Zhang L, Lv P, Yang T, Gao J, et al. Long non-coding RNA AC023115.3 suppresses chemoresistance of glioblastoma by reducing autophagy. Biochim Biophys Acta. 2017;1864:1393–404.
9. Lee YJ, Jang BK. The role of autophagy in hepatocellular carcinoma. Int J Mol Sci. 2015;16:26629–43.
10. Liang XH, Kleeman LK, Jiang HH, Gordon G, Goldman JE, Berry G, et al. Protection against fatal Sindbis virus encephalitis by beclin, a novel Bcl-2-interacting protein. J Virol. 1998;72:8586–96.
11. Kang R, Zeh HJ, Lotze MT, Tang D. The Beclin 1 network regulates autophagy and apoptosis. Cell Death Differ. 2011;18:571–80.
12. He Y, Zhao X, Subahan NR, Fan L, Gao J, Chen H. The prognostic value of autophagy-related markers beclin-1 and microtubule-associated protein light chain 3B in cancers: a systematic review and meta-analysis. Tumour Biol. 2014;35:7317–26.
13. Yue Z, Jin S, Yang C, Levine AJ, Heintz N. Beclin 1, an autophagy gene essential for early embryonic development, is a haploinsufficient tumor suppressor. Proc Natl Acad Sci U S A. 2003;100:15077–82.
14. Qiu DM, Wang GL, Chen L, Xu YY, He S, Cao XL, et al. The expression of beclin-1, an autophagic gene, in hepatocellular carcinoma associated with clinical pathological and prognostic significance. BMC Cancer. 2014;14:327.
15. Ding ZB, Shi YH, Zhou J, Qiu SJ, Xu Y, Dai Z, et al. Association of autophagy defect with a malignant phenotype and poor prognosis of hepatocellular carcinoma. Cancer Res. 2008;68:9167–75.
16. Wu DH, Jia CC, Chen J, Lin ZX, Ruan DY, Li X, et al. Autophagic LC3B overexpression correlates with malignant progression and predicts a poor prognosis in hepatocellular carcinoma. Tumour Biol. 2014;35:12225–33.
17. Zeng X, Zhang Y, Kwong JS, Zhang C, Li S, Sun F, et al. The methodological quality assessment tools for preclinical and clinical studies, systematic review and meta-analysis, and clinical practice guideline: a systematic review. J Evid Based Med. 2015;8:2–10.
18. Lu L, Wu M, Zhao F, Fu W, Li W, Li X, et al. Prognostic and clinicopathological value of Gli-1 expression in gastric cancer: a meta-analysis. Oncotarget. 2016;7:69087–96.
19. Tierney JF, Stewart LA, Ghersi D, Burdett S, Sydes MR. Practical methods for incorporating summary time-to-event data into meta-analysis. Trials. 2007;8:16.
20. Moher D, Liberati A, Tetzlaff J, Altman DG. Preferred reporting items for systematic reviews and meta-analyses: the PRISMA statement. Ann Intern Med. 2009;151:264–9. w64
21. Kang KF, Wang XW, Chen XW, Kang ZJ, Zhang X, Wilbur RR, et al. Beclin 1 and nuclear factor-kappaBp65 are upregulated in hepatocellular carcinoma. Oncol Lett. 2013;5:1813–8.
22. Lee YJ, Hah YJ, Kang YN, Kang KJ, Hwang JS, Chung WJ, et al. The autophagy-related marker LC3 can predict prognosis in human hepatocellular carcinoma. PLoS One. 2013;8:e81540.
23. Osman NA, Abd El-Rehim DM, Kamal IM. Defective Beclin-1 and elevated hypoxia-inducible factor (HIF)-1alpha expression are closely linked to tumorigenesis, differentiation, and progression of hepatocellular carcinoma. Tumour Biol. 2015;36:4293–9.
24. Al-Shenawy HA. Expression of Beclin-1, an autophagy-related marker, in chronic hepatitis and hepatocellular carcinoma and its relation with apoptotic markers. APMIS. 2016;124:229–37.
25. Zhou Y, Wu PW, Yuan XW, Li J, Shi XL. Interleukin-17A inhibits cell autophagy under starvation and promotes cell migration via TAB2/TAB3-p38 mitogen-activated protein kinase pathways in hepatocellular carcinoma. Eur Rev Med Pharmacol Sci. 2016;20:250–63.
26. Guo XD, Gao YJ, Wan W, Li RS, Zhou YX, Zhao JM, et al. Expression and clinical significance of Beclin 1 in patients with hepatocellular carcinoma. Progress in Modern Biomedicine. 2013;13:85–7.
27. Yang W, Yang HJ, Mo RX, Li XR, Liao WS, Zhang HM, et al. Expression of Beclin1 in human hepatocellular carcinoma and effects of TGF-β on proliferation of hepatocellular carcinoma cells. Int J Lab Med. 2015;36:108–9.
28. Xia P, Wang JJ, Zhao BB, Song CL. The role of beclin-1 expression in patients with gastric cancer: a meta-analysis. Tumour Biol. 2013;34:3303–7.
29. Wang TT, Cao QH, Chen MY, Xia Q, Fan XJ, Ma XK, et al. Beclin 1 deficiency correlated with lymph node metastasis, predicts a distinct outcome in intrahepatic and extrahepatic cholangiocarcinoma. PLoS One. 2013;8:e80317.
30. Liu GH, Zhong Q, Ye YL, Wang HB, Hu LJ, Qin ZK, et al. Expression of beclin 1 in bladder cancer and its clinical significance. Int J Biol Markers. 2013;28:56–62.
31. Cai M, Hu Z, Liu J, Gao J, Liu C, Liu D, et al. Beclin 1 expression in ovarian tissues and its effects on ovarian cancer prognosis. Int J Mol Sci. 2014;15:5292–303.
32. Lee S, Kim H, Jin Y, Choi A, Ryter S. Beclin 1 deficiency is associated with increased hypoxia-induced angiogenesis. Autophagy. 2011;7:829–39.
33. Koneri K, Goi T, Hirono Y, Katayama K, Yamaguchi A. Beclin 1 gene inhibits tumor growth in colon cancer cell lines. Anticancer Res. 2007;27:1453–7.
34. Mathew R, Kongara S, Beaudoin B, Karp CM, Bray K, Degenhardt K, et al. Autophagy suppresses tumor progression by limiting chromosomal instability. Genes Dev. 2007;21:1367–81.
35. Tang J, Fang Y, Hsi E, Huang Y, Hsu N, Yang W, et al. Immunopositivity of Beclin-1 and ATG5 as indicators of survival and disease recurrence in oral squamous cell carcinoma. Anticancer Res. 2013;33:5611–6.
36. Wan X, Fan X, Chen M, Xiang J, Huang P, Guo L, et al. Elevated Beclin 1 expression is correlated with HIF-1alpha in predicting poor prognosis of nasopharyngeal carcinoma. Autophagy. 2010;6:395–404.
37. Ko Y, Cho Y, Won H, Jeon E, An H, Hong S, et al. Prognostic significance of autophagy-related protein expression in resected pancreatic ductal adenocarcinoma. Pancreas. 2013;42:829–35.

8

Surgical excision and oncoplastic breast surgery in 32 patients with benign phyllodes tumors

Jie Ren[1†], Liyan Jin[1,2†], Bingjing Leng[1], Rongkuan Hu[1] and Guoqin Jiang[1*]

Abstract

Background: The purpose of this study was to assess the effectiveness and safety in patients with benign phyllodes after performing local excision and following with intra-operative breast flap reconstruction.

Methods: Patients ($n = 32$) with eligible breast cystosarcoma phyllodes underwent wide local excision followed by intra-operative breast flap reconstruction. Primary outcome measures included average operative time, length of in-hospital stay, postoperative recurrence, and intra-operative and postoperative complications.

Results: Thirty-two patients who underwent surgical excision and oncoplastic breast surgery were evaluated using the BCCT.core software. A satisfactory symmetrical breast shape was achieved. The average operative time was 56.3 ± 8.2 min. The average postoperative duration of hospitalization was 3.7 ± 1.2 days. While there was no breast disease recurred during the 1 to 8-year follow-up period.

Conclusions: Wide local excision accompanied by intra-operative breast flap reconstruction could be adopted for removing benign phyllodes tumors while retaining the basic shape of the breast.

Keywords: Phyllodes tumor, Core needle biopsy, Oncoplastic breast surgery, Breast reconstruction

Background

Phyllodes tumor is a very rare breast tumor that comprises 0.3–1% of all primary breast tumors. Phyllodes tumors are often misdiagnosed as fibroadenomas, and the masses are usually so large that surgical resection may cause breast deformity.

Patients and methods

Patients

From January 2005 to January 2016, 32 patients who were referred to our institution (the Second Affiliated Hospital of Soochow University) for management of breast benign phyllodes tumors were retrospectively studied. All patients were well informed and signed informed consent prior to surgery. This study was approved by the ethics committee at the Second Affiliated Hospital of Soochow University. The diameter of the

breast tumor was determined by preoperative ultrasonography and magnetic resonance imaging (MRI) in all patients (Fig. 1). Biopsies and pathological evaluations were performed with all patients before the surgery. Table 1 shows the baseline characteristics of the patients. Primary outcome measures included average operative time, length of in-hospital stay, postoperative recurrence, and intra-operative and postoperative complications.

Methods

Wide local excision

We created a conventional incision around the areola, with a radial incision in the mass, forming a T-shaped incision. Areola-nipple complex dissection was performed in one patient involving an areola with skin damage. After dissecting the skin and subcutaneous tissue, the tumor was resected using a wide local dissection, removing the mass and approximately 10 mm of the surrounding tissue.

* Correspondence: jiang_guoqin@163.com
†Jie Ren and Liyan Jin contributed equally to this work.
[1]Department of General Surgery, The Second Affiliated Hospital of Soochow University, Suzhou 215006, China
Full list of author information is available at the end of the article

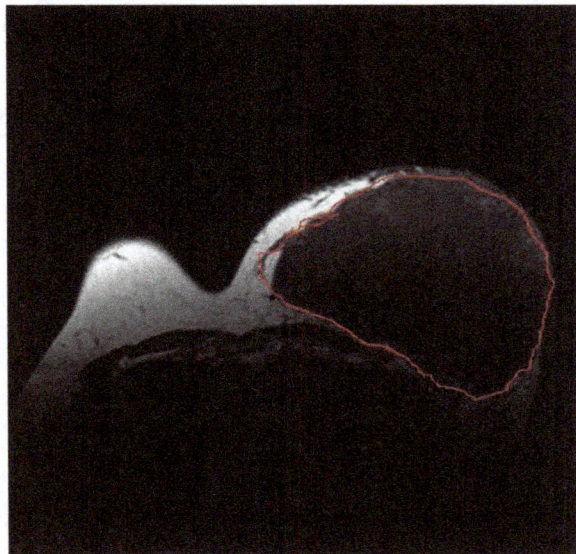

Fig. 1 The presence or absence of breast tumor and the diameter of the tumor were determined by preoperative MRI

Breast flap reconstruction

Before surgery, we measured the distance from the midpoint of the clavicle to the nipple and then to the lowest point of the inframammary fold (Fig. 2). The remaining breast tissue and subcutaneous fat layer were assessed

Table 1 Baseline characteristics of the patients

Parameter	No(%)
Lump location	
Left	16 (50.0)
Right	15 (46.9)
Both	1 (3.1)
Diameter of the lump (cm)	
≤ 5	1 (3.1)
> 5,≤10	13 (40.6)
> 10,≤15	15 (46.9)
> 15	3 (9.4)
Proportion of tumor in breast (%)	
≤ 20	3 (9.4)
> 20,≤ 50	20 (62.5)
> 50	9 (28.1)
Symptoms	
Breast lump	32 (100)
Pain	3 (9.4)
Local ulceration and bleeding	1 (3.1)
Nipple retraction	0 (0)
Orange peel-like change	0 (0)
Breast operation history	
Fibroadenoma	13 (40.6)

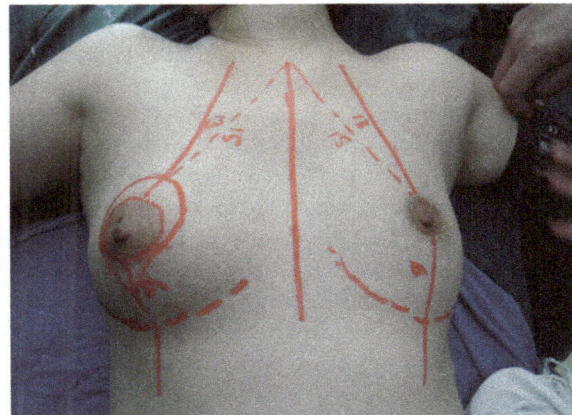

Fig. 2 The measurement of one patient before surgery

after the wide local excision, and glands with more than one lobe were rotated or overlapped and then fixed to the pectoralis major fascia at the second intercostal space. We removed extra skin before suturing to ensure symmetry of both sides (Fig. 3). We sutured the incision with absorbable threads and placed a drainage tube under the incision.

Postoperative follow-up care

All patients received routine care and resumed oral food intake at 6 h after surgery. The drainage tube in patients was removed after the drainage volume was less than 10 ml. An elastic bandage was applied for one month.

Photographs of all 32 women, taken 1 year after surgery, were evaluated using the BCCT.core software (INSEC Porto, the University of Porto).

Results

Wide local excision and breast flap reconstruction were completed in all patients. The average operative time

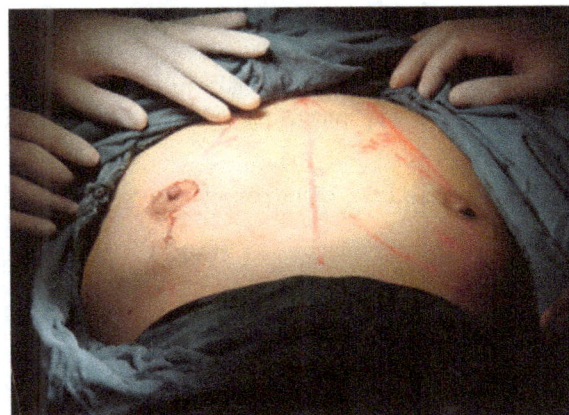

Fig. 3 Symmetry of both sides after surgery

was 56.3 ± 8.2 min. The average postoperative duration of hospitalization was 3.7 ± 1.2 days. All 32 cases were pathologically confirmed as benign phyllodes tumors with no margin of tumor involvement in any patient. There was no mortality, postoperative bleeding, severe breast deformity, or intra-operative complications in any of the cases (Table 2). The cosmetic outcome of the surgical excision and oncoplastic breast surgery was evaluated by BCCT.core software with 18.8% excellent, 65.6% good, and 15.6% fair. No patients experienced poor cosmetic outcomes.

There was no patient experienced breast lump recurrence after a mean follow-up period of 18 months.

Discussion

Phyllodes tumors also known as cystosarcoma phyllodes and phylloides tumor are a set of large and fast-growing masses of the breast which were first described in 1838 [1]. This rare type of breast cancer was accounted for less than 1% of all breast neoplasms and was originally considered benign; in 1931, Lee and Pack first indicated that this type of tumor also contained a malignant variant [2]. The terminology of phyllodes tumors has been adopted by the World Health Organization (WHO), which recommends that the tumors be classified as benign, malignant, or borderline according to their pathological features [3]. Though the phyllodes tumors always occur in females, but several cases were found in male patients that were diagnosed with gynecomastia [4].

As shown in this study, there were no patients that experienced postoperative bleeding, severe breast deformity, or intra-operative complications. Furthermore, we used BCCT.core to evaluate the outcome. The BCCT.core software (INSEC Porto) is an appropriate tool that is both simple and objective, and its feasibility was previously reported [5, 6]. In our opinion, surgical excision and oncoplastic breast surgery have some advantages for patients with benign phyllodes tumor.

(1) The diagnosis of phyllodes tumor mainly relies on ultrasound, mammography, and MRI [7]. In mammograms, the mass usually presents as a solid, non-interrupted parenchyma with micro-calcifications.

Table 2 Surgical outcomes of the patients

	No (%)
Mean operative time (min)	56.3 ± 8.2
Postoperative stay (days)	3.7 ± 1.2
Operative complication (n)	
Postoperative bleeding	0
Breast severely deformed	0
Intra-operative complications	0

It is difficult to distinguish phyllodes tumor using MRI due to the absence of unique features. The sarcoma of phyllodes tumor is similar to undifferentiated breast cancer in intra-operative frozen sections, which often leads to a misdiagnosis of fibro-adenoma and unnecessary over-treatment. As a result, frozen sections of the breast tissue have limited value for phyllodes tumors' diagnosis [8]. In this study, all patients underwent multi-point ultrasound-guided BARD core needle biopsy, providing sufficient tissue for routine pathological sections and immune-pathological examination.

(2) Preoperative core needle biopsy of large masses may also be beneficial for developing rational surgical plans, such as local excision, wide local excision, or simple mastectomy. The biological behavior and pathological features of phyllodes tumors can vary, as histologically benign phyllodes tumors can recur and metastasize, with a recurrence rate of 10–40%. Conversely, some histologically malignant phyllodes tumors may have good clinical outcomes. In a previous study, Putti TC reported that the extent of the surgical procedure remarkably affected the rate of local recurrence [9]. Thus, the goal for the treatment of phyllodes tumors should be complete tumor removal with margins free from small lesions. Since patients in our group were preoperatively diagnosed as having benign phyllodes tumors, we used a wide (10 mm) local removal strategy. No margin of tumor involvement was pathologically detected in any patient, and no breast disease recurred during follow-up.

(3) With the pursuit of increased quality of life, retention of an acceptable breast shape after the removal of large masses is a priority. In this series, even after the removal of large masses (10 mm of normal tissue), enough tissue was retained for breast reconstruction. As the breast often had a defect due to tumor resection, we made full use of the free fat layer under the entire breast and created breast tissue flaps by internal rotation or overlapping. Large breast masses can induce deformation and compression of surrounding glands as well as lead to a degree of breast displacement after lumpectomy. Thus, we outlined the breast shape, fixed remaining glands on the pectoralis major fascia at the second intercostal space, and used elastic bandages for 1 month to reconstruct a relatively intact breast shape.

Some scholars believe that benign phyllodes tumor can be cured by ultrasound-guided vacuum-assisted biopsy (UGVAB). The relapse-free survival (RFS) in patients underwent surgical excision is good than those received

UGVAB alone [10]. Moreover, several previous studies mentioned that it is possible to choose an ideal prosthesis to reconstruct the tissues [11]. These can also be regarded as good methods to keep breast shape.

Conclusions

Surgical excision and oncoplastic breast surgery are a safe and feasible procedure for patients with benign phyllodes tumors, in which rational surgical plans are developed based on preoperative multi-point ultrasound-guided BARD core needle biopsy. Utilizing wide (10 mm) local excision, making full use of the free fat layer under the entire breast, and creating breast tissue flaps can reduce recurrence and retain a good breast shape.

Abbreviations
MRI: Magnetic resonance imaging; RFS: Relapse-free survival; UGVAB: Ultrasound-guided vacuum-assisted biopsy

Funding
The project was supported by the Second Affiliated Hospital of Soochow University's Preponderant Clinic Discipline Group Project Funding (XKQ2015008).

Authors' contributions
All authors have contributed significantly. JR, LJ, and BL performed the surgery. RH and GJ analyzed the data, supervised the study, and wrote the manuscript. All authors read and approved the final manuscript.

Competing interests
The authors declare that they have no competing interests.

Author details
[1]Department of General Surgery, The Second Affiliated Hospital of Soochow University, Suzhou 215006, China. [2]Department of Thyroid and Breast Surgery, Traditional Chinese Medicine Hospital of Kunshan, Suzhou 215006, China.

References
1. Reich T, Solomon C. Bilateral cystosarcoma phyllodes, malignant variant, with 14-year follow-up; a case report. Ann Surg. 1958;147:39–43.
2. Lee BJ, Pack GT. Giant intracanalicular myxoma of the breast: the so-called cystosarcoma phyllodes mammae of Johannes Muller. Ann Surg. 1931;93:250 68.
3. Fiks A. Cystosarcoma phyllodes of the mammary gland—Muller's tumor. For the 180th birthday of Johannes Muller. Virchows Arch A Pathol Anat Histol. 1981;392:1–6.
4. Bumpers HL, Tadros T, Gabram-Mendola S, Rizzo M, Martin M, Zaremba N, Okoli J. Phyllodes tumors in African American women. Am J Surg. 2015;210:74–9.
5. Heil J, Carolus A, Dahlkamp J, Golatta M, Domschke C, Schuetz F, Blumenstein M, Rauch G, Sohn C. Objective assessment of aesthetic outcome after breast conserving therapy: subjective third party panel rating and objective BCCT.core software evaluation. Breast. 2012;21:61–5.
6. Preuss J, Lester L, Saunders C. BCCT.core - can a computer program be used for the assessment of aesthetic outcome after breast reconstructive surgery? Breast. 2012;21:597–600.
7. Jacklin RK, Ridgway PF, Ziprin P, Healy V, Hadjiminas D, Darzi A. Optimising preoperative diagnosis in phyllodes tumour of the breast. J Clin Pathol. 2006;59:454–9.
8. Putti TC, Pinder SE, Elston CW, Lee AH, Ellis IO. Breast pathology practice: most common problems in a consultation service. Histopathology. 2005;47:445–57.
9. Bhargav PR, Mishra A, Agarwal G, Agarwal A, Verma AK, Mishra SK. Phyllodes tumour of the breast: clinicopathological analysis of recurrent vs. non-recurrent cases. Asian J Surg. 2009;32:224–8.
10. Ouyang Q, Li S, Tan C, Zeng Y, Zhu L, Song E, Chen K, Su F. Benign Phyllodes tumor of the breast diagnosed after ultrasound-guided vacuum-assisted biopsy: surgical excision or wait-and-watch? Ann Surg Oncol. 2016;23:1129–34.
11. Ciancio F, Innocenti A, Cagiano L, Portincasa A, Parisi D. Skin-reducing mastectomy and direct-to-implant reconstruction in giant phyllodes tumour of breast: case report. Int J Surg Case Rep. 2017;41:356–9.

9

Reconstruction options following pancreaticoduodenectomy after Roux-en-Y gastric bypass

William F. Morano[1][*] ⓘ, Mohammad F. Shaikh[1], Elizabeth M. Gleeson[1], Alvaro Galvez[2], Marian Khalili[1], John Lieb II[3], Elizabeth P. Renza-Stingone[2] and Wilbur B. Bowne[1]

Abstract

Background: Obesity is a risk factor for pancreatic cancer which may be treated with Roux-en-Y gastric bypass and represents an increasing morbidity. Post-RYGB anatomy poses considerable challenges for reconstruction after pancreaticoduodenectomy (PD), a growing problem encountered by surgeons. We characterize specific strategies used for post-PD reconstruction in the RYGB patient.

Methods: PubMed search was performed using MeSH terms "Gastric Bypass" and "Pancreaticoduodenectomy" between 2000 and 2018. Articles reporting cases of pancreaticoduodenectomy in post-RYGB patients were included and systematically reviewed for this study.

Results: Three case reports and five case series (25 patients) addressed PD after RYGB; we report one additional case. The typical post-gastric bypass PD patient is a woman in the sixth decade of life, presenting most commonly with pain (69.2%) and/or jaundice (53.8%), median 5 years after RYGB. Five post-PD reconstructive options are reported. Among these, the gastric remnant was resected in 18 cases (69.2%), with reconstruction of biliopancreatic drainage most commonly achieved using the distal jejunal segment of the pre-existing biliopancreatic limb (73.1%). Similarly, in the eight cases where the gastric remnant was spared (30.8%), drainage was most commonly performed using the distal jejunal segment of the biliopancreatic limb (50%). Among the 17 cases reporting follow-up data, median was 27 months.

Conclusion: Reconstruction options after PD in the post-RYGB patient focus on resection or preservation gastric remnant, as well as creation of new biliopancreatic limb. Insufficient data exists to make recommendations regarding the optimal reconstruction option, yet surgeons must prepare for the possible clinical challenge. PD reconstruction post-RYGB requires evaluation through prospective studies.

Keywords: Roux-en-Y gastric bypass, Pancreaticoduodenectomy, Whipple, Pancreatic cancer, Bariatrics

Background

Morbid obesity, a known risk factor for the development of pancreatic cancer, may be treated surgically with Roux-en-Y gastric bypass (RYGB). The post-bypass anatomy can make reconstruction after pancreaticoduodenectomy more complex, with multiple surgical options. Although uncommon, this situation will be encountered more frequently as the post-RYGB population increases in size. Few reported cases exist to provide evidence-based guidelines for options for reconstruction of the post-pancreaticoduodenectomy anatomy in a patient with prior Roux-en-Y gastric bypass.

Introduction

Obesity is a growing problem in the USA and known risk factor for development of pancreatic malignancy [1–3]. The Roux-en-Y gastric bypass (RYGB) has proven to be an effective, long-term solution for obesity and its associated morbidities [4–6]. RYGB addresses the problem of obesity in two ways: a restrictive component involving the

* Correspondence: Morano.william@gmail.com
[1]Division of Surgical Oncology, Department of Surgery, Drexel University College of Medicine, 245 N. 15th Street, Suite 7150, Philadelphia, PA 19102, USA
Full list of author information is available at the end of the article

creation of a gastric pouch with alimentary limb, and a malabsorptive component bypassing the proximal portion of the small intestine. The resultant configuration is a significant reconstruction and poses potential future diagnostic and therapeutic challenges [7–11]. In the case of pancreatic malignancy requiring pancreaticoduodenectomy (PD), the surgeon must consider whether or not to resect the gastric remnant, as well as the method of reconstruction of the biliopancreatic and alimentary limbs [12]. To date, few case reports or series of post-RYGB pancreaticoduodenectomies have directly addressed this challenging clinical scenario. With the growing prevalence of obese patients undergoing RYGB, surgeons will be facing similar issues more frequently in the future. We present such a case and systematically review the existing literature to report management strategies and discuss relevant considerations for reconstruction.

Methods

PubMed search was performed using MeSH terms "Gastric Bypass" and "Pancreaticoduodenectomy" between 2000 and 2018. We systematically reviewed and extracted data from included cases such as patient-related demographics, diagnosis, operative techniques, and outcomes. Articles in which no patient data was provided, operative technique-specific, and reports in which PD was not performed after RYGB were excluded from this review (Fig. 1). Qualitative variables are reported as proportions. Continuous quantitative variables are provided as medians with interquartile ranges.

Results

Our search returned 55 English language articles. Eight of these articles were found to specifically address PD after RYGB. In the included articles, 25 patient cases were reported; our institution included an additional case, for a total of 26 cases (Fig. 1) [13–20]. Table 1 contains a synopsis of all reported cases with regard to clinicopathological characteristics. Tables 2 and 3 summarize patient pre-operative, operative, and post-operative characteristics, respectively. Briefly, the patients were predominantly female, in the sixth decade of life (median age 54 years, IQR 52–61). Median interval between gastric bypass and PD was 5 years (IQR 2–11). Patients initially presented with abdominal/back pain [18], jaundice [14], weight loss [9], nausea/vomiting [5], as an incidental finding [4], diarrhea [2], and fever/chills [1]. Computed tomography (CT) was the diagnostic modality of choice in all patients. Pathological diagnoses included pancreatic adenocarcinoma [15], neuroendocrine tumors [3], chronic pancreatitis [3], bile duct fibrosis [2], intraductal papillary mucinous neoplasm [1], duodenal adenocarcinoma [1], and ampullary adenocarcinoma [1]. Procedures included pancreaticoduodenectomy [21],

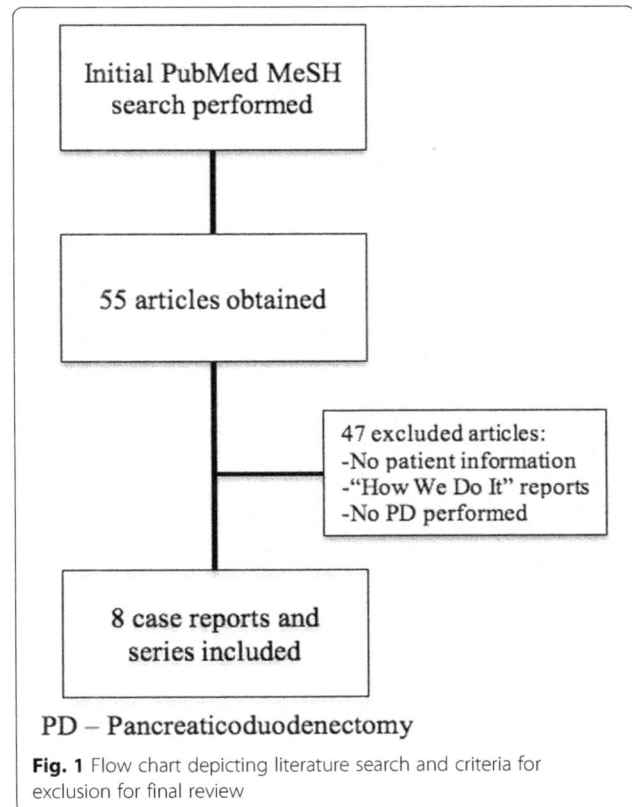

Fig. 1 Flow chart depicting literature search and criteria for exclusion for final review

pylorus-preserving pancreaticoduodenectomy [1], and total pancreatectomy [1]. Report of resection margin status [13] and histologic lymph node examination [4] for malignancies were infrequently provided. The gastric remnant was resected in majority of patients [18]. Few surgeons resected the entire biliopancreatic limb [3]. Reconstruction of biliopancreatic drainage was achieved by using distal jejunal segment of the old biliopancreatic limb [22], a new limb raised from the old common channel [3], a new limb raised from the old alimentary limb [1], and creation of a hepaticojejunostomy and pancreaticojejunostomy in-continuity with the old common channel and gastric pouch [1] (Fig. 2). In the reported cases, margin status was reported in 65% of patients with a diagnosis of malignancy. Three post-operative complications were reported: two pancreatic fistulas, one enterocutaneous fistula, and one bile leak from gastrojejunostomy anastomotic breakdown. Of the 17 cases reporting follow-up data (median 27 months), 10 patients had no evidence of disease at last follow-up, 8 died of malignancy.

Discussion

Obesity is a known risk factor for pancreatic cancer [1, 2]. As in our patient, the diagnosis of a resectable

Table 1 Overview of all relevant clinicopathological characteristics in the 26 cases reviewed of post-RYGB patients who underwent pancreaticoduodenectomy

Author	Year	Sex	Age	Diagnosis	Imaging/ diagnostic modalities	Years from RYGB	RYGB type	Presenting complaint(s)	Resection specimen	Gastric remnant	Biliary drainage	Pancreatic drainage	Gastric remnant drainage	Feeding access	OR time (min)	EBL (cc)	N staging	Margins	Complications	Oncological Outcome	Follow-up (moths)
Helmick	2010	M	71	IPMN	CT	4	NR	Pain	SPDS	Spared	BL	BL	BL	BL	GT	NR	NR	NR	NR	Bile leak	NED	NR
	2010	F	58	CP	CT	5	NR	Pain, jaundice	SPDS	Spared	BL	BL	BL	BL	GT	NR	NR	NR	N/A	NR	N/A	NR
Swain	2010	F	50	PDAC	CT	1.75	Open	Jaundice, weight loss	SPDS, GR	Resected	BL	BL	N/A	N/A	NR	NR	NR	NR	NR	NR	NED	12
		F	55	NET	CT	2	Lap	Incidental finding	SPDS, GR	Resected	BL	BL	N/A	N/A	NR	NR	NR	NR	NR	Pancreatic leak	NED	12
		F	61	PDAC	CT	25	Open loop	Incidental finding	SPDS, GR	Resected	BL	BL	N/A	N/A	NR	NR	NR	NR	NR	NR	NED	36
		F	56	Ampullary Ca	CT	0.75	Lap	Fever/chills, jaundice	SPDS, GR, BL	Resected	AL	AL	N/A	N/A	NR	NR	NR	NR	NR	NR	NED	84
Cruz-Muñoz		M	51	NET	CT, Perc	10	Open	Pain	PPPDS, BL	Spared	CC	CC	CC	NR	NR	NR	NR	NR	NR	ECF	NED	NR
	2011	M	61	NET	CT	0.18	Lap	Incidental finding	SPDS, GR	Resected	BL	BL	N/A	NR	NR	410	250	0	Neg	Pancreatic leak	NED	NR
Khithani	2009	F	60	PDAC	CT	NR	NR	Jaundice, pain	SPDS, GR	Resected	BL	BL	N/A	JT	NR	NR	NR	NR	NR	NR	NED	NR
	2009	F	57	PDAC	CT	NR	NR	Incidental finding	SPDS	Resected	BL	BL	N/A	JT	NR	NR	NR	NR	NR	NR	NED	NR
Rutkoski	2008	F	49	PDAC	CT, US, MRCP	5	Lap	Pain, nausea/ vomiting, jaundice	SPDS	Spared	CC	CC	BL	BL	NR	NR	NR	1	Neg	NR	DOD	9
Theodoropoulos	2012	F	53	PDAC	CT	14	Open	Pain	SPDS, BL	Spared	CC distal to J-J	CC distal to J-J	CC distal to J-J	NR	NR	NR	1	Neg	NR	NED	NR
Nikfarjam	2009	F	46	FDBDF	CT, PTC	3	Lap	Jaundice	SPDS, GR	Resected	BL	BL	N/A	NR	NR	480	100	N/A	N/A	NR	N/A	12
	2009	F	72	FDBDF	CT, PTC	5	Open	Jaundice, weight loss	SPDS, GR	Resected	BL	BL	N/A	NR	NR	300	950	N/A	N/A	NR	N/A	12
Peng	2018			PDAC	CT, Perc		Open		SPDS	Spared	AL	AL	CC	NR				NR	Pos	NR	DOD	81
				PDAC	CT		Open		SPDS, GR	Resected	BL	BL	N/A	NR				NR	Pos	NR	DOD	50
				IPMN	CT, PTC		Lap		SPDS, GR	Resected	BL	BL	N/A	NR				NR	Neg	NR	DOD	18
				PDAC	CT		NR		SPDS, GR	Resected	BL	BL	N/A	NR				NR	Pos	NR	DOD	37
				PDAC	CT, PTC		Open		SPDS, GR	Resected	BL	BL	N/A	NR				NR	Pos	NR	AWD	53
				CP	CT, PTC		Open		SPDS, GR, GJ	Resected	BL	BL	N/A	NR				N/A	N/A	NR	N/A	NR
				Duodenal Ca	CT, PTC, Endo		Open		SPDS	Spared	BL	BL	BL	NR				NR	Neg	NR	AWD	57
				PDAC	CT, Perc		Lap		SPDS, GR	Resected	BL	BL	N/A	NR				NR	Neg	NR	AWD	34
				CP	CT, PTC, Endo		Open		SPDS, GR	Resected	BL	BL	N/A	NR				N/A	N/A	NR	N/A	NR
				PDAC	CT, PTC		Open		SPDS, GR, Spleen	Resected	BL	BL	N/A	NR				NR	Neg	NR	DOD	16
				PDAC	CT, PTC		Lap		Pancreas, GR	Resected	BL	BL	N/A	NR				NR	Neg	NR	DOD	27

Table 1 Overview of all relevant clinicopathological characteristics in the 26 cases reviewed of post-RYGB patients who underwent pancreaticoduodenectomy (*Continued*)

Author	Year	Sex	Age	Diagnosis	Imaging/ diagnostic modalities	Years from RYGB	RYGB type	Presenting complaint(s)	Resection specimen	Gastric remnant	Biliary drainage	Pancreatic drainage	Gastric remnant drainage	Feeding access	OR time (min)	EBL (cc)	N staging	Margins	Complications	Oncological Outcome	Follow-up (mths)
Mean			64			10									361	500					
Current report	2015	F	63	PDAC	CT	12	Open	Pain, nausea/ vomiting	SPDS, BL	Spared	CC	CC	CC	GT	765	400	2	Neg	Pancreatic fistula	DOD	23

NR not reported, N/A not applicable, RYGB Roux-en-Y Gastric Bypass, PDAC pancreatic ductal adenocarcinoma, NET neuroendocrine tumor, FDBDF focal distal bile duct fibrosis, CP chronic pancreatitis, CT computed tomography, US ultrasound, MRCP magnetic resonance cholangiopancreatography, PTC percutaneous transhepatic cholangiography, Perc percutaneous biopsy, Lap laparoscopic, Endo endoscopic biopsy, SPDS standard pancreaticoduodenectomy specimen (pancreatic head, duodenum, antrum, common bile duct, and gallbladder, if present), PPPDS pylorus-preserving pancreaticoduodenectomy specimen (pancreatic head, distal duodenum, common bile duct), GR gastric remnant, BL biliopancreatic limb, CC common channel, AL alimentary limb, jejjej jejunojejunostomy, JT feeding jejunostomy tube placed, GT feeding gastrostomy tube, ECF enterocutaneous fistula, NED no evidence of disease, DOD dead of disease, AWD alive with disease

Table 2 Patient, diagnostic, and pathologic characteristics of post-RYGB patients undergoing pancreaticoduodenectomy in reviewed cases (N = 26)

Parameter	Proportion or median	Percentage (%) or IQR
Patient demographics		
Sex (female)	12/15	80
Age (years)	54	52–61
Years from RYGB*	5	2–10
Presenting complaint**		
Pain	18/26	69.2
Jaundice	14/26	53.8
Weight loss	9/26	34.6
Nausea/vomiting	5/26	19.2
Incidental finding	4/26	15.4
Diarrhea	2/26	7.7
Fever/chills	1/26	3.9
Preoperative diagnostic modality**		
CT	26/26	100
PTC	9/26	34.6
Percutaneous biopsy	3/26	11.5
Endoscopic biopsy	2/26	7.7
US	1/26	3.9
MRCP	1/26	3.9
Pathologic diagnosis		
PDAC	14/26	53.8
NET	3/26	11.5
CP	3/26	11.5
FDBDF	2/26	7.7
IPMN	1/26	3.9
Duodenal Ca	1/26	3.9
Ampullary Ca	1/26	3.9

IQR interquartile range, RYGB Roux-en-Y Gastric Bypass, PDAC pancreatic ductal adenocarcinoma, NET neuroendocrine tumor, FDBDF focal distal bile duct fibrosis, CP chronic pancreatitis, IPMN intraductal papillary mucinous neoplasm, CT computed tomography, US ultrasound, MRCP magnetic resonance cholangiopancreatography, PTC percutaneous transhepatic cholangiography

*Only 11 cases with reported RYGB details

**Possible for one patient to have multiple presenting symptoms or diagnostic modalities

Table 3 Operative and post-operative characteristics of post-RYGB patients undergoing pancreaticoduodenectomy in reviewed cases (N = 26)

Parameter	Proportion	Percentage (%)
Pancreatic resection performed		
Pancreaticoduodenectomy	24/26	92.3
Pylorus-preserving pancreaticoduodenectomy	1/26	3.8
Total pancreatectomy	1/26	3.8
Resection specimen (in addition to standard PD specimen)		
Gastric remnant	18/26	69.2
Old biliopancreatic limb	3/26	11.5
Reconstruction of biliopancreatic drainage		
Biliopancreatic limb	21/26	73.1
New limb from common channel	3/26	19.2
New limb from alimentary limb	1/26	3.8
Common channel (limb in continuity)	1/26	3.8
Drainage of gastric remnant		
Biliopancreatic limb	4/8	50
New limb from common channel	3/8	37.5
Common channel (limb in continuity)	1/8	12.5
Enteral feeding access		
Gastrostomy tube	3/26	11.5
Jejunostomy tube	2/26	7.7
Oncologic outcome		
NED	10/21	84.6
DOD	8/21	7.7
AWD	3/21	7.7
Median follow-up (months)	17/26	27

PD pancreaticoduodenectomy, IQR interquartile range, NED no evidence of disease, DOD dead of disease, AWD alive with disease

preoperative planning to identify resectable disease are paramount [22].

Classically, the RYGB reconstruction involves creating an anastomosis of the jejunal alimentary limb to the gastric pouch, which is connected to a separate biliopancreatic limb. This reconstructed anatomy produces both restrictive and malabsorptive components for weight loss. A subsequent PD requires reconstruction of biliary and pancreatic drainage which had previously been achieved by the biliopancreatic limb. If there remains sufficient length on this limb, most authors recommend using the distal jejunal segment of this limb to accomplish drainage [12]. In certain cases, the entire biliopancreatic limb may need to be resected, requiring construction of a new limb. The source of this new biliopancreatic limb may arise from the old common channel distal to the jejunojejunostomy (Fig. 2a) or from the amputated alimentary limb, the distal part of which becomes utilized for a hepaticojejunostomy and

pancreatic head mass requires a PD, classically involving en bloc resection of the pancreatic head, distal stomach and duodenum, common bile duct, and gallbladder. Reconstruction is typically achieved by creation of a pancreaticojejunostomy, hepaticojejunostomy, and gastrojejunostomy, in series. However, given the anatomical alterations, post-PD reconstruction requires greater forethought in the post-RYGB population. Although infrequently reported, these procedures can be longer in duration with a greater potential for morbidity. All potential reconstruction options found in the literature are summarized in Fig. 2. Patient selection and

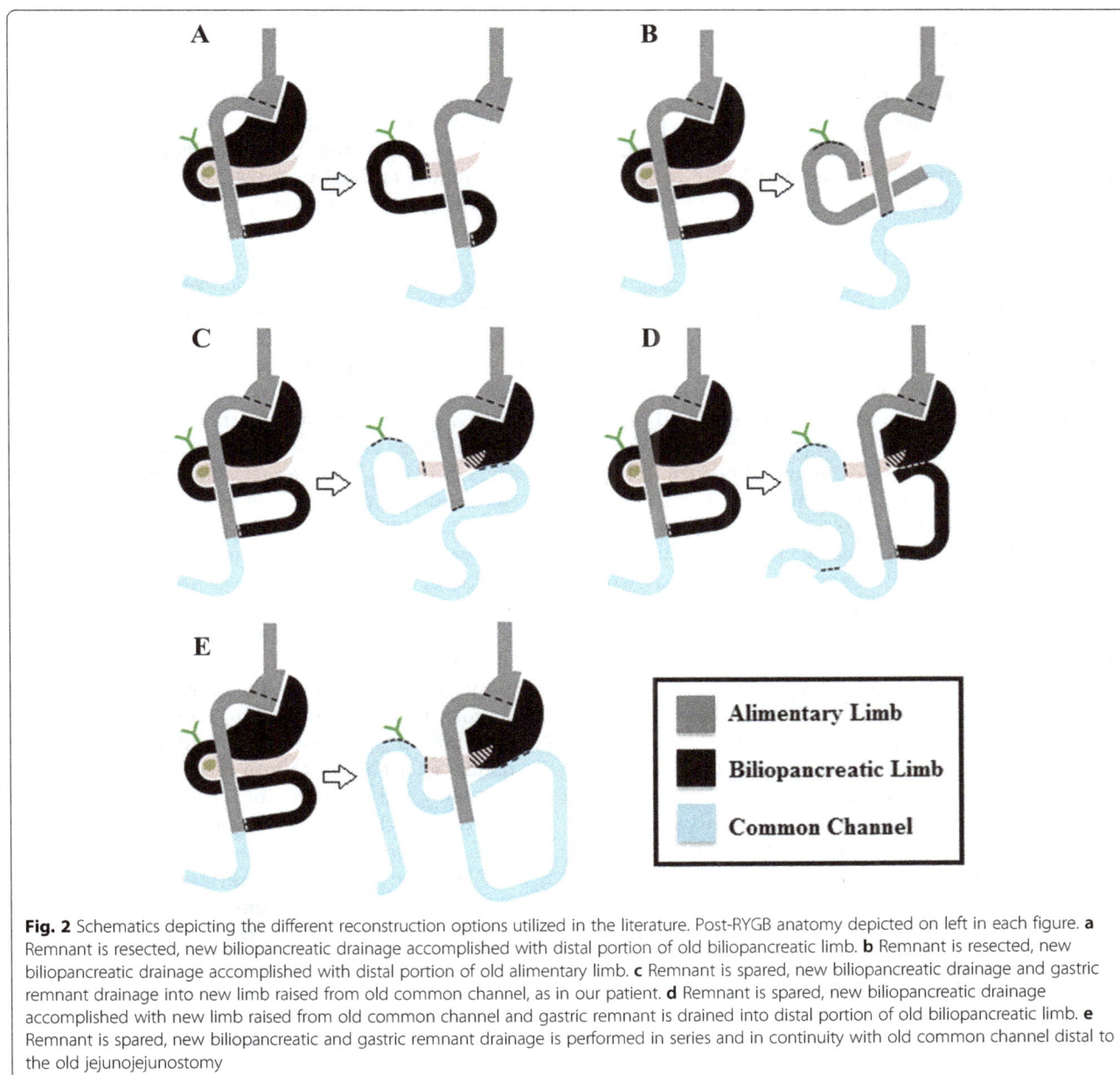

Fig. 2 Schematics depicting the different reconstruction options utilized in the literature. Post-RYGB anatomy depicted on left in each figure. **a** Remnant is resected, new biliopancreatic drainage accomplished with distal portion of old biliopancreatic limb. **b** Remnant is resected, new biliopancreatic drainage accomplished with distal portion of old alimentary limb. **c** Remnant is spared, new biliopancreatic drainage and gastric remnant drainage into new limb raised from old common channel, as in our patient. **d** Remnant is spared, new biliopancreatic drainage accomplished with new limb raised from old common channel and gastric remnant is drained into distal portion of old biliopancreatic limb. **e** Remnant is spared, new biliopancreatic and gastric remnant drainage is performed in series and in continuity with old common channel distal to the old jejunojejunostomy

pancreaticojejunostomy (Fig. 2b). In both circumstances, a separate jejunojejunal anastomosis will need to occur.

If the gastric remnant is not resected, drainage of this channel must be factored into the reconstruction. The more commonly reported reconstruction consists of using a new limb from the old common channel for hepaticojejunostomy, pancreaticojejunostomy, and remnant gastrojejunostomy (Fig. 2c). Our patient underwent a PD with resection of the old biliopancreatic limb, sparing the gastric remnant and placement of a feeding gastrostomy tube (pre-operative albumin 2.6 g/dL). We recreated the biliopancreatic limb from the prior common channel. Since the gastric remnant was left in situ,

we performed a jejuno-gastric remnant anastomosis in series with this same limb. Alternatively, another author reported using the old biliopancreatic limb for the remnant gastrojejunostomy while raising a new limb from the old common channel for the hepaticojejunostomy and pancreaticojejunostomy (Fig. 2d) [19]. While physiologically appropriate, this does increase the number of anastomoses and possibility of morbidity. Of interest, one author reported construction of a hepaticojejunostomy and pancreaticojejunostomy with the common channel far distal to the jejunojejunostomy and in continuity with the gastric pouch and alimentary limb (Fig. 2e) [20]. This is inadvisable, as there is risk for reflux of enteric contents into the biliary tree, increasing the incidence of cholangitis [12]. Each of these reconstruction methods reflects surgeon preference, as well as anatomic considerations posed by individual patients.

Though less commonly performed in the reviewed cases (30.8%), there may be advantages to retaining the gastric remnant during PD in the post-RYGB patient including retained physiologic function, nutritional support, and ease of future diagnostic and therapeutic interventions. Since the first gastric bypass reported by Ito and Mason in 1967, interest in gastrointestinal tract physiologic changes brought on by altered surgical anatomy persists [23]. Particular focus was paid to the importance of the excluded stomach (remnant) for motility and secretory function, plus the impact of surgical discontinuity of the gastric pouch. Printen et al. and Mason et al. published studies in which pre- and post-operative gastric pH and secretions were found to be identical [21, 24]. Both studies pointed to retention of vagal innervation to the gastric remnant. Given that motor migratory complex (MMC) initiates mainly from the interstitial cells of Cajal at the gastric antrum, peristalsis remains present in the gastric remnant. The propulsion of gastric, biliary, and pancreatic secretions into the common channel after bypass is evidence of this [25].

The gastric remnant also retains importance in the body's endocrine and exocrine functions in the post-RYGB anatomy. The increase in levels of incretin hormones in the post-RYGB, such as glucagon-like peptide-1 (GLP—1) and gastric inhibitory peptide (GIP), is well studied [26, 27]. Severe hypogylcemia after RYGB is an increasingly recognized complication, possibly due to hyperinsulinemia and β-cell proliferation from increased GLP-1 activity, or failure of islet cell regression in diabetic patients post-RYGB [28]. McLaughlin et al. successfully treated medically refractory hypoglycemia after RYGB with enteral feeds through a gastrostomy tube placed in the gastric remnant. This corrected post-surgical derangements in glucose, insulin, GLP-1, glucagon, and GIP after oral food intake [29].

Additionally, 16% of partial gastrectomy patients develop B12 deficiency and this rate increases with elapsed-time post-surgery, with some patients presenting with B12 deficiency 10 years or more after partial gastrectomy [30, 31]. This effect is, in part, due to both the restrictive and malabsorptive aspects of the procedure. The early satiety induced by gastric restriction leads to reduction in hydrochloric acid and pepsin production. Reduction of available B12 from food and decreased exposure to intrinsic factor (IF) producing cells subsequently leads to B12 malabsorption [32]. B12 deficiency can have profound implications on overall health, anemia, and neurologic disorders [33]. Recently, Sala et al. demonstrated that post-RYGB risk of B12 deficiency

may also be the result of changes in upregulation of B12 pathway-encoding genes [32]. The gastric remnant may also be capable of reasserting its function for intrinsic factor production, as well as modulating secondary measures of intestinal B12 absorption via increased production of transcobalamin II, which binds B12 after its release from IF in the ileum [32].

Delayed gastric emptying (DGE) is a common post-operative complication of PD, occurring in 15–40% of patients [34, 35]. Suspected causes of DGE include removal of the motilin-secreting duodenum, gastric irritation from bile, and interruption of the myoneural pathways in the bowel wall [36]. Furthermore, DGE has been associated with deep space infection and leak, although causal relationships remain poorly defined [37]. Regardless of etiology, DGE interferes with resumption of normal diet and post-operative nutrition. In the post-RYGB patient, this complication may be amplified due to the altered physiology. A study by Dutra et al. on Wistar rats previously showed that increased length of the biliopancreatic limb could serve as a functional barrier to gastric emptying while offering no advantages in preventing enterogastric reflux [38]. Gustavsson et al. analyzed outcomes of 234 patients who underwent total or subtotal gastrectomy with Roux-en-Y reconstruction, demonstrating that those with gastric dysmotility had longer roux-limbs (mean 41 cm), and shortening these limbs improved symptoms [39]. Additional studies of dysmotility after RYGB focus on reconstruction of intestinal anatomy and disruption of MMCs, displacement of the native pacemaker cells of the gut by slower ectopic signals, and changes in the metabolic and endocrine regulation of these events [40]. Preservation of the gastric remnant with subsequent reconstruction in this patient population may allow for improved physiologic parameters, and diagnostic and therapeutic interventions.

Intolerance to oral intake is multi-factorial in the PD-RYGB population and can sufficiently compromise patient nutrition, requiring further intervention for enteral supplementation. An intact gastric remnant provides the opportunity to leave a remnant gastrostomy tube for post-operative decompression and enteral nutrition post-PD [41]. In our patient, we placed a feeding gastrostomy tube in the gastric remnant, as malnutrition is associated with adverse outcomes following PD, especially in a patient who has already had significant weight loss and hypoalbuminemia [42, 43]. These complications include sepsis, impaired wound healing, and pancreatic fistula formation [44–46]. A recent systematic analysis of different enteral routes of nutrition (15 articles, 3474 patients) found that gastrojejunostomy feeding was associated with the shortest hospital stay (mean 15 days) and lowest incidence of delayed gastric emptying (6%) [47]. Barbour et al. published an experience with five patients requiring pancreatic resections after RYGB in which a gastrostomy tube in the gastric remnant was successfully used for decompression and, later, to supplement with enteral nutrition [41]. This may be particularly significant in the post-RYGB patient as hypoalbuminemia (< 3.5 mg/dL) may occur in up to 13% [48]. Remnant gastrojejunostomy placement may help overcome these issues.

Preservation of the gastric remnant also aids in post-PD diagnostic and therapeutic intervention. Performing ERCP in the altered anatomy post-PD can be technically challenging even with an intact stomach. Many endoscopists favor anterograde EUS access for pancreatic duct interventions post-PD. Such interventions may be difficult, from a small gastric pouch. Chalal et al. demonstrated only a 51% success rate in 88 ERCPs performed in post-PD patients at the Mayo Clinic (2002–2005) [49]. Laparoscopic-assisted ERCP to access the remnant stomach, as opposed to the jejunum or gastric pouch, may provide a number of advantages, especially in terms of supporting access in a position similar to native anatomy [50]. Several investigators described success with EUS access of the remnant stomach to allow for laparoscopic-assisted ERCP through the remnant in post-Roux-en-Y anatomy [51].

While reversal of RYGB is an uncommon procedure, the related literature demonstrates improvement in post-operative morbidities related to the post-RYGB anatomy, lending support to the concept that the gastric remnant retains much of its physiologic function [52, 53]. In cases in which the post-RYGB patient develops severe complications (acute hypoglycemia, weight regain, intractable diarrhea, extreme dumping syndrome, cachexia), reversal of the bypass to normal anatomy commonly leads to resolution of symptoms [52]. Vilallonga et al. published an experience with 20 patients in which they describe laparoscopic reversal of RYGB with resolution of most complications, although few patients did develop gastroesophageal reflux disease (three patients) and diarrhea (one patient), secondary to damage of the vagus nerves [54]. Similarly, Pernar et al. showed resolution of the predominant symptoms in 15 of 19 patients, including 6 weaned from total parenteral nutrition (TPN). Given that the gastric remnant retains its function, this procedure remains an option, though it should only be considered in select patients.

Despite the benefits of leaving the gastric remnant in situ, there may be technical advantages to resecting the gastric remnant en bloc with the specimen [55–57]. First, it obviates the need for a jejuno-gastric remnant anastomosis and associated potential complications. However, an important consideration, a prospectively collected, multicenter study by Smith et al. of nearly 4500 gastric bypass patients, found only 1% clinically significant gastrojejunostomy leak rate [57]. In turn,

other recent series report anastomotic stricture rates between 4.8 and 7.3% [55, 56]. Therefore, by resecting the remnant and avoiding additional anastomoses, the surgeon may simplify the subsequent reconstruction while avoiding potential morbidity. In contrast, preserving the gastric remnant may also allow for future development of bleeding, ulceration, or undetected malignancy, although the overall risk of developing gastric and esophageal malignancies is reportedly rare in the post-RYGB patient [58–60].

This systematic review has limitations. Few publications exist interrogating this particular area; therefore, there remains a paucity of data with which to develop clear, evidence-based guidelines for reconstruction options. Indeed, with both the increasing incidence of pancreatic cancer and number of patients undergoing bariatric procedures, this clinical scenario will become more prevalent, making discussions of the surgical options more frequent and relevant. Furthermore, gastric remnant preservation, while currently performed less frequently, may be advantageous from a multidisciplinary standpoint, but clearly requires further investigation [61]. Although not discussed, decisions regarding preoperative diagnostic modalities or perioperative neoadjuvant and adjuvant treatments for this unique, but expanding, patient population deserves further review.

Conclusions

Pancreaticoduodenectomy after Roux-en-Y gastric bypass is a complex procedure that is rarely performed. Varying practice patterns reflect the complexity of the surgery and diversity of surgeon preference. Few publications exist to develop recommendations, yet there is a growing need to provide evidence for the safest and most effective method of resection and reconstruction in this growing population. Regardless of reconstruction used, the most important goal should be definitive resection (R0), followed by consideration for the patient's future quality of life and further treatment.

Abbreviations

CT: Computed tomography; DGE: Delayed gastric emptying; ERCP: Endoscope retrograde cholangiopancreatography; IQR: Inter-quartile range; MMC: Motor migratory complex; PD: Pancreaticoduodenectomy; RYGB: Roux-en-Y gastric bypass; TPN: Total parenteral nutrition

Acknowledgements

The authors would like to acknowledge the late Dr. Andres E. Castellanos, MD, FACS, whose leadership and experience within our department was vital to the development of the bariatric surgery program and resident education.

Funding

Funding for manuscript publication is provided by the Drexel University College of Medicine Departments of Surgery and Medicine.

Authors' contributions

WFM, MFS, AG, JL, and WBB wrote the manuscript. WFM, MFS, EMG, MK, and ERS conducted the literature search and assisted with the data acquisition and analysis. WBB supervised the work conducted by all co-authors. All authors read and approved the final manuscript.

Competing interests

The authors declare that they have no competing interests.

Author details

[1]Division of Surgical Oncology, Department of Surgery, Drexel University College of Medicine, 245 N. 15th Street, Suite 7150, Philadelphia, PA 19102, USA. [2]Division of Minimally Invasive Surgery, Department of Surgery, Drexel University College of Medicine, 245 N. 15th St, Suite 7150, Philadelphia, PA 19102, USA. [3]Division of Gastroenterology & Hepatology, Department of Medicine, Drexel University College of Medicine, 219 N Broad St, 5th Floor, Philadelphia, PA 19107, USA.

References

1. Flegal KM, Carroll MD, Ogden CL. Prevalence and trends in obesity among US adults, 1998-2008. JAMA. 2010;303(3):235–41.
2. Rebours V, Gaujoux S, d'Assignies G, Sauvanet A, Ruszniewski P, Lévy P, et al. Obesity and fatty pancreatic infiltration are risk factors for pancreatic precancerous lesions (PanIN). Clin Cancer Res. 2015;21(15):3522–8.
3. Nimptsch K, Pischon T. Body fatness, related biomarkers and cancer risk: epidemiological perspective. Horm Mol Biol Clin Investig. 2015;22(2):39–51.
4. O'Brien PE, McPhail T, Chaston TB, Dixon JB. Systematic review of medium-term weight loss after bariatric operations. Obes Surg. 2006;16(8):1032–40.
5. Buchwald H, Avidor Y, Braunwald E, Jensen MD, Pories W, Fahrbach K, et al. Bariatric surgery: a systematic review and meta-analysis. JAMA. 2004;292(14): 1724–37.
6. Korenkov M, Sauerlan S, Junginger T. Surgery for obesity. Curr Opin Gastroenterol. 2005;21(6):679–83.
7. Khashab MA, Okolo PI. Accessing the pancreatobiliary limb and ERCP in the bariatric patient. Gastrointest Endosc Clin N Am. 2011;21(2):305–13.
8. Schreiner MA, Chang L, Gluck M, Irani S, Gan S, Brandabur JJ, et al. Laparoscopy-assisted versus balloon enteroscopy-assisted ERCP in bariatric post-Roux-en-Y gastric bypass patients. Gastrointest Endosc. 2012;75(4):748–56.
9. Lopes TL, Clements RH, Wilcox CM. Laparoscopy-assisted ERCP: experience of a high-volume bariatric surgery center (with video). Gastrointest Endosc. 2009;70(6):1254–9.
10. Saleem A, Levy MJ, Petersen BT, Que FG, Baron TH. Laparoscopic-assisted ERCP in Roux-en-Y gastric bypass (RYGB) surgery patients. J Gastrointest Surg. 2012;16(1):203–8.
11. Baron TH, Song LM, Ferreira LE, Smyrk TC. Novel approach to therapeutic ERCP after long-limb Roux-en-Y gastric bypass surgery using transgastric self-expandable metal stents: experimental outcomes and first human case study (with videos). Gastrointest Endosc. 2012;75(6):1258–63.
12. Hatzaras I, Sachs TE, Weiss M, Wolfgang CL, Pawlik T. Pancreaticoduodenectomy after bariatric surgery: challenges and available techniques for reconstruction. J Gastrointest Surg. 2014;18(4):869–77.
13. Helmick R, Singh R, Welshhans J, Fegelman EJ, Shahid H. Pancreaticoduodenectomy after Roux-en-Y gastric bypass: a single institution retrospective series. IJHPD. 2013;3:17–21.
14. Swain JM, Adams RB, Farnell MB, Que FG, Sarr MG. Gastric and pancreatoduodenal resection for malignant lesions after previous gastric bypass—diagnosis and methods of reconstruction. Surg Obes Relat Dis. 2010;6(6):670–5.
15. de la Cruz-Muñoz N, Hartnett S, Sleeman D. Laparoscopic pancreatoduodenectomy after laparoscopic gastric bypass. Surg Obes Relat Dis. 2011;7(3):326–7.
16. Peng JS, Corcelles R, Choong K, Gandhi N, Walsh RM, Hardacre JM, et al. Pancreatoduodenectomy after Roux-en-Y gastric bypass: technical considerations and outcomes. HPB (Oxford). 2018;20(1):34–40.
17. Khithani AS, Curtis DE, Galanopoulos C, Jeyarajah DR. Pancreaticoduodenectomy after a Roux-en-Y gastric bypass. Obes Surg. 2009;19(6):802–5.
18. Nikfarjam M, Staveley-O'Carroll KF, Kimchi ET, Hardacre JM. Pancreaticoduodenectomy in patients with a history of Roux-en Y gastric bypass surgery. Journal of the Pancreas. 2009;10(2):169–73.

19. Rutkoski JD, Gagne DJ, Volpe C, Papasavas PK, Hayetian F, Caushaj PF. Pancreaticoduodenectomy for pancreatic cancer after laparoscopic Roux-en-Y gastric bypass. Surg Obes Relat Dis. 2008;4(4):552–4.
20. Theodoropolous I, Franco C, Gervasoni JE. Pancreaticoduodenectomy for pancreatic carcinoma after complicated open Roux-en-Y gastric bypass surgery: an alternative approach to reconstruction. Surg Obes Relat Dis. 2012;8(5):648–50.
21. Mason EE, Munns JR, Kealey GP, Wangler R, Clarke WR, Cheng HF, et al. Effect of gastric bypass on gastric secretion. Am J Surg. 1976;131(2):162–8.
22. Raut CP, Tseng JF, Sun CC, Wang H, Wolff RA, Crane CH, et al. Impact of resection status on pattern of failure and survival after pancreaticoduodenectomy for pancreatic adenocarcinoma. Ann Surg. 2007; 246(1):52–60.
23. Bray GA. Obesity and surgery for a chronic disease. Obes Res. 1996;4(3):301–3.
24. Printen KJ, Owensby M. Vagal innervation of the bypassed stomach following gastric bypass. Surgery. 1978;84(4):455–6.
25. Deloose E, Janssen P, Depoortere I, Tack J. The migrating motor complex: control mechanisms and its role in health and disease. Nat Rev Gastroenterol Hepatol. 2012;9(5):271–85.
26. Patti ME, McMahon G, Mun EC, Bitton A, Holst JJ, Goldsmith J, et al. Severe hypoglycemia post-gastric bypass requiring partial pancreatectomy: evidence for inappropriate insulin secretion and pancreatic islet hyperplasia. Diabetologia. 2005;48(11):2236–40.
27. Borg CM, Le Roux CW, Ghatei MA, Bloom SR, Patel AG, Aylwin SJ. Progressive rise in gut hormone levels after Roux-en-Y gastric bypass suggests gut adaptation and explains altered satiety. Br J Surg. 2006;93(2):210–5.
28. Service GJ, Thompson GB, Service FJ, Andrews JC, Collazo-Clavell ML, Lloyd RV. Hyperinsulinemic hypoglycemia with nesidioblastosis after gastric-bypass surgery. N Engl J Med. 2005;353(3):249–54.
29. McLaughlin T, Peck M, Holst J, Deacon C. Reversible hyperinsulinemic hypoglycemia after gastric bypass: a consequence of altered nutrient delivery. J Clin Endocrinol Metab. 2010;95(4):1851–5.
30. Hu Y, Kim HI, Hyung WJ, Lee JH, Kim YM, Noh SH. Vitamin B(12) deficiency after gastrectomy for gastric cancer: an analysis of clinical patterns and risk factors. Ann Surg. 2013;258(6):970–5.
31. Weir DG, Temperley IJ, Gatenby PBB. Vitamin B12 deficiency following partial gastrectomy. Ir J Med Sci. 1966;41(3):97–102.
32. Sala P, Belarmino G, Torrinhas RS, Machado NM, Fonseca DC, Ravacci GR, et al. Gastrointestinal transcriptomic response of metabolic vitamin B12 pathways in Roux-en-Y gastric bypass. Clin Transl Gastroenterol. 2017;8(1):e212.
33. Nielse MJ, Rasmussen MR, Andersen CB, Nexø E, Moestrup SK. Vitamin B12 transport from food to the body's cells—a sophisticated, multistep pathway. Nat Rev Gastroenterol Hepatol. 2012;9(5):345–54.
34. Mon RA, Cullen JJ. Standard Roux-en-Y gastrojejunostomy vs. "uncut" Roux-en-Y gastrojejunostomy: a matched cohort study. J Gastrointest Surg. 2000; 4(3):298–303.
35. Fabre JM, Burgel JS, Navarro F, Boccarat G, Lemoine C, Domergue J. Delayed gastric emptying after pancreaticoduodenectomy and pancreaticogastrostomy. Eur J Surg. 1999;165(6):560–5.
36. Wayne MG, Jorge IA, Cooperman AM. Alternative reconstruction after pancreaticoduodenectomy. World J Surg Oncol. 2008;6(9). https://doi.org/10.1186/1477-7819-6-9.
37. Parmar MD, Sheffield KM, Vargas GM, Pitt HA, Kilbane EM, Hall BL, et al. Factors associated with delayed gastric emptying after pancreaticoduodenectomy. HPB (Oxford). 2013;15(10):763–72.
38. Dutra RA, Araújo WM, Andrade JI. The effects of Roux-en-Y limb length on gastric emptying and enterogastric reflux in rats. Acta Cir Bras. 2008;23(2):179–83.
39. Gustavsson S, ilstrup DM, Morrison P, Kelly KA. Roux-en-Y stasis syndrome after gastrectomy. Am J Surg. 1988;155(3):490–4.
40. Quercia I, Dutia R, Kotler DP, Belsley S, Laferrère B. Gastrointestinal changes after bariatric surgery. Diabetes Metab. 2014;40(2):87–94.
41. Barbour JR, Thomas BN, Morgan KA, Byrne TK, Adams DB. The practice of pancreatic resection after Roux-en-Y gastric bypass. Am Surg. 2008;74(8): 729–34.
42. Gleeson EM, Shaikh MF, Shewokis PA, Clarke JR, Meyers WC, Pitt HA, et al. Whipple-ABACUS, a simple, validated risk score for 30-day mortality after pancreaticoduodenectomy developed using the ACS-NSQIP database. Surgery. 2016;160(5):1279–87.
43. Gleeson EM, Clarke JR, Morano WF, Shaikh MF, Bowne WB, Pitt HA. Patient-specific predictors of failure to rescue after pancreaticoduodenectomy. HPB. 2018;In-press.

44. M FA, Feliciano DV, Andrassy RJ, AH MA, Booth FV, Morgenstein-Wagner TB, et al. Early enteral feeding, compared with parenteral, reduces postoperative septic complications. The results of a meta-analysis. Ann Surg. 1992;216(2):172–83.

45. Zaloga GP, Bortenschlager L, Black KW, Prielipp R. Immediate postoperative enteral feeding decreases weight loss and improves wound healing after abdominal surgery in rats. Crit Care Med. 1992;20(1):115–8.

46. Aranha GV, Aaron JM, Shoup M, Pickleman J. Current management of pancreatic fistula after pancreaticoduodenectomy. Surgery. 2006;140(4):561–8.

47. Gerritsen A, Besselink MG, Gouma DJ, Steenhagen E, Borel Rinkes IH, Molenaar IQ. Systematic review of five feeding routes after pancreatoduodenectomy. Br J Surg. 2013;100(5):589–98.

48. Faintuch J, Matsuda M, Cruz ME, Silva MM, Teivelis MP, Garrido AB, et al. Severe protein-calorie malnutrition after bariatric procedures. Obes Surg. 2004;14(2):175–81.

49. Chalal P, Baron TH, Topazian MD, Petersen BT, Levy MJ, Gostout CJ. Endoscopic retrograde cholangiopancreatography in post-Whipple patients. Endoscopy. 2006;38(12):1241–5.

50. Ross AS. Techniques for performing ERCP in Roux-en-Y gastric bypass patients. Gastroenterol Hepatol (NY). 2012;8(6):390–2.

51. Attam R, Leslie D, Arain MA, Freeman ML, Ikramuddin S. EUS-guided sutured gastropexy for transgastric ERCP (ESTER) in patients with Roux-en-Y gastric bypass: a novel, single-session, minimally invasive approach. Endoscopy. 2015;47(7):646–9.

52. Pucher PH, Lord AC, Sodergren MH, Ahmed AR, Darzi A, Purkayastha S. Reversal to normal anatomy after failed gastric bypass: systematic review of indications, techniques, and outcomes. Surg Obes Relat Dis. 2016;12(7):1351–6.

53. Pernar LIM, Kim JJ, Shikora SA. Gastric bypass reversal: a 7-year experience. Surg Obes Relat Dis. 2016;12:1492–8.

54. Vilallonga R, Van De Vrande S, Himpens J. Laparoscopic reversal of Roux-en-Y gastric bypass into normal anatomy with or without sleeve gastrectomy. Surg Endosc. 2013;27(12):4640–8.

55. Carrodeguas L, Szomstein S, Zundel N, Lo Menzo E, Rosenthal R. Gastrojejunal anastomotic strictures following laparoscopic Roux-en-Y gastric bypass surgery: analysis of 1291 patients. Surg Obes Relat Dis. 2006;2(2):92–7.

56. Ibele AR, Bendewald FP, Mattar SG, McKenna DT. Incidence of gastrojejunostomy stricture in laparoscopic Roux-en-Y gastric bypass using an autologous fibrin sealant. Obes Surg. 2014;24(7):1052–6.

57. Smith MD, Adeniji A, Wahed AS, Patterson E, Chapman W, Courcoulas AP, et al. Technical factors associated with anastomotic leak after Roux-en-Y gastric bypass. Surg Obes Relat Dis. 2015;11(2):313–20.

58. Jawad A, Bar AH, Merianos D, Zhou J. MALT lymphoma of the gastric remnant after Roux-en-Y gastric bypass. Gastrointest Cancer. 2012;43(Supple(s1)):194–7.

59. Khitin L, Roses RE, Birkett DH. Cancer in the gastric remnant after gastric bypass: a case report. Curr Surg. 2003;60(5):521–3.

60. Raghavendra RS, Kini D. Benign, premalignant, and malignant lesions encountered in bariatric surgery. JSLS. 2012;16(3):360–72.

61. Younan G, Tsai S, Evans DB, Christians KK. A novel reconstruction technique during pancreaticoduodenectomy after Roux-en-Y gastric bypass: how I do it. J Gastrointest Surg. 2017;21(17):1186–91.

10

Serum magnesium levels and lung cancer risk

Xinghui Song[1], Xiaoning Zhong[1*], Kaijiang Tang[2], Gang Wu[3] and Yin Jiang[2]

Abstract

Background: Whether serum magnesium levels were lower in patients with lung cancer than that in healthy controls is controversial. The aim of this study was to identify and synthesize all citations evaluating the relationship between serum magnesium levels and lung cancer.

Methods: We searched PubMed, WanFang, China National Knowledge Internet (CNKI), and SinoMed databases for relevant studies before December 31, 2017. Two authors independently selected studies, extracted data, and assessed risk of bias.

Results: Eleven citations comprising 707 cases with lung cancer and 7595 healthy controls were included in our study. Serum magnesium levels were not significantly lower in patients with lung cancer [summary SMD = 0.193, 95%CI = $-$ 1.504 to 1.890] when compared to health controls, with significant heterogeneity (I^2 = 99.6%, $P < 0.001$) found. Negative associations were found among Asian populations [summary SMD = 0.229, 95%CI = $-$ 1.637 to 2.094] and European populations [summary SMD = $-$ 0.168, 95%CI = $-$ 0.482 to 0.147]. No publication bias was found using the test of Egger and funnel plot.

Conclusions: Our study suggested that serum magnesium levels had no significant association on lung cancer risk.

Keywords: Magnesium level, Lung cancer, Meta-analysis, Healthy controls

Background

Lung cancer is the leading cause of death from cancer, resulting 1.38 million people deaths each year [1]. Its 5-year survival rate is still as low as 15%, and it is poor while compared with those in high incidence of other cancer [2]. Previous studies pointed out that lung cancer is the most common cancer among men and women, and both developed and developing countries bear a huge social and economic burden [3]. Previous publications proved that both genetic and environment factors were related to lung cancer risk [4–7]. Furthermore, trace-heavy elements also played a significant role on human health and disease [8, 9], as well as lung cancer [10].

Magnesium is one of the trace elements in our bodies, and to date, some papers had been published to investigate the association between serum magnesium levels and lung cancer risks. Two papers [11, 12] reported a higher of serum magnesium level in cases with lung cancer, while six papers [13–18] found a lack of significant association. Conversely, three papers [19–21] suggested that it is lower in lung cancer cases when compared to the healthy controls. Therefore, the aim of this study was to identify and synthesize all citations evaluating the relationship between serum magnesium levels and lung cancer risk.

Methods

Study selection

A comprehensive literature search was conducted in platforms of PubMed, WanFang, China National Knowledge Internet (CNKI), and SinoMed databases up to December 31, 2017. Free words adopted were as follows: "magnesium" or "Mg" combined with "lung cancer" or "lung carcinoma" without restrictions. Reference lists of the studies retrieved were also examined to find any additional study potentially unidentified. The course of study selection was completed by two investigators independently. Any resulting discrepancies were resolved by a third reviewer.

* Correspondence: xnzhong101@sina.com
[1]Department of respiration, the First Affiliated Hospital of Guangxi Medical University, N0.6 Shuangyong Road, Nanning 530021, Guangxi, China
Full list of author information is available at the end of the article

The inclusion criteria were as follows: (i) having a prospective design or a case-control design or a cross-sectional study; (ii) evaluating the association between serum magnesium levels and risk of lung cancer; (iii) reporting mean and standard deviation (SD) of magnesium levels (or sufficient data to compute them) both in lung cancer patients and healthy controls; and (iv) studies published in English language or Chinese language. If more than one article referred to the same populations, only the study that included the most lung cancer cases or the latest publication was included.

Data extraction and quality assessment of studies

Two investigators independently extracted the following data: (1) first author's last name; (2) publication year; (3) study design; (4) country; (5) number of lung cancer cases and participants; (6) sex of cases; (7) age range or mean age of the cases; (8) mean and SD of magnesium levels both in lung cancer patients and healthy controls; and (9) method used for detection of magnesium. Any resulting discrepancies were resolved by a third reviewer.

The methodological quality of studies was evaluated independently by two researchers using the Newcastle-Ottawa Quality Assessment Scale [22]. The three components were as follows: (1) patient selection (4 points); (2) comparability (2 points); and (3) outcome (3 points) for a total score of 9 points.

Statistical analysis

Standardized mean difference (SMD) and their 95% confidence interval (CI) were calculated for relationship between serum magnesium levels and lung cancer risk. A random effect model was used in our meta-analysis [23]. The heterogeneity among studies was evaluated with I^2 and Q tests. [24]. $P < 0.05$ in Q test and $I^2 > 50\%$ indicated statistically significant heterogeneity [25]. Meta-regression was adopted to assess the between-study heterogeneity. Egger's regression asymmetry test [26] and funnel plot [27] were used to visually examine publication bias on study outcome. Statistical analyses were performed using STATA version 12.0 (Stata Corporation, College Station, TX, USA). A two-sided $P < 0.05$ was defined as statistical significance.

Results

Study characteristics

As shown in Fig. 1, the initial 486 articles screened through databases of PubMed, WanFang, China National Knowledge Internet (CNKI), and SinoMed databases searching and 1 additional record identified through other sources. There are 372 articles that were reviewed in the title and abstract while excluding the duplications from different databases. Three hundred and forty two of

372 articles were excepted when screened on the basis of title and abstract; 30 articles were examining full texts. Nineteen studies were further excluded (reviews, not report mean or SD, animal studies, letter to the editors). Finally, 11 articles [11–21] were eligible to be included in the analysis comprising 707 patients with lung cancer and 7595 healthy controls. All the included studies were case-control studies. Nine studies were carried out from China, 1 from Spain, and 1 from Turkey. Ten of the included studies used the methods of atomic absorption spectrophotometer measurements for detection of magnesium. In the study quality assessment, all the included studies were with a score greater or equal to 6. The basic features of all citations are shown in Table 1.

Serum magnesium levels and lung cancer risk

Pooled results suggested that magnesium levels in patients with lung cancer was not significantly lower than healthy controls [summary SMD = 0.193, 95%CI = − 1.504 to 1.890, I^2 = 99.6%, $P_{\text{for heterogeneity}} < 0.001$] (Fig. 2). When we performed the subgroup analysis by geographic location, the association was not significant either in Asian populations [summary SMD = 0.229, 95%CI = − 1.637 to 2.094] or in European populations [summary SMD = − 0.168, 95%CI = − 0.482 to 0.147].

Sources of heterogeneity and meta-regression

Meanwhile, I^2 was 99.6% ($p < 0.001$) for the pooled sensitivity, suggesting high heterogeneity in the sample of studies. Univariate meta-regression was then carried out to determine the reason of heterogeneity. However, there were no significant contributions about publication year, case number, geographic location, sex, and different methods on this high between-study heterogeneity.

Sensitivity analysis and publication bias

Sensitivity analysis conducted while removing one study at the time revealed that no single study had essential effect on the whole result. Figure 3 showed that no publication was considered by the funnel plot method on the basis of data, as well as the Egger's test ($P = 0.586$).

Discussion

In this study, we assessed the association between serum magnesium levels and risk of lung cancer. We did not find a positive association between serum magnesium levels and lung cancer risk. Through our subgroup analysis, we further found no significant association among Asian and European populations. Significant heterogeneity between studies observed in this meta-analysis should be considered as a major limitation of these findings; however, heterogeneity was mainly related to strength of the association rather than the direction of risk estimate,

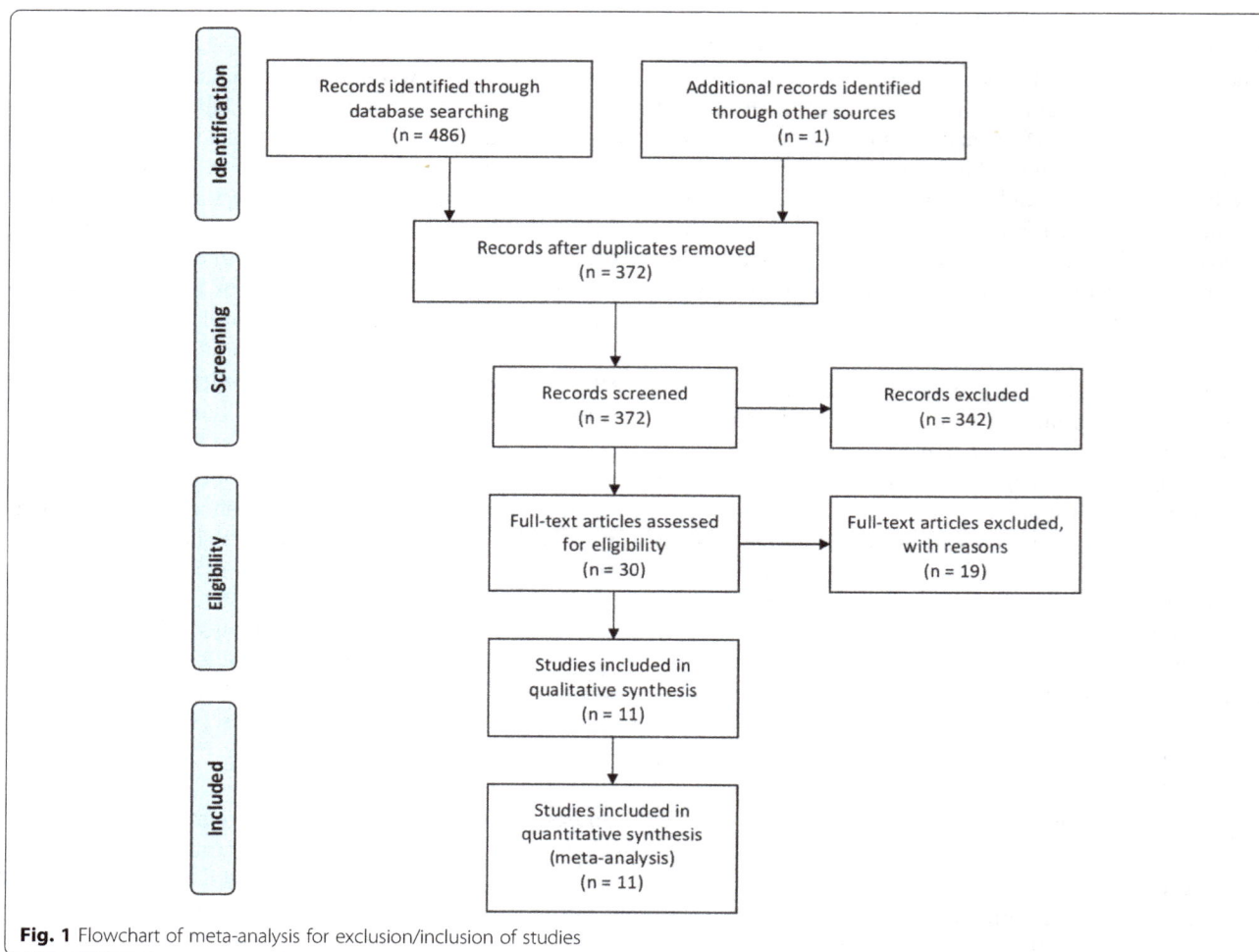

Fig. 1 Flowchart of meta-analysis for exclusion/inclusion of studies

suggesting overall promising findings on the outcome investigated in the present study.

Two previous prospective cohort studies concluded that higher category of dietary magnesium intake had no significant association on lung cancer risk among German population and China population [28, 29]. However, a report [30] had been resulting that higher magnesium levels in drinking water could reduce the risk of lung cancer deaths in women. To our knowledge, no comprehensive analysis had been published to assess the serum magnesium levels on lung cancer risk. In our study, we did not find significant association of lower serum magnesium levels in patient with lung cancer. However, level of magnesium in other disease may be in the normal range, and that magnesium can have an effect on this disease [31].

The existence of heterogeneity among the studies, which is common in meta-analyses [32], may affect the pooled results. Meta-regression was performed to find the potential covariates (publication year, case number, geographic location, sex, and different methods to detect

magnesium levels) which may cause this high heterogeneity. However, no covariate was found to significantly contribute to heterogeneity. In our study, most of the included studies obtained nonsignificant association between serum magnesium levels and lung cancer risk. Only one study [12] reported that serum magnesium level in patient with lung cancer is extremely higher than that in healthy controls. We reviewed the article again and confirmed the data exacted from the study; no error was made. Sensitivity analysis was performed, and no study had essential effect to the significant between-study heterogeneity and the whole result. On the other hand, we used a random effect model to combine the results. As we all know, random effect model had wider rage about 95%CI than fix effect model and could obtain more accurate results. Furthermore, only three studies [12, 13, 17] reported the types and staging of lung cancer, which may also be a factor on the between-study heterogeneity. Therefore, studies with detailed information of types and staging of lung cancer are wanted to further explore this association.

Table 1 Characteristics of all included studies

Study, year	Country	Age (range or Mean ± SD)	Study type	Lung cancer cases			Controls		Methods of measured magnesium
				n	Female (%)	Magnesium: Mean ± SD	n	Magnesium: Mean ± SD	
Cobanoglu U et al., 2010	Turkey	54 ± 8.29	Case-control	30	33.33	156.21 ± 22.21 µg/L	20	185.8 ± 4.05 µg/L	Atomic Absorption Spectrophotometer measurements (UNICAM-929 spectrophotometer)
Diez M et al., 1989	Spain	60 ± 7	Case-control	64	7.81	20.6 ± 3.2 µg/L	100	21.7 ± 8 µg/L	Perkin-Elmer 5.000 atomic absorption spectrophotometer
Jin ZJ et al., 2001	China	45–70	Case-control	40	7.50	1300 ± 390 µmol/L	46	1320 ± 310 µmol/L	Atomic Absorption Spectrophotometer measurements
Xu ZF et al., 1993	China	56 ± 7.5	Case-control	42	9.52	804.63 ± 71.29 µmol/L	40	936.83 ± 93.31 µmol/L	Atomic Absorption Spectrophotometer measurements
He WD et al., 1995	China	34–72	Case-control	143	39.16	940.88 ± 116.95 µmol/L	50	871.24 ± 96.88 µmol/L	Atomic Absorption Spectrophotometer measurements
Huang ZY et al., 1998	China	25–65	Case-control	136	19.12	1.8275 ± 0.375 µmol/L	7101	0.8254 ± 0.1778 µmol/L	Atomic Absorption Spectrophotometer measurements (Japan Shimadzu-AA670/C2H2)
Wang ZL et al., 2003	China	28–69	Case-control	50	40.00	68.29 ± 35.26 µg/L	60	114.1 ± 52.12 µg/L	Atomic Absorption Spectrophotometer measurements and 721 spectrophotometer
Du FL et al., 1996	China	22–73	Case-control	73	31.51	1100 ± 300 µmol/L	63	1100 ± 100 µmol/L	Atomic Absorption Spectrophotometer measurements
Guo XH et al., 1994	China	55.1	Case-control	26	26.92	20.88 ± 6.72 µg/mL	26	18.84 ± 5.86 µg/mL	Atomic Absorption Spectrophotometer measurements (Varian Spectr AA-40p, USA)
Wang FJ et al., 2014	China	17–77	Case-control	68	44.12	880 ± 60 µmol/L	60	860 ± 90 µmol/L	Xylene blue method
Fang JQ et al., 1998	China	55–65	Case-control	35	5.71	1.34 ± 0.35 µmol/L	29	1.36 ± 0.29 µmol/L	Atomic Absorption Spectrophotometer measurements

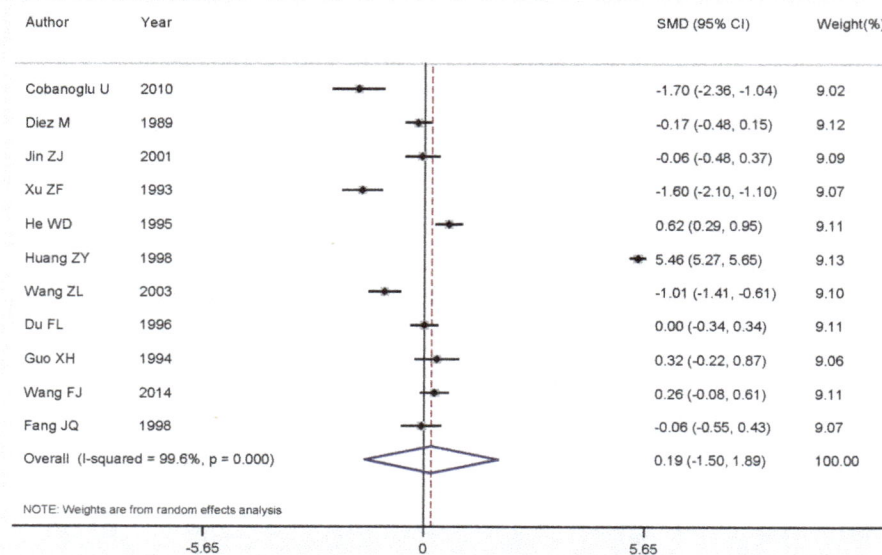

Fig. 2 The forest plot of the relationship between serum magnesium levels and lung cancer risk

Some advantages existed in our study. Firstly, a comprehensive literature search was performed to investigate the relationship between serum magnesium levels and lung cancer risk. Secondly, most of the included studies involved large numbers of patients and healthy controls, and this may strengthen the power of the pooled results. Thirdly, there was no significant publication when tested by Egger and funnel plot, which indicates that our results are stable.

The present study has some limitations. Firstly, the individual studies may have failed to control for potential confounders, which may introduce bias in an unpredictable direction. Secondly, ten of 11 studies were from Asia, and 9 were from China, and thus, more related researches from other countries are wanted to verify the association between geographic location and lung cancer risk.

Conclusions

Based on the obtained results, we concluded that serum magnesium levels may have no significant association in patients with lung cancer. As we experienced some limitations in our study, such as more studies were from Asia, further studies are wanted to confirm this finding.

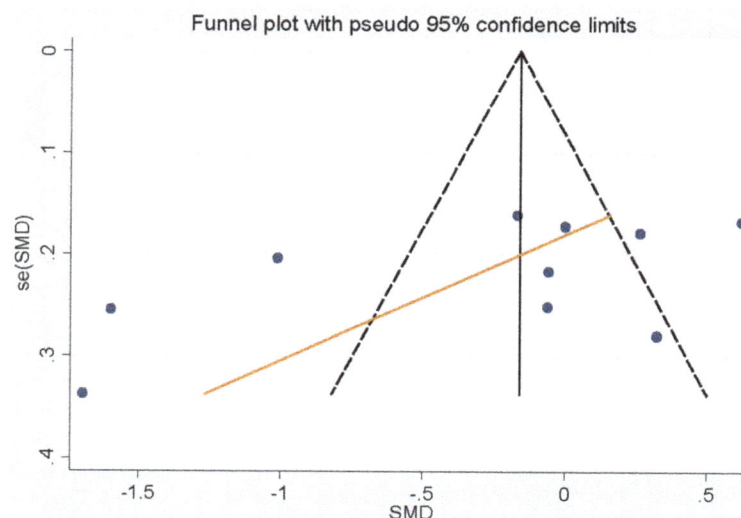

Fig. 3 Funnel plot for the analysis of publication bias between serum magnesium levels and lung cancer risk

Abbreviations

CI: Confidence intervals; SD: Standard deviation; SMD: Standard mean differences

Authors' contributions

XNZ was the guarantor of integrity of the entire study and was responsible for the definition of intellectual content and manuscript editing. XHS contributed to the study concepts, study design, and data analysis and was responsible for the manuscript preparation. KJT and GW were responsible for the literature research. GW carried out the experimental studies. KJT and YJ were responsible for the data acquisition. All authors read and approved the final manuscript.

Competing interest

The authors declare that they have no competing interests.

Author details

[1]Department of respiration, the First Affiliated Hospital of Guangxi Medical University, N0.6 Shuangyong Road, Nanning 530021, Guangxi, China. [2]Department of rheumatism, Liuzhou Worker's Hospital, Liuzhou 545005, Guangxi, China. [3]Department of neurosurgery, Liuzhou General Hospital, Liuzhou 545006, Guangxi, China.

References

1. Torre LA, Bray F, Siegel RL, et al. Global cancer statistics, 2012. CA Cancer J Clin. 2015;65(2):87–108.
2. Tsao AS, Scagliotti GV, Bunn PA Jr, et al. Scientific advances in lung cancer 2015. J Thorac Oncol. 2016;11(5):613–38.
3. Minguet J, Smith KH, Bramlage P. Targeted therapies for treatment of non-small cell lung cancer—recent advances and future perspectives. Int J Cancer. 2016;138(11):2549–61.
4. Liu C, Cui H, Gu D, et al. Genetic polymorphisms and lung cancer risk: evidence from meta-analyses and genome-wide association studies. Lung Cancer. 2017;113:18–29.
5. Wang J, Liu Q, Yuan S, et al. Genetic predisposition to lung cancer: comprehensive literature integration, meta-analysis, and multiple evidence assessment of candidate-gene association studies. Sci Rep. 2017;7(1):8371.
6. Papadopoulos D, Papadoudis A, Kiagia M, et al. Nonpharmacologic interventions for improving sleep disturbances in patients with lung Cancer: a systematic review and meta-analysis. J Pain Symptom Manag. 2018;55(5): 1364–81.
7. Poinen-Rughooputh S, Rughooputh MS, Guo Y, et al. Occupational exposure to silica dust and risk of lung cancer: an updated meta-analysis of epidemiological studies. BMC Public Health. 2016;16(1):1137.
8. Demir N, Basaranoglu M, Huyut Z, et al. The relationship between mother and infant plasma trace element and heavy metal levels and the risk of neural tube defect in infants. J Matern Fetal Neonatal Med. 2017. Epub ahead of print.
9. Wu T, Bi X, Li Z, et al. Contaminations, sources, and health risks of trace metal (loid) s in street dust of a Small City impacted by artisanal Zn smelting activities. Int J Environ Res Public Health. 2017;14(9):961.
10. Zablocka-Slowinska K, Placzkowska S, Prescha A, et al. Serum and whole blood Zn, Cu and Mn profiles and their relation to redox status in lung cancer patients. J Trace Elem Med Biol. 2018;45:78–84.
11. He WD. Detection and analysis of some trace elements in serum of patients with lung cancer. Jiujiang Med J. 1995;10(2):69–71.
12. Huang ZY, Hu FD. Comparative study of serum trace elements in patients with lung cancer. Shanxi Clin Med J. 1998;17(2):114–6.
13. Diez M, Arroyo M, Cerdan FJ, et al. Serum and tissue trace metal levels in lung cancer. Oncology. 1989;46(4):230–4.
14. Jin ZJ, Qian LQ, Dong GQ, et al. Measurement and analysis of serum copper, zinc and magnesium in patients with lung cancer and gastric cancer. Shaanxi Med J. 2001;30(3):165–6.
15. Du FL, Li ZM, Cao MJ, et al. Determination of serum copper, zinc, magnesium and iron in patients with pulmonary tuberculosis, chronic bronchitis, pulmonary heart disease and lung cancer. J of Xi'an Med University. 1996;17(3):348–50.
16. Guo XH, Li PF, Peng FK, et al. Relationship between serum zinc, copper, manganese and lung cancer. Chin Pub Heal. 1994;10(4):156–7.
17. Wang FJ, Zhao ZE, Wen JB, et al. Levels of some major elements in patients with lung cancer: a retrospective analysis. Chin J Gen Pract. 2014;12(4):528–30.
18. Fang JQ, Mei YL, Li LJ, et al. Analysis of selenium, copper, magnesium, magnesium and selenium contents in elderly patients with lung cancer. Ningxia Med J. 1998;20(4):247–8.
19. Cobanoglu U, Demir H, Sayir F, et al. Some mineral, trace element and heavy metal concentrations in lung cancer. Asian Pacific journal of cancer prevention : APJCP. 2010;11(5):1383–8.
20. Xu ZF, Sun YC, Zhang CW, et al. Clinical significance of changes of serum copper, zinc and magnesium contents in patients with lung cancer. J of Second Mil Med Univ. 1993;14(2):195–6.
21. Wang ZL, Zhang W, Zhang HY, et al. Determinat ion of serum trace elements and their clinical value in patients with lung cancer. Clin Focus. 2003;18(4):183–5.
22. Stang A. Critical evaluation of the Newcastle-Ottawa scale for the assessment of the quality of nonrandomized studies in meta-analyses. Eur J Epidemiol. 2010;25(9):603–5.
23. DerSimonian R, Laird N. Meta-analysis in clinical trials. Control Clin Trials. 1986;7(3):177–88.
24. Higgins JP, Thompson SG, Deeks JJ, et al. Measuring inconsistency in meta-analyses. BMJ. 2003;327(7414):557–60.
25. Higgins JP, Thompson SG. Controlling the risk of spurious findings from meta-regression. Stat Med. 2004;23(11):1663–82.
26. Egger M, Davey Smith G, Schneider M, et al. Bias in meta-analysis detected by a simple, graphical test. BMJ. 1997;315(7109):629–34.
27. Begg CB, Mazumdar M. Operating characteristics of a rank correlation test for publication bias. Biometrics. 1994;50(4):1088–101.
28. Li K, Kaaks R, Linseisen J, et al. Dietary calcium and magnesium intake in relation to cancer incidence and mortality in a German prospective cohort (EPIC-Heidelberg). Cancer Causes Control. 2011;22(10):1375–82.
29. Takata Y, Shu XO, Yang G, et al. Calcium intake and lung cancer risk among female nonsmokers: a report from the Shanghai Women's Health Study. Cancer Epidemiol Biomarkers Prev. 2013;22(1):50–7.
30. Cheng MH, Chiu HF, Tsai SS, et al. Calcium and magnesium in drinking-water and risk of death from lung cancer in women. Magnes Res. 2012; 25(3):112–9.
31. Srebro DP, Vučković SM, Dožić IS, et al. Magnesium sulfate reduces formalin-induced orofacial pain in rats with normal magnesium serum levels. Pharmacol Rep. 2018;70(1):81–6.
32. Munafo MR, Flint J. Meta-analysis of genetic association studies. Trends Genet. 2004;20(9):439–44.

11

Systematic review of single-incision versus conventional multiport laparoscopic surgery for sigmoid colon and rectal cancer

Xin Liu, Ji-bin Li, Gang Shi, Rui Guo and Rui Zhang*

Abstract

Objectives: To explore whether single-incision laparoscopic surgery (SILS) has the better short-term clinical and pathological outcomes than conventional multiport laparoscopic surgery (CLS) for sigmoid colon and rectal cancer.

Methods: A literature investigation of MEDLINE, PubMed, Ovid, Embase, Cochrane Library, Web of Science, Chinese National Knowledge Infrastructure (CNKI), Chinese Biological Medicine (CBM), and Wanfang databases for relevant researches was performed. Fixed effects and random effects models were used to calculate the corresponding outcomes. Standardized mean difference and risk ratio were calculated for continuous and dichotomous variables separately.

Results: Nine clinical controlled trials were composed of two randomized clinical trials and seven non-randomized clinical trials with a total of 829 patients. Two hundred ninety-nine (36.1%) patients underwent SILS, and 530 (63.9%) patients underwent CLS. The meta-analysis showed that SILS had more lymph node resection (SMD − 0.25, 95% CI − 0. 50 to − 0.002) and less defecation time (SMD − 0.46, 95% CI − 0.75 to − 0.17), exhaust time (SMD − 0.46, 95% CI − 0.75 to − 0.18), and hospital stay (SMD − 0.30, 95% CI − 0.45 to − 0.15 than CLS. SILS was also accompanied with shorter incision length (SMD − 2.46, 95% CI − 4.02 to − 0.90), less pain score (SMD − 0.56, 95% CI − 0.91 to − 0.21), and lower complication rate (RR 0.66, 95% CI 0.47 to 0.91). Blood loss, operative time, distal margin, conversion rate, anastomotic fistula, readmission, local recurrence, and distant metastasis showed no statistical differences in two groups. In all subgroup analysis, SILS also had advantages of incision length, operative time, defecation time, exhaust time, and hospitalization time than CLS.

Conclusion: SILS could be a more safe and reliable surgical technique than CLS for sigmoid colon and rectal cancer. However, further high-quality studies between these two techniques need to be further developed.

Keywords: Single-incision, Meta-analysis, Laparoscopic surgery, Sigmoid colon and rectal cancer

Background

Conventional multiport laparoscopy (CLS) is increasingly being used in colorectal surgery. CLS had the advantages of faster recovery, reduced morbidity, and blood loss, but also had incision-related complications. Since single-incision laparoscopic surgery (SILS) was developed in 2008, incision-related complications of hemorrhage, incision rupture, and organ damage have

been greatly reduced [1–3]. There were different opinions about the clinical efficacy between SILS and CLS.

Several published meta-analyses evaluating SLIS versus CLS have shown that short-term clinical and oncological outcomes of SILS are better than that of CLS [4]. Li et al. had very fully confirmed that SILS had less blood loss, shorter incision length, shorter and hospital stay but longer operative time for colorectal disease [5]. However, laparoscopic sigmoid and rectal surgery based on these two techniques has rarely been studied by meta-analysis. Here we comprehensively compared the clinical outcomes of two techniques for treatment of sigmoid and rectal cancer.

* Correspondence: zhangrui612006@sina.com
Department of Colorectal Surgery, Cancer Hospital of China Medical University, Liaoning Cancer Hospital and Institute, No 44 Xiaoheyan Road, Dadong District, Shenyang 110042, Liaoning Province, People's Republic of China

Methods

Literature search

We had systematically collected useful studies from MEDLINE, PubMed, Embase, Cochrane Library, and Wanfang from 2010 to 2018. Search terms included "laparoscopy," "single incision," "single port," "single site," "SILS," "CLS," "sigmoid cancer," "rectal cancer," and "TME (total mesenteric resection)." Manual searches of references from relevant articles were performed when necessary. We increased the scope of the research by "related articles" option. Included studies were English or Chinese human researches with the abstracts, scope, and reference checked.

Eligibility criteria

One hundred seventy-nine studies searched from the Internet were separately screened by three investigators according to the following inclusion criteria: (1) comparing the outcomes of SILS versus CLS for sigmoid or rectal cancer, (2) one outcome mentioned at least, and (3) randomized clinical trials (RCTs), non-randomized controlled trail (NRCTs), or comparative observational (cohort and case-control) studies.

Additionally, the exclusion criteria were as follows: (1) related research was not about sigmoid colon or rectal disease, (2) the relevant data were not specifically reported, and (3) conference articles, case, letters, and other unqualified articles.

Types of interventions

Laparoscopic surgery was performed through a laparoscope with special instruments by a small incision length. CLS always had three or more ports, while SLIS had only one port for surgery.

Outcome of interest

We used the following results to compare SILS and CLS: (1) intraoperative data based on operative time, incision length, amount of bleeding, conversion, lymph node resection, and distal surgical edge; (2) postoperative data including complication, anastomotic fistula rate, defecation time, exhaust time, pain score, and hospitalization time; and (3) short-term follow-up data including readmission, local recurrence, and distant metastasis. Subgroup analysis of tumor location (sigmoid colon and rectal cancer), region (eastern and western), and language (Chinese and English) were conducted.

Data extraction

The literatures were searched according to the above criteria by two reviewers independently. The following data were collected: (1) the first author(s) and publication data, (2) the study area, (3) the characteristics of patients in each group, and (4) the quality of the study. A third reviewer was introduced to resolve all disagreements about the articles until a consensus was reached.

We contacted the authors of all studies with incomplete data but did not get any additional information. As referred to in the missing data of means and SDs, we calculated them based on medians and ranges according to availability [6, 7].

Risk of bias evaluation

Two RCT qualities were assessed by the Cochrane Reviewers' Handbook with the Jadad score in three metrics: randomization, double blindness, and control.

The quality of NRCTs was assessed with the Newcastle-Ottawa Scale from three aspects: patient selection, confirmation of exposure, and comparability of both groups [8].

Statistical analysis

This study followed the Preferred Reporting Items for Systematic reviews and Meta-Analysis (PRISMA) guidelines. We used Stata 11.0 to compare two groups by standardized mean differences (SMD) with 95% confidence intervals (95% CIs) for continuous data and relative risks (ORs or RRs) with 95% CIs for dichotomous outcomes. The statistical heterogeneity was estimated by I^2 statistic and χ^2 test.

When $I^2 > 50\%$ and $I^2 < 50\%$, random effects and fixed effects models were utilized separately. $P < 0.05$ indicated statistical differences. Begg's test was used to evaluate publication bias. Sensitivity analyses were conducted by sequentially excluding studies one by one to decrease the impact of single study.

Results

Study characteristics

We identified 179 publications and found 80 relevant eligible studies. We removed 71 studies (non-SILS or CLS, sigmoid or rectal cancer, RCTs or NRCTs), and finally, nine of these studies met our inclusion criteria, which included two RCTs and seven NRCTs with a total of 829 patients included. Of the nine studies, two studies evaluated sigmoid colon cancer, five studies evaluated rectal cancer, one study evaluated rectosigmoid junction cancer, and one study contained both sigmoid and rectal cancer. This study included three western researches and six eastern researches. This study also contained seven English articles and two Chinese articles. All patients who underwent SILS or CLS were confirmed pathologically for sigmoid colon or rectal cancer [9–17] (Fig. 1).

Of the patients evaluated by these studies, 299 (36.1%) patients underwent SILS and 530 (63.9%) patients underwent CLS. Table 1 shows the baseline characteristics and quality assessment of these nine researches; there was no statistical difference for each study.

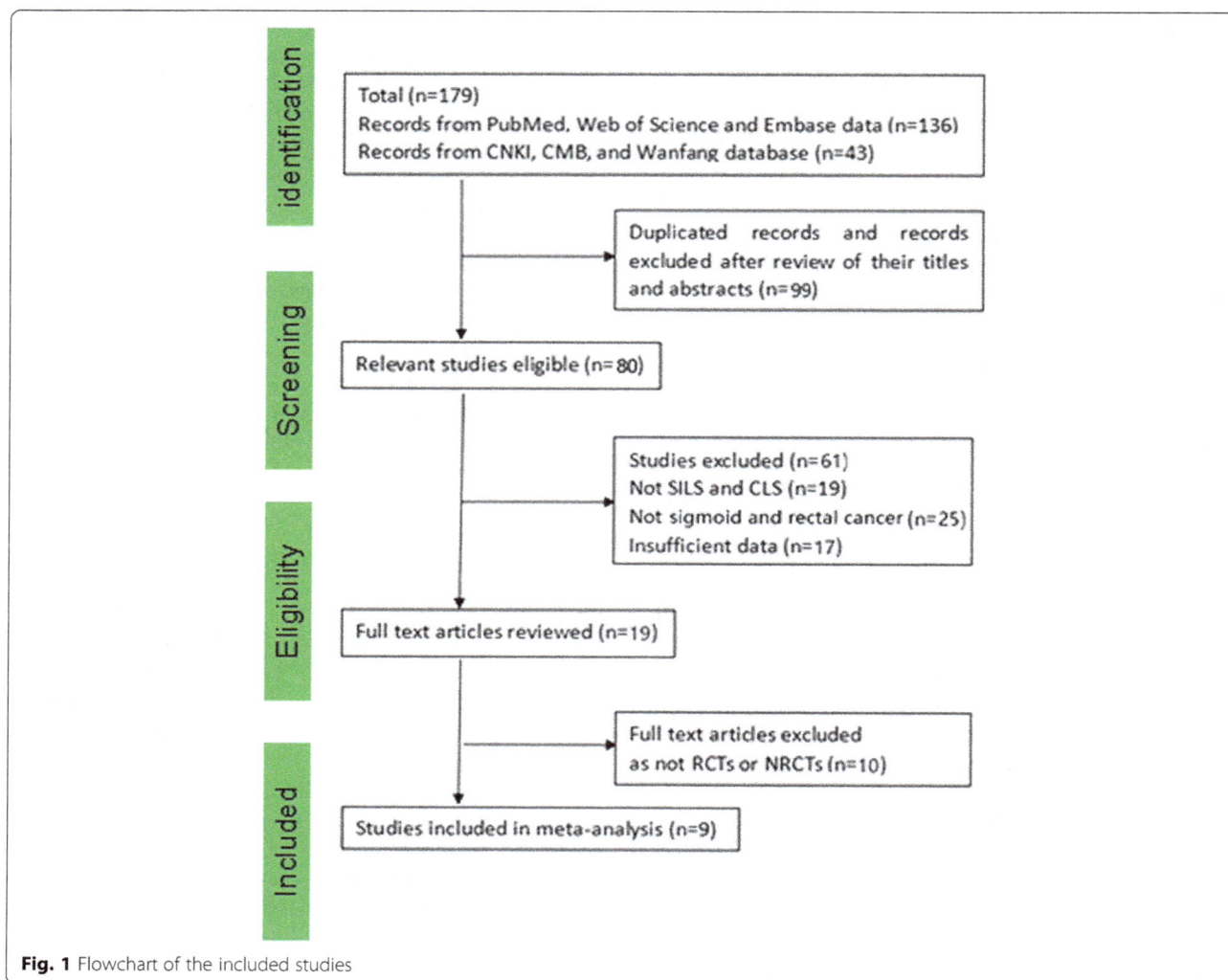

Fig. 1 Flowchart of the included studies

Table 1 Characteristics of the included studies in the meta-analysis

First author	Year	Study area	Type	Patients (n) SILS/CLS	BMI SILS	BMI CLS	Tumor size (cm) SILS	Tumor size (cm) CLS	Sex (M/F) SILS	Sex (M/F) CLS	Age SILS	Age CLS	Tumor location	Score
Liu [7]	2016	China	NRCT	16/32	21.9	22.4	3.6	3.6	13/3	23/9	56.4	55.6	Sigmoid and rectum	5
Hong [8]	2016	China	RCT	43/43	NR	NR	NR	NR	23/20	26/17	52.3	54.1	Rs	3
Bulut [9]	2015	Denmark	RCT	20/20	24	24	2.5	4.0	12/8	12/8	69	73	Rectum	3
Kim [10]	2014	Korea	NRCT	67/49	23.1	23.5	4.3	5.3	44/23	28/21	63.8	61.3	Rectum	7
Levic [11]	2014	Denmark	NRCT	36/194	23.8	25	NR	NR	17/19	133/61	69	68	Rectum	8
Tei [12]	2018	Japan	NRCT	44/49	23.6	22	3.9	4.1	29/15	29/20	66	63	Rectum	8
Kwag [13]	2013	Korea	NRCT	24/48	24.4	24	2.6	3.4	9/15	18/30	59.5	59	Sigmoid	7
Park [14]	2012	Korea	NRCT	37/54	24.7	23.9	NR	NR	21/16	26/28	63.8	59.9	Sigmoid	7
Nerup [15]	2018	Denmark	NRCT	12/41	23.5	25	NR	NR	7/5	13/28	76	69	Rectum	6

F female, *M* male, *NR* no record, *RCT* randomized controlled trials, *NRCT* non-randomized controlled trials, *SILS* single-port laparoscopic surgery, *CLS* conventional multi-port laparoscopic surgery, *Rs* rectosigmoid junction cancer

Quality assessment

According to the modified Jadad rating scale for assessing RCTs, scores between 1 and 3 were considered low quality and scores between 4 and 7 were considered high quality. Due to single blinding and unclear method of randomization, two RCTs got scores of 3 with low quality.

According to NRCT evaluation criteria, scores between 1 and 3 were considered low quality, scores between 4 and 6 were considered moderate quality, and scores between 7 and 9 points were considered high quality. The included NRCTs all had moderate or high quality. The specific scores of RCTs and NRCTs are shown in Table 1.

Meta-analysis results

Intraoperative index

The incision length was shorter in SILS than CLS (SMD − 2.46, 95% CI − 4.02 to − 0.90), with large heterogeneity in random effects model ($P = 0$, $I^2 = 95.6\%$, Fig. 2a). SILS had more lymph node resection than CLS in random effects model (SMD − 0.25, 95% CI − 0.50 to − 0.002, $P = 0$, $I^2 = 61.5\%$, Fig. 2b) Two groups had similar results in operative time with CLS (SMD 0.23, 95% CI − 0.27 to 0.73, Fig. 2c), amount of bleeding (SMD − 0.01, 95% CI − 0.32 to 0.31, Fig. 2d), conversion rate (RR 1.69, 95% CI 0.93 to 3.05, Fig. 2e), and distal surgical edge (SMD − 0.03, 95% CI − 0.24 to 0.19, Fig. 2f). All studies had significant heterogeneity in random effects model, except conversion rate without significant heterogeneity in fixed effects model. In subgroup analysis, RCTs had shorter incision length, but higher conversion rate than NRCTs, and other index in RCTs and NRCTs were similar. The detailed values are shown in Table 2.

Postoperative data

This study showed SILS had obvious advantages over CLS in complication (RR 0.66, 95% CI 0.47 to 0.91, Fig. 3e), defecation time (SMD − 0.46, 95% CI − 0.75 to − 0.18, Fig. 3a), exhaust time (SMD − 0.46, 95% CI − 0.75 to − 0.18, Fig. 3b), pain score (SMD − 0.56, 95% CI − 0.91 to − 0.21, Fig. 3c), and hospitalization time (SMD − 0.30, 95% CI − 0.45 to − 0.15, Fig. 3d). No significant heterogeneity was discovered in two groups except for hospitalization time with high heterogeneity. There was no obvious difference in anastomotic fistula rate between SILS and CLS groups (RR 0.752, 95% CI 0.46 to 1.23, Fig. 3f). SILS mainly contributed to the part of postoperative recovery. The detailed values are shown in Table 3.

Follow-up outcomes

There were no significant differences in readmission (RR 1.46, 95% CI 0.71 to 3.02, Fig. 4a), local recurrence (RR 0.40, 95% CI 0.07 to 2.20, Fig. 4b), and distant metastasis (RR 0.82, 95% CI 0.27 to 2.52, Fig. 4c) between SILS and CLS groups. Readmission and local recurrence used fixed effect model with no significant heterogeneity, while distant metastasis used random effect model with significant heterogeneity. The detailed values are shown in Table 3.

Subgroup analysis

Sigmoid colon cancer versus rectal cancer

For rectal cancer, subgroup analysis showed SILS had a lower complication rate (RR 0.66, 95% CI 0.45 to 0.97, Fig. 4d) than CLS. However, SILS had shorter incision length (SMD − 3.69, 95% CI − 5.72 to − 1.67, Fig. 4e), shorter operative time (SMD − 0.45, 95% CI − 0.78 to − 0.13, Fig. 4e), and shorter hospitalization time (SMD − 0.47, 95% CI − 0.80 to − 0.15, Fig. 4e) than CLS for sigmoid colon cancer patients.

Eastern versus western patients

Subgroup analyses related to the region were conducted in further research. In eastern research, SILS had lower complication rate (RR 0.65, 95% CI 0.42 to 0.98, Fig. 5a), faster defecation time (SMD − 0.46, 95% CI − 0.75 to − 0.18, Fig. 5b), faster exhaust time (SMD − 0.47, 95% CI − 0.75 to 0.18, Fig. 5b), and shorter incision length (SMD − 2.26, 95% CI − 4.08 to 0.43, Fig. 5b) than CLS, accompanied with lower pain score (SMD − 0.56, 95% CI − 0.91 to − 0.21, Fig. 5b) and shorter hospital stay (SMD − 0.34, 95% CI − 0.52 to − 0.16, Fig. 5b). But SILS had more lymph node resection (SMD − 0.37, 95% CI − 0.66 to − 0.09, Fig. 5b) than CLS in western research. SILS and CLS had similar results in other indexes.

English versus Chinese articles

Seven English articles indicated SILS had a lower complication rate (RR 0.68, 95% CI 0.48 to 0.98, Fig. 5c), more lymph node resection (SMD − 0.34, 95% CI − 0.63 to − 0.04, Fig. 5d), shorter incision length (SMD − 3.56, 95% CI − 4.84 to − 2.29, Fig. 5d), and shorter hospital stay (SMD − 0.25, 95% CI − 0.42 to − 0.08, Fig. 5d), but a higher conversion rate (RR 2.13, 95% CI 1.06 to 4.26, Fig. 5c) compared to CLS. Two Chinese articles contained defecation and exhaust time data and indicated SILS had a shorter defecation time (SMD − 0.43, 95% CI − 0.78 to − 0.08, Fig. 5e) and exhaust time (SMD − 0.39, 95% CI − 0.74 to − 0.04, Fig 5e) than CLS, accompanied with a better distal surgical edge (SMD − 0.40, 95% CI − 0.75 to − 0.05, Fig. 5e) and hospital stay (SMD − 0.51, 95% CI − 0.86 to − 0.15, Fig. 5e).

Sensitivity analysis

Begg's correlation test (complication, $P = 0.639$) revealed there was no obvious publication bias. Quality of

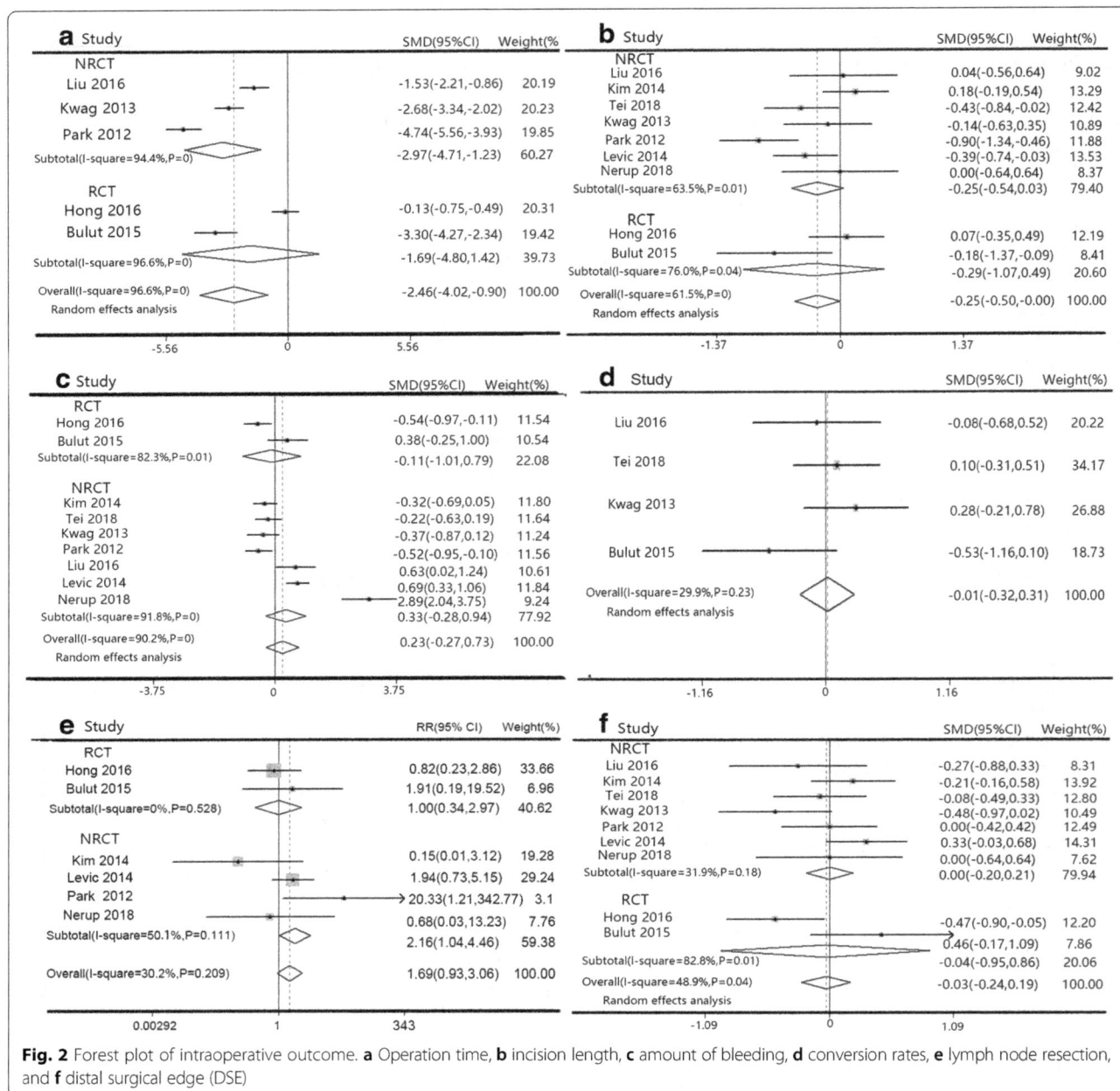

Fig. 2 Forest plot of intraoperative outcome. **a** Operation time, **b** incision length, **c** amount of bleeding, **d** conversion rates, **e** lymph node resection, and **f** distal surgical edge (DSE)

researches after sensitivity analysis would not impact the final results.

Discussion

Laparoscopic colorectal surgery has become the trend of the times in modern colorectal surgery. CLS is the traditional laparoscopic surgery; it has become a routine procedure in many hospitals. However, some disadvantages of CLS also existed, such as poor three-dimensional (3D) visualization, limited dexterity of movements, and high conversion rate to open surgery. With the development of medical science, new devices have prompted the wide use

of SILS in colorectal surgery. Some studies have demonstrated that SILS is more accurate, effective, and less invasive than CLS in colorectal cancer. However, whether SILS is better than CLS for sigmoid and rectal cancer still remains unclear.

In this meta-analysis, we aimed to collect evidence-based data to compare intraoperative data, postoperative indexes, and short-term follow-up outcomes between SILS with CLS in sigmoid and rectal cancer. We utilized the latest studies to compare outcomes between SILS and CLS for laparoscopic resection in sigmoid colon and rectal cancer; we also carried out subgroup analysis in

Table 2 Comparison of intraoperative index between SILS and CLS for the included studies

First author	Operation time (min)		Incision length (cm)		Amount of bleeding (ml)		Conversion		Lymph node resection		Distal surgical edge (cm)	
	SILS	CLS	SILS	CLS	SILS	CLS	SILS	CLS	SILS	CLS	SILS	CLS
Liu [7]	126.9±40.3	106.9±26.7	4.8±1.5	6.8±1.2	46.3±61.1	50.3±39.3	NR	NR	21.3±8.1	21±7.5	5.8±2.3	6.6±3.2
Hong [8]	122.3±23.4	137.6±32.4	4.4±3.5	4.8±2.8	NR	NR	4	5	18.2±8.1	17.6±8.9	5.8±1.9	6.8±2.3
Bulut [9]	295 (108–465)	264 (125–421)	4 (2.5–12.5)	13.3 (7–19.5)	33 (0–300)	100 (0–650)	2	1	14 (4–33)	19 (7–33)	3.2 (0.5–7.5)	2.5 (1–6.5)
Kim [10]	277±106	309±93	NR	NR	NR	NR	0	2	23.4±15.3	20.9±12.6	6.9±5.5	5.8±4.9
Levic [11]	295 (108–465)	248 (51–431)	NR	NR	35 (0–400)	100 (0–3142)	5	13	13 (3–33)	16 (1–48)	3 (0.5–7.5)	2.5 (0–9.5)
Tei [12]	198±52.8	210±55	NR	NR	34.5±106	24.8±85	1	0	23±10	28±13	2.97±0.85	3.04±0.88
Kwag [13]	135±28	144±22	3.4±1.1	7.3±1.6	251±50	237±49	0	0	19.6±10.7	20.8±7.7	7.5±2.5	9.2±4
Park [14]	118.1±41.5	140±42.2	3.3±0.9	9.1±1.4	NR	NR	8	0	14.6±6.8	23.4±11.4	5.1±2.5	5.1±2.6
Nerup [15]	316.5 (294–323.3)	269 (236.5–309)	NR	NR	50 (0–200)	150 (62.5–250)	0	2	12 (9–17)	12 (7–15)	4 (3.5–5)	4 (2–5)

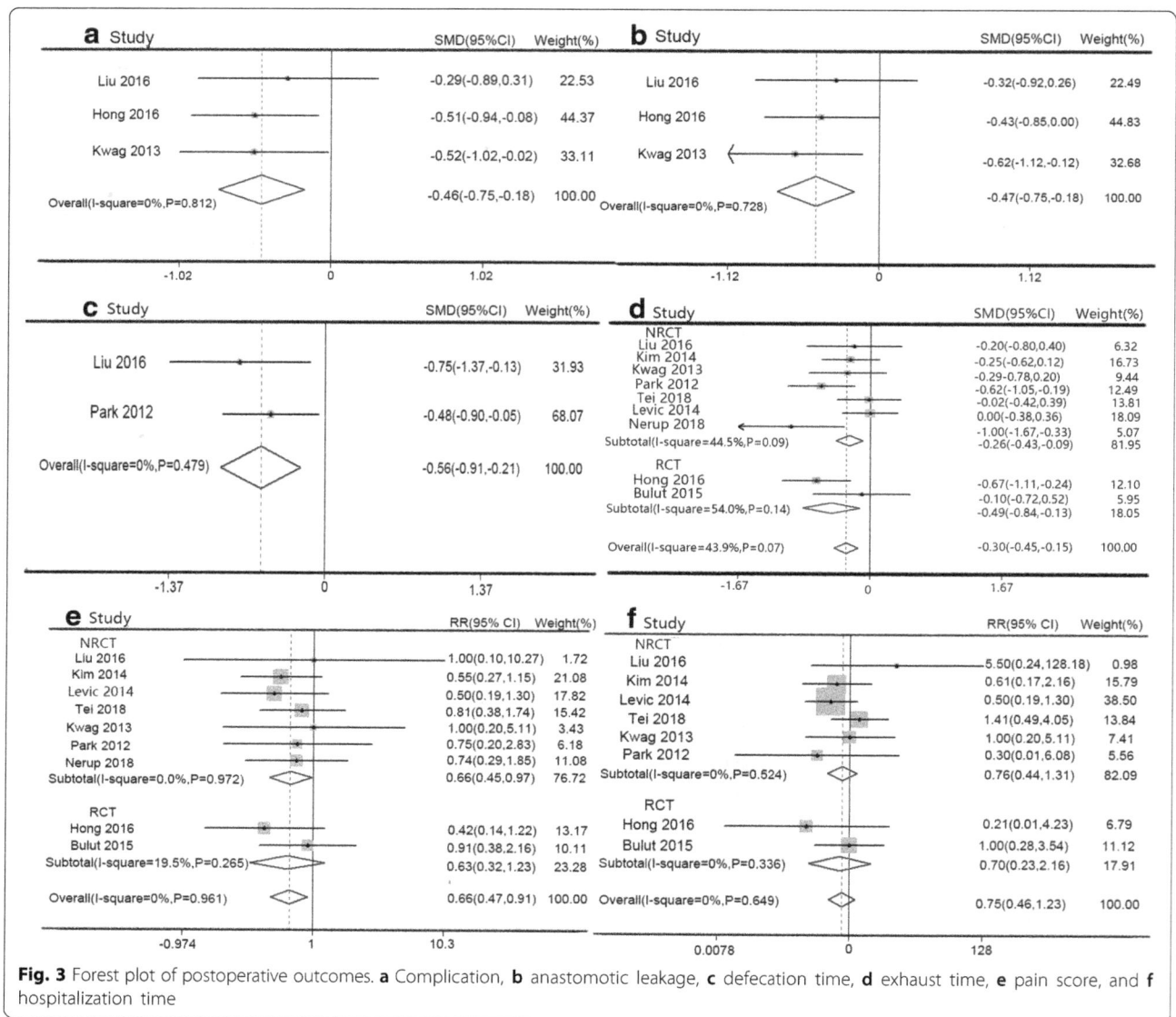

Fig. 3 Forest plot of postoperative outcomes. **a** Complication, **b** anastomotic leakage, **c** defecation time, **d** exhaust time, **e** pain score, and **f** hospitalization time

tumor location, region, and language. Two moderate-quality RCTs and seven moderate- to high-quality NRCTs involving total 829 patients were analyzed for the final results. Our selected studies included moderate sample sizes and provided reliable data to compare the outcomes of the two groups. Among all of the searched articles, two relevant articles were very similar both in background and recruited patients written by Tei et al., so we chose the latest article with long-term follow-up outcomes for our study [18].

The results revealed that SILS had an advantage over CLS in incision length, lymph node resection, complication rate, defecation time, exhaust time, pain score, and hospital stay. No statistical difference was observed in other data. Our results were partially same with that of Li et al. They made a meta-analysis in comparing the effects of SILS with CLS for colorectal cancer and also found that SILS had advantages in incision length, pain score, and hospital stay compared with CLS. Meanwhile, Li et al. also reported SILS with fewer blood transfusion and less blood loss than CLS. Although we did not compare blood transfusion and extra port rate due to incomplete data, SILS still had better outcome than CLS in the above index. Besides, there were some opposite results including lymph node resection, complication rate, operative time, and blood loss between our study and Li et al.'s. In our study, SILS had more lymph node resection and lower complication rate than CLS. We thought that this was due to the different tumor location. Our study focused on sigmoid and rectal cancer and Li et al.'s study focused on colorectal cancer. Different tumor locations could cause more lymph node resection

Table 3 Comparison of postoperative data and follow-up outcomes between SILS and CLS for the included studies

First author	Complication		Anastomotic fistula		Defection time (days)		Exhaust time (days)		Pain score		Hospitalization time (days)		Readmission		Recurrence		Metastasis	
	SILS	CLS	SILS	CLS	SILS	CLS	SILS	CLS	SILS	CLS	SILS	CLS	SILS	CLS	SILS	CLS	SILS	CLS
Liu [7]	1	2	1	0	3.3±0.9	3.6±1.1	2.4±1	2.7±0.9	4.3±1.4	5.2±1.1	8.4±5.3	9.2±3.1	NR	NR	NR	NR	2	2
Hong [8]	4	11	0	2	4.8±2.1	5.9±2.2	2.5±2.3	3.4±1.9	NR	NR	6.7±3.7	8.8±2.4	NR	NR	NR	NR	NR	NR
Bulut [9]	7	8	4	4	NR	NR	NR	NR	NR	NR	7 (3–51)	8 (4–30)	4	1	NR	NR	NR	NR
Kim [10]	10	15	4	5	NR	NR	NR	NR	NR	NR	12.6±11.2	15.3±10.1	NR	NR	NR	NR	NR	NR
Levic [11]	4	49	4	49	NR	NR	NR	NR	NR	NR	7 (3–51)	7 (3–80)	5	22	0	3	2	29
Tei [12]	9	13	6	6	NR	NR	NR	NR	NR	NR	13.5±11.2	13.7±11.6	NR	NR	1	4	1	7
Kwag [13]	2	4	2	4	1.7±0.6	2.2±1.1	2.8±1	3.6±1.4	NR	NR	7.1±3.4	8.1±3.5	NR	NR	NR	NR	NR	NR
Park [14]	3	6	0	2	NR	NR	NR	NR	2.6±1.3	3.4±1.9	5.5±2.3	7.7±4.2	NR	NR	NR	NR	NR	NR
Nerup [15]	4	21	NR	NR	NR	NR	NR	NR	NR	NR	7 (7–9)	8 (7–11.5)	2	5	NR	NR	4	8

NR no record

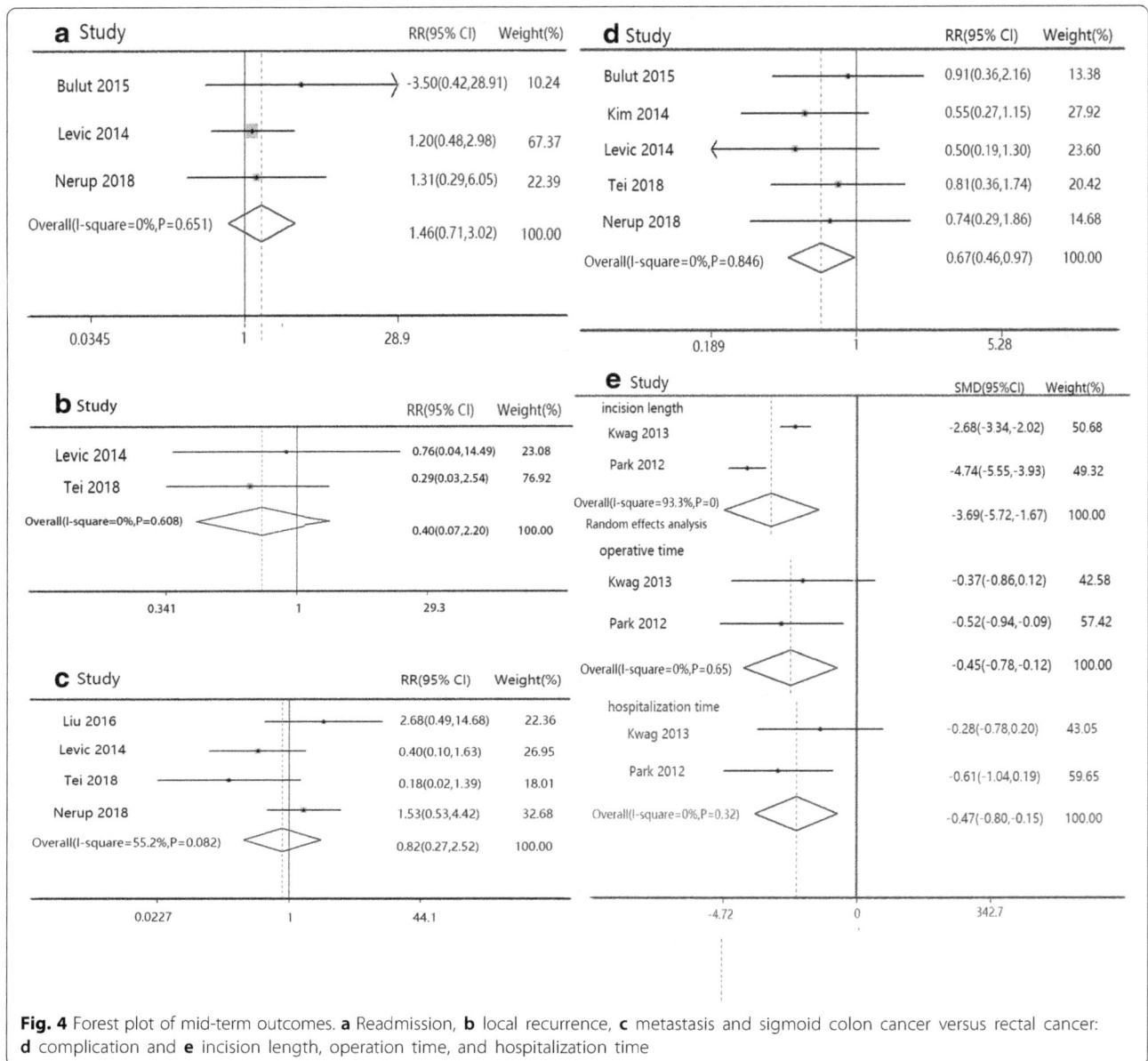

Fig. 4 Forest plot of mid-term outcomes. **a** Readmission, **b** local recurrence, **c** metastasis and sigmoid colon cancer versus rectal cancer: **d** complication and **e** incision length, operation time, and hospitalization time

and lower complication rate in our study [19]. Li et al. indicated SILS had less blood loss and longer operative time compared with our study. We think a surgeon could increase operative time due to variation of blood vessels in the right colon [20].

With respect to the conversion rate to open surgery, SILS is similar with CLS. The main reasons could impact conversion rate including obesity, narrow pelvis, important vascular variation, vascular injury, and hypertrophic mesentery [21]. But for sigmoid colon cancer, SILS had a shorter operation time, operative time, and hospital stay than CLS due to good location of sigmoid colon cancer. These results could be affected by the substantial

learning curve inherent in performing SILS. The skill of the surgeon could also influence the conversion rate.

The heterogeneity of lower postoperative complication rates especially for rectal cancer in SILS was likely attributable to hospital stay, defecation time, and exhaust time. The complication rate is the main contributor to surgical technique and operative time. SILS with a short incision length could reduce postoperative pain, promote early activities, and cut down the incidence of complication [22]. The heterogeneity of proximal surgical edge might be attributed to variation in surgical skills and experience of surgeons, but with more lymph node resection in SILS. We imaged SILS could cut off enough

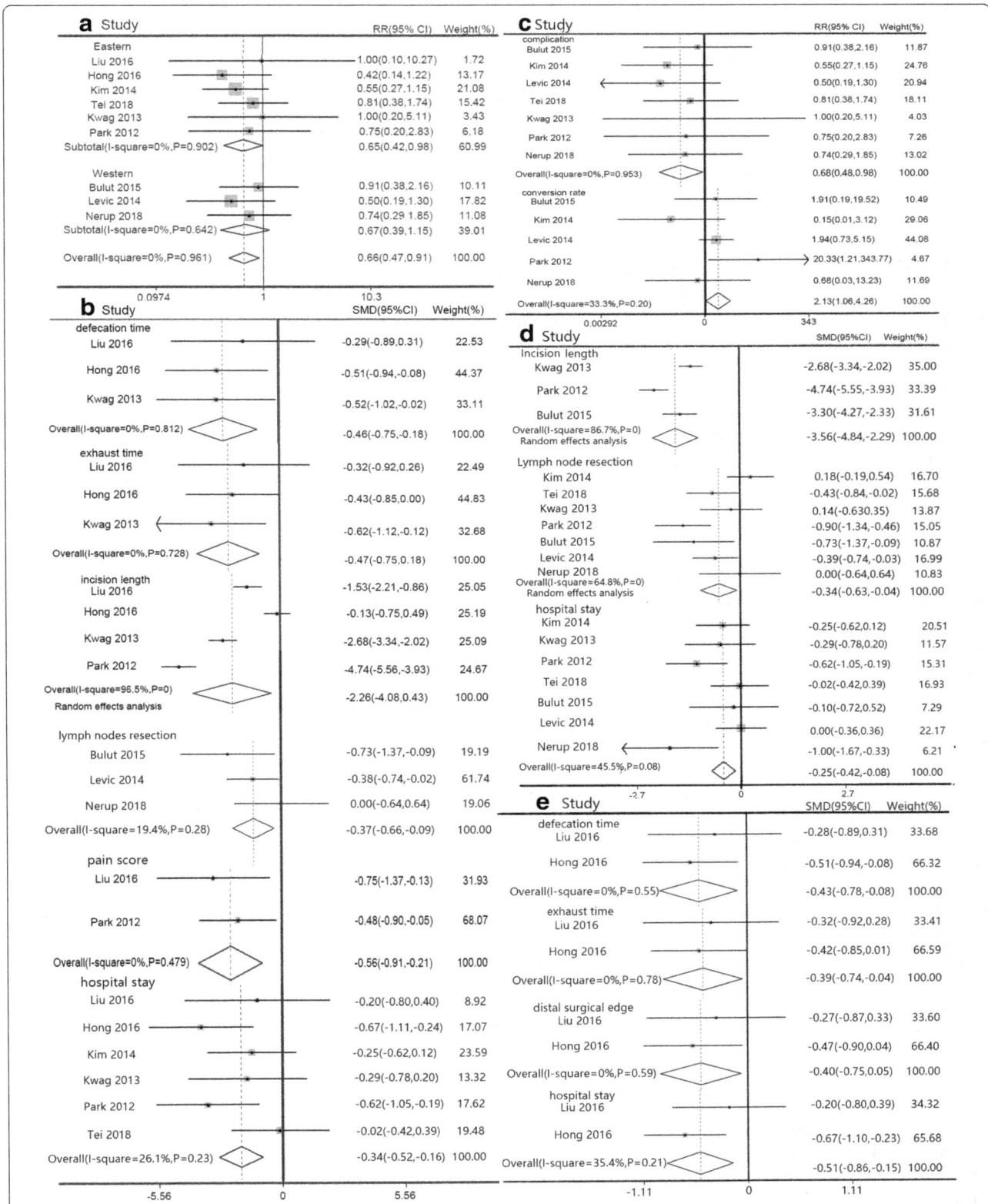

Fig. 5 Forest plot of eastern versus western patients. **a** Complication, **b** defecation time, exhaust time, incision length, lymph node resection, pain score, and hospital stay. English versus Chinese studies: **c** complication and conversion; **d** incision length, lymph node resection, and hospital stay; and **e** defecation time, exhaust time, distal surgical edge, and hospital stay

mesentery to get more lymph nodes, especially with the technique of TME.

Three studies evaluated readmission, two studies evaluated local recurrence, and four studies evaluated distant metastase; SILS and CLS had similar results. Due to the short development time of SILS, lack of clinical data might impact the results of readmission, local recurrence, and distal metastasis. We expect more clinical research to further illuminate the relationship between the groups [23].

In subgroup analysis of region, SILS had better outcomes than CLS, including complication rate, incision length, defecation time, exhaust time, and hospital stay for eastern patients, and SILS had more lymph node resection for western patients than CLS. Western patients had a particularly difficult surgery with high body mass and narrow operation space. Although all surgeries were performed by experienced surgical teams, we still found SILS with a short incision length could reduce the suture time and pain sensation. This finding was the same to some clinical reports [24]. The benefits of minimally invasive surgery could be reflected by incision length, defecation time, exhaust time, and hospital stay [25].

In the subgroup analysis of language, seven English articles had indicated SILS have better results of complication, incision length, lymph node resection, and hospital stay than CLS except for conversion rate. However, two Chinese articles supplied additional data of superior defecation time and exhaust time, accompanied with better distal surgical edge and shorter hospital stay. English articles included more patients' data than Chinese articles, but Chinese articles added some available data of intestinal movement.

The results of the article could be subjected to some interference due to several limitations. First, nine studies with only a modest number of patients were a limitation that might affect the outcomes and induce bias. Only two RCTs had been published on this subject, while seven retrospective studies had been published, which were not the highest quality of evidence. Second, although the majority of the assessed outcomes across all papers had no dramatic conflicts in the findings between units, variation between different units could influence the outcomes. Third, SILS technique which is not yet popular due to its long learning curve and high cost could affect the results. Additionally, insufficient postoperative follow-up time might also produce a performance bias. In the near future, more large-scale RCTs with complete follow-up data will emerge to reveal the clinical and prognostic effects of SILS [26]. All countries should invest a great deal of financial and material resources to promote SILS for colorectal surgery. With the improving of the equipment, the SILS port could hold more holes which make it easier to contain more forceps to accelerate the operation.

Our meta-analysis provided current information on the role of SILS compared with CLS. We incorporated research into strict standards and used a number of methods to ensure the quality of the included studies. We used Begg's test to evaluate publication bias. Our study focused on sigmoid colon and rectal cancer and minimized bias for a broad range of colorectal surgery.

Conclusions

In conclusion, this study confirmed the feasibility and compared the advantages and disadvantages of two techniques. SILS had some advantages, such as shorter hospital stay, smaller incision length, more rapid time to return to bowel function, slighter pain score, and a lower complication rate. SILS and CLS had several similar clinical outcomes, such as blood loss, rate of conversion to open surgery, anastomotic fistula rate, readmission, local recurrence, and distal metastases. With the continuing development of professional technology, future evidence in long-term outcomes could promote widespread use of SILS for sigmoid colon and rectal cancer.

Abbreviations
BMI: Body mass index; CLS: Conventional multi-port laparoscopic surgery; HR: Hazard ratios; NRCT: Non-randomized controlled trials; OR: Odds ratio; OS: Overall survival; RCTs: Randomized clinical trails; SD: Standard deviation; SILS: Single-port laparoscopic surgery; WMD: Weighted mean difference

Acknowledgements
We thank the Department of Colorectal Surgery of the Cancer Hospital of China Medical University, Liaoning Cancer Hospital and Institute for technical assistance.
We are grateful to Dr. Sufang Li from Peking University People's Hospital for her help in carefully revising the manuscript.

Funding
This work was supported by the Cancer Hospital of China Medical University. The funding project is the National Natural Science Fund from the National Natural Science Foundation of China (grant nos.81672427).

Authors' contributions
All authors participated in the study. JBL and GS performed the literature search and the acquisition of data. XL and RG performed the data analysis. RZ participated in the interpretation of data and revised the article for important intellectual content. All authors approved the final version of the article. The authors thank BioMed Proofreading Company for the help in editing the manuscript.

Competing interests
The authors declare that they have no competing interests.

References

1. Osborne AJ, Lim J, Kj G, et al. Comparison of single-incision laparoscopic high anterior resection with standard laparoscopic high anterior resection. Color Dis. 2013;15:329–33.
2. Linden YT, Govaert JA, Fiocco M, et al. Single center cost analysis of single-cost and conventional laparoscopic surgical treatment in colorectal malignant diseases. Int J Color Dis. 2017;32:233–9.
3. Sulu B, Gorgun E, Aytac E, et al. Comparison of hospital costs for single-port and conventional laparoscopic colorectal resection: a case-matched study. Tech Coloproctol. 2014;18:835–9.
4. Brockhaus AC, Sauerland S, Saad S. Single-incision versus standard multi-incision laparoscopic colectomy in patients with malignant or benign colonic disease: a systematic review, meta-analysis and assessment of evidence. BMC Surg. 2016;16:71.
5. Li HJ, Huang L, Li TJ, et al. Short-term outcomes of single-incision versus conventional laparoscopic surgery for colorectal diseases: meta-analysis of randomized and prospective evidence. J Gastrointest Surg. 2017;21:1931–45.
6. Wan X, Wang W, Liu J, et al. Estimating the sample mean and standard deviation from the sample size, median, range and/or interquartile range. BMC Med Res Methodol. 2014;14:135.
7. Hozo SP, Djulbegovic B, Hozo I. Estimating the mean and variance from the median, range, and the size of a sample. BMC Med Res Methodol. 2005;5:13.
8. Wells GA, Shea B, O'Connell D, et al. The Newcastle-Patent Scale (NOS) for assessing the quality of nonrandomised studies in meta-analyses. 2007. Available at: http://www.ohri.ca/programs/clinical_epidemiology/oxford.htm 2008.
9. Liu R, Wang Y, Xiong W, et al. Efficacy analysis of suprapubic single-incision laparoscopy in the treatment of rectosigmoid cancer. Zhonghua Wei Chang Wai Ke Za Zhi. 2016;19:647–53.
10. Hong W. Application effect of single port laparoscopic surgery above the pubic symphysis for rectosigmoid junction cancer. J laparosc Surg. 2016;21:757–9.
11. Bulut O, Aslak KK, Levic K, et al. A randomized pilot study on single-port versus conventional laparoscopic rectal surgery: effects on postoperative pain and the stress response to surgery. Tech Coloproctol. 2015;19:11–22.
12. Kim SJ, Choi BJ, Lee SC. Successful total shift from multiport to single-port laparoscopic surgery in low anterior resection of colorectal cancer. Surg Endosc. 2014;28:2920–030.
13. Levic K, Bulut O. The short-term outcomes of conventional and single-port laparoscopic surgery for rectal cancer: a comparative non-randomized study. Minim Invasive Ther Allied Technol. 2014;23:214–22.
14. Tei M, Otsuka M, Suzuki Y, et al. Safety and feasibility of single-port laparoscopic low anterior resection for upper rectal cancer. Am J Surg. 2018. https://doi.org/10.1016/j.amjsurg.2018.03.022. [Epub ahead of print].
15. Kwag SJ, Kim JG, Oh ST, et al. Single incision vs conventional laparoscopic anterior resection for sigmoid colon cancer: a case-matched study. Am J Surg. 2013;206:320–5.
16. Park SJ, Lee KY, Kang BM, et al. Initial experience of single-port laparoscopic surgery for sigmoid colon cancer. World J Surg. 2012;37:652–6.
17. Nerup N, Rosenstock S, Bulut O. Comparison of single-port and conventional laparoscopic abdominoperineall resection. J Minim Access Surg. 2018;14:27–32.
18. Tei M, Wakasugi M, Akamatsu H. Comparison of short-term surgical results of single-port and multi-port laparoscopic rectal resection for rectal cancer. Am J Surg. 2015;210:309–14.
19. Shen XF, Jiang LJ, Ma DH, et al. Influencing factor analysis of the number of lymph nodes harvest after radical resection of colorectal cancer. Chin J Dig Surg. 2017;16:731–5.
20. Tokuoka M, Ide Y, Takeda M, et al. Single-port versus multi-port laparoscopic surgery for colon cancer in elderly patients. Oncol Lett. 2016;12:1465–70.
21. Yu H, Shin JY. Short-term outcomes following reduced-port, single-port, and multi-port laparoscopic surgery for colon cancer: tailored laparoscopic approaches based on tumor size and nodal status. Int J Color Dis. 2016;31:115–22.
22. Marker SR, Wiggins T, Penna M, et al. Single-incision versus conventional multiport laparoscopic colorectal surgery-systematic review and pooled analysis. J Gastrointest Surg. 2014;18:2214–7.
23. Hirano Y, Hattori M, Douden K, et al. Single-incision laparoscopic surgery for colorectal cancer. World J Gastrointest Surg. 2016;8:95–100.
24. Keller DS, Ibarra S, Flores GJ, et al. Outcomes for single-incision laparoscopic colectomy surgery in obese patients: a case-matched study. Surg Endosc. 2016;30:739–44.
25. Cianchi F, Staderini F, Badii B. Single-incision laparoscopic colorectal surgery for cancer: state of art. World J Gastroenterol. 2014;20:6073–80.
26. Kim CW, Kim WR, Kim HY, et al. Learning curve for single-incision laparoscopic anterior resection for sigmoid colon cancer. J Am Coll Surg. 2015;221:397–403.

12

The role of definitive chemoradiotherapy versus surgery as initial treatments for potentially resectable esophageal carcinoma

Ming-Wei Ma[1], Xian-Shu Gao[1*], Xiao-Bin Gu[1], Mu Xie[1], Ming Cui[1], Min Zhang[1], Ling Liu[1], Huan Yin[2] and Long-Qi Chen[3*]

Abstract

Background: We performed a meta-analysis to compare the efficacy of definitive chemoradiotherapy (dCRT) and esophagectomy as initial treatments for potentially resectable esophageal cancer.

Methods: To assess both strategies, the combined odds ratios (ORs) and 95% confidence intervals (CIs) were calculated. Thirteen studies ($N = 2071$; dCRT = 869 and surgery = 1202) were included. In all, 90.39% of the patients were diagnosed with esophageal squamous cell carcinoma (ESCC).

Results: The 2-year (OR = 1.199, 95% CI 0.922–1.560; $P = 0.177$) and 5-year overall survival (OS) rates (OR = 0.947, 95% CI 0.628–1.429; $P = 0.796$) were not significantly different. No significant differences were identified in the 2-year OS among patients with stage I disease (OR = 1.397, 95% CI 0.740–2.638; $P = 0.303$) or stage II–III (OR = 0.418, 95% CI 0.022–7.833; $P = 0.560$). Patients with lymph node metastases tended to have a better 5-year OS when treated with dCRT than with surgery (OR = 0.226, 95% CI 0.044–1.169; $P = 0.076$); however, the difference between the two methods was not significant. Western patients who received dCRT had poorer prognoses than patients who underwent surgery (OR = 1.522, 95% CI 1.035–2.238; $P = 0.033$). dCRT and surgery led to similar 5-year progression-free survival rates (OR = 1.06, 95% CI 0.79–1.42; $P = 0.70$).

Conclusions: dCRT and surgery are equally effective as initial treatments for potentially resectable esophageal cancer. These results apply primarily to Asian populations as they have an increased incidence of ESCC.

Keywords: Esophageal cancer, Definitive chemoradiotherapy, Esophagostomy, Survival, Meta-analysis

Background

Among all malignancies, esophageal cancer is the sixth most common cause of cancer-related death [1]. Esophageal squamous cell carcinoma (ESCC) is the dominant type of esophageal cancer in Asia [2]. While preoperative chemoradiotherapy can improve survival and local control [3, 4], surgery increases the risk of comorbidities and mortality, and patients who undergo surgery may

experience a poor quality of life [5–8]. It has been reported that even in high-volume centres, surgery alone may lead to a 5% surgical mortality rate and a 10% mortality rate overall [9]. Furthermore, older patients are at a greater risk for surgical mortality following esophagectomy [10], and the safety and therapeutic effect of preoperative chemoradiation cannot be guaranteed in centres with little experience.

In clinical practice, surgery alone is frequently used as the primary treatment modality for esophageal cancer treatment modality, especially for less advanced esophageal tumours in patients in Asian countries [1]. One study showed that the rate of pathological complete response after chemoradiotherapy was 29% for all patients

* Correspondence: doctorgaoxs@126.com; drchenlq@scu.edu.cn
[1]Department of Radiation Oncology, Peking University First Hospital, No.7 Xishiku Street, Beijing 100034, People's Republic of China
[3]Department of Thoracic Surgery, West China School of Medicine/West China Hospital of Sichuan University, No. 37 Guoxue Alley, Chengdu 610041, Sichuan, People's Republic of China
Full list of author information is available at the end of the article

and was as high as 49% for ESCC patients [4]. Definitive chemoradiotherapy (dCRT) is used as the initial treatment in selected patients to avoid surgical mortality [11]. In patients with persistent or recurrent disease, salvage esophagectomy may be performed. Additionally, for stage I esophageal cancer patients in Japan, studies using chemoradiotherapy have demonstrated high rates of complete response and high survival rates with mild toxicity [12]. However, data on the comparative efficacies of dCRT and surgery are insufficient.

We therefore performed a meta-analysis to compare the therapeutic effects of dCRT and esophagectomy as initial treatments for resectable esophageal cancer. Subgroup analyses based on tumour stage, lymph node metastasis, and ethnicity were also conducted.

Methods

Search strategy

This study was conducted according to the Preferred Reporting Items for Systematic Reviews and Meta-Analyses (PRISMA) guidelines [13]. Two reviewers performed an independent systematic literature search. Databases were searched for studies as follows: PubMed (1985 to May 2016) and Web of Science (1992 to June 2018). The following search terms were used: (esophageal cancer or esophageal neoplasms) and (chemoradiotherapy or chemoradiotherapy) and (esophagectomy OR surgery).

Inclusion and exclusion criteria

Studies were included if (1) they were randomised clinical trials (RCTs) or non-randomised clinical trials (nRCTs) that compared dCRT with surgery as the primary treatment in patients with resectable esophageal carcinoma, (2) they reported data on overall survival (OS) and progression-free survival (PFS) or if this information could be extracted from survival curves, and (3) the language of publication was English or Chinese. Studies that recruited patients who received neoadjuvant chemotherapy were excluded. Articles in which non-standardised scoring systems were used and those that reported insufficient data were also excluded.

Data extraction

Each study was evaluated and classified by two independent investigators. Discrepancies were resolved by discussion and/or a third reviewer. The following data were extracted and listed: first author, year of publication, demographic characteristics, treatment regimen, OS, and PFS.

Data analysis

This meta-analysis was conducted using STATA software version 12 (StataCorp, College Station, TX, USA).

The primary endpoint was OS. We assessed and quantified statistical heterogeneity using Cochran's C statistic and the I^2 statistic. If heterogeneity was detected ($I^2 <$ 50% and $P > 0.10$), a fixed-effects model was adopted; otherwise, a random-effects model was used. A pooled analysis was performed with the combined odds ratio (OR) and 95% confidence intervals (CIs) using the Z-test. To assess potential publication bias, Begg's test and Egger's test were performed using STATA version 12. Data were considered statistically significant when $P < 0.05$.

Results

Characteristics of the studies

The characteristics of the patient populations from all eligible studies are listed in Table 1. The selection process for eligible studies is shown in Fig. 1; we identified a total of 13 studies conducted between 1985 and 2015 that included 2071 patients and that compared dCRT ($N = 869$) with surgery ($N = 1202$). Of these 13 studies, 2 [14, 15] were randomised trials. The sample sizes ranged from 49 to 299 patients. Nine studies were restricted to patients with ESCC only, while 4 [16–19] enrolled patients with both ESCC and patients with adenocarcinoma; the predominant tumour histology of these 4 studies was ESCC ($N = 1872$ patients, 90.39%). Only 189 patients (9.13%) were diagnosed with adenocarcinoma, and 0.48% of the patients were diagnosed with cancer of other histological types. Overall, 712 (34%) patients had stage I disease. Most of the studies [14–16, 19–26] were performed in East Asia, including Korea, Japan, and China, while 2 studies [17, 18] were performed in Western countries.

The radiotherapy dose, scheduling, and different chemotherapy regimens are presented in Table 1. All radiation treatments delivered in each study were definitive doses, and total doses ranged from 50 to 71.4 Gy. A platinum-based chemotherapy protocol was administered in most studies [14, 16, 17, 19–26]. The overall R0 resection rate, which was reported in 10 studies [14, 18–26], ranged from 83 to 100%.

Effect of dCRT and surgery on OS

Figure 2 shows pooled estimates for OS in the randomised and non-randomised studies that compared dCRT with surgery. One study [16] was ineligible for the analysis of OS as only the PFS was reported. Both the short-term and long-term OS of patients treated with dCRT versus surgery were not significantly different. The pooled ORs for the 2-year and 5-year OS were 1.199 (95% CI 0.922–1.560; $P = 0.177$) and 0.947 (95% CI 0.628–1.429; $P = 0.796$), respectively.

Table 1 Characters and treatment regimens in trials included in the meta-analysis

Study	Study period	Country	Study design	Group	SCC, n(%)	EAC, n(%)	TN stage	Location	Treatment regimen	N	R0 rate %	Follow-up (months)
Chan 1999 [18]	1984–1994	Canada	nRCT	CRT	68(83)	14(17)	T1-3Nany	Thoracic/EGJ	RT 50-60 Gy concurrent with mitomycin C + 5-FU	82		U
				S	24(30)	57(70)			Transhiatal/thoracoabdominal esophagectomy	81	83	
Hironaka 2003 [22]	1992–1999	Japan	nRCT	CRT	53(100)	0	T2-3Nany	Thoracic	RT 60 Gy (2-week break) + PF (weekly, 5 weeks*2)	53		43
				S	45(100)	0			Total or subtotal thoracic esophagectomy with 3-field resection	45	98	
Sun 2006 [15]	1998–2002	China	RCT	CRT	134(100)	0	T1-3N0	Thoracic	RT (LCAF) 68.4-71 Gy	134		57
				S	135(100)	0			U	135		
Toh 2006 [21]	1995–2003	Japan	nRCT	CRT	25(100)	0	T1N0-1	Thoracic	RT 60 Gy + PF (5 days a week, 4 weeks)	25		32
				S	24(100)	0			Right transthoracic subtotal esophagectomy with 2/3-field dissection	24	88	
Yamashita 2009 [16]	2000–2009	Japan	nRCT	CRT	65(90)	5(7)*	T1N1 or T2-4N0-1	Cervical/thoracic	RT 50.4 Gy, 1.8 Gy/f, nedaplatin + 5-FU*4	72		37.8
				S	54(96)	0			Total/subtotal thoracic esophagectomy with at least 2-field lymphadenectomy.	56		
Yamashita 2008 [25]	2000–2005	Japan	nRCT	CRT	33(100)	0	T1-3Nany	Cervical/thoracic	RT 50.4 Gy + PF*2-4	33		36
				S	49(100)	0			Left thoracotomy by total or subtotal thoracic esophagectomy + least a 2-field lymphadenectomy	49	98	
Ariga 2009 [23]	2001–2005	Japan	nRCT	CRT	51(100)	0	T1-3N0-1	Thoracic	RT 60 Gy (including a 2-week break) + PF	51		49.7
				S	48(100)	0			Thoracoscopy + 2/3-field lymph node dissection.	48	91	36.4
Morgan 2009 [17]	1998–2005	UK	nRCT	CRT	93(53.8)	80(46.2)	T1-4Nany	Thoracic	RT 50 Gy, 2 Gy/f, PF*4	173		U
				S	18(14.3)	108(85.7)			2-phase method described by Lewis and Tanner.	126		
Yamamoto 2011 [26]	1995–2008	Japan	nRCT	CRT	54(100)	0	T1N0	Cervical/thoracic	RT 60 Gy concurrently with PF*2 cycles	54		30
				S	116(100)	0			Right thoracotomy + 2/3-field lymphadenectomy	116	100	67
Motoori 2012 [24]	1995–2007	Japan	nRCT	CRT	71(100)	0	T1bN0	Thoracic	RT ≥ 50 Gy concurrently with 5-FU and cisplatin-based chemotherapy	71		U
				S	102(100)	0			Subtotal esophagectomy via right thoracotomy with 2/3-field lymphadenectomy	102	100	
Teoh 2013 [14]	2000–2004	Hong Kong(China)	RCT	CRT	36(100)	0	T1-4N0-1	Mid/lower thoracic	RT 50-60 Gy, 2 Gy/f PF*3 weekly cycles	36		93
				S	44(100)	0			2- or 3-stage esophagectomy with 2-field lymphadenectomy	44	86.4	
Park 2014 [19]	2003–2012	Korea	nRCT	CRT	20(100)	0	T1N0	Thoracic	Induction XP + RT 54 Gy concurrently with XP/PF or RT alone	20		49
				S	256(97)	2(0.8)**			Ivor Lewis or McKeown, or a transhiatal esophagectomy, with 2/3-field lymph node dissection	264	98.9	
Matsuda 2015 [20]	2002–2011	Japan	nRCT	CRT	65(100)	0	T1-3N0-2	Thoracic	RT > 50 Gy + PF	65		46
				S	112(100)	0			Transthoracic esophagectomy with 2/3-field lymphadenectomy	112	87	

RCT randomised clinical trials, nRCT non-randomised clinical trials, EGJ esophagogastric junction, RT radiation therapy, 5-FU 5-fluorouracil, PF fluorouracil and cisplatin, LCAF late course accelerated fractionation, U unavailable, XP cisplatin + capecitabine

*Two (3%) patients from dCRT group and three (4%) patients from surgery group had esophageal cancer with other pathological types other than ESCC or EAC

**Six (2.2%) patients from the surgery group had esophageal cancer with other pathological types other than ESCC or EAC

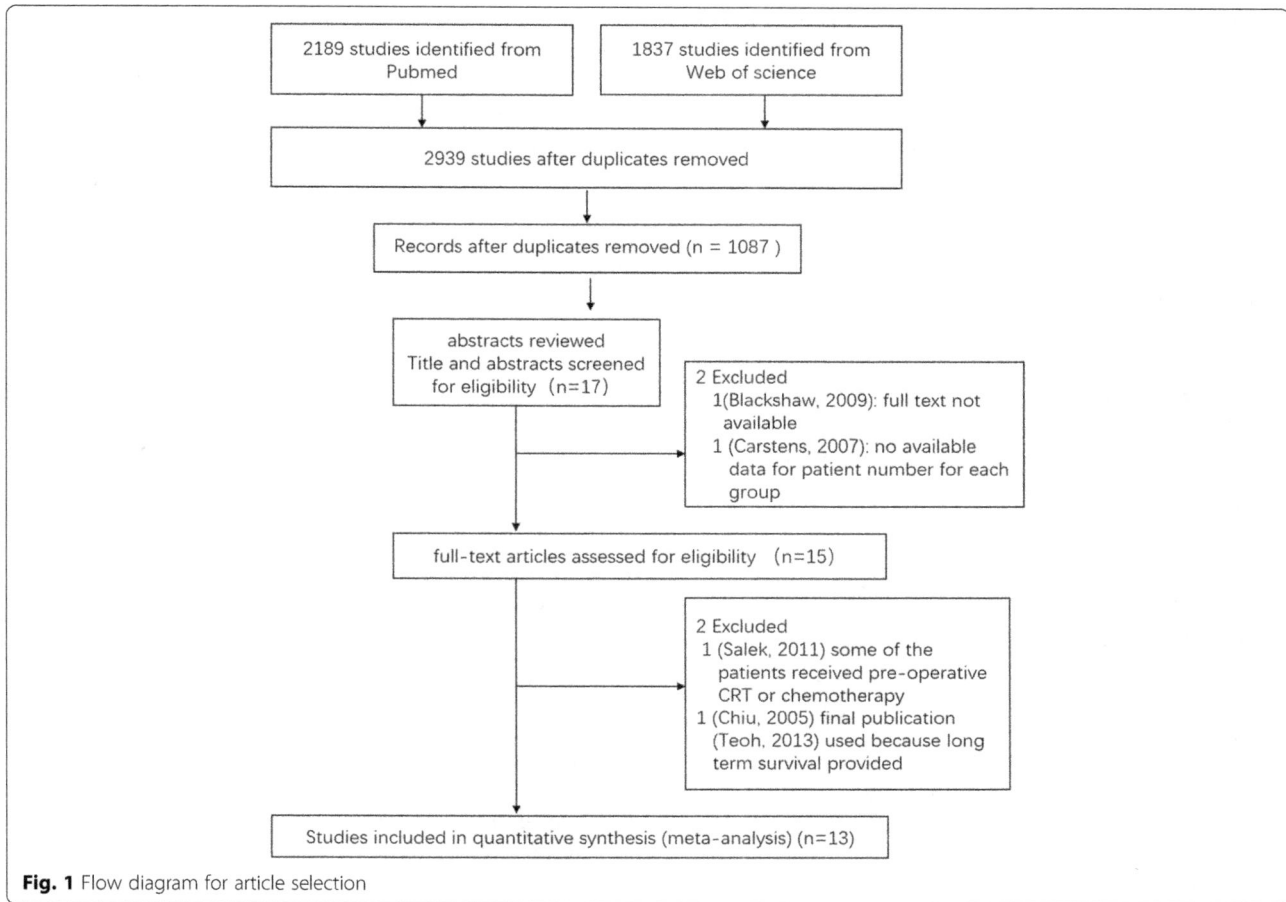

Fig. 1 Flow diagram for article selection

Flow diagram content:

2189 studies identified from Pubmed

1837 studies identified from Web of science

2939 studies after duplicates removed

Records after duplicates removed (n = 1087)

abstracts reviewed
Title and abstracts screened for eligibility (n=17)

2 Excluded
1(Blackshaw, 2009): full text not available
1 (Carstens, 2007): no available data for patient number for each group

full-text articles assessed for eligibility (n=15)

2 Excluded
1 (Salek, 2011) some of the patients received pre-operative CRT or chemotherapy
1 (Chiu, 2005) final publication (Teoh, 2013) used because long term survival provided

Studies included in quantitative synthesis (meta-analysis) (n=13)

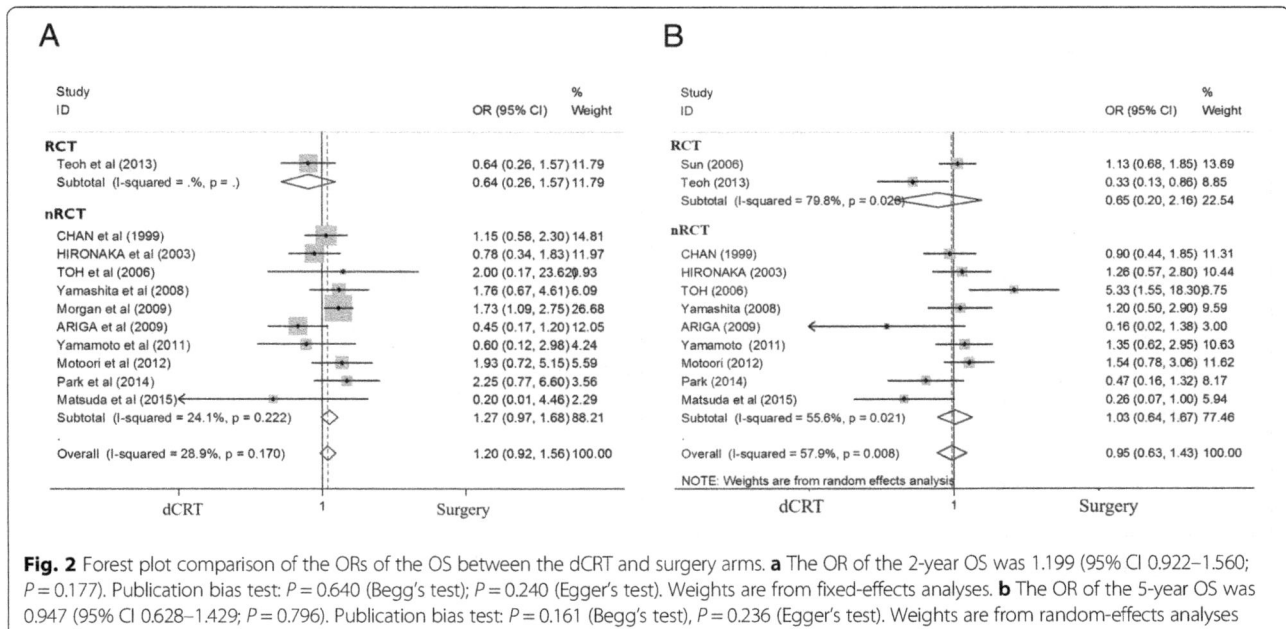

A

Study ID	OR (95% CI)	% Weight
RCT		
Teoh et al (2013)	0.64 (0.26, 1.57)	11.79
Subtotal (I-squared = .%, p = .)	0.64 (0.26, 1.57)	11.79
nRCT		
CHAN et al (1999)	1.15 (0.58, 2.30)	14.81
HIRONAKA et al (2003)	0.78 (0.34, 1.83)	11.97
TOH et al (2006)	2.00 (0.17, 23.62)	0.93
Yamashita et al (2008)	1.76 (0.67, 4.61)	6.09
Morgan et al (2009)	1.73 (1.09, 2.75)	26.68
ARIGA et al (2009)	0.45 (0.17, 1.20)	12.05
Yamamoto et al (2011)	0.60 (0.12, 2.98)	4.24
Motoori et al (2012)	1.93 (0.72, 5.15)	5.59
Park et al (2014)	2.25 (0.77, 6.60)	3.56
Matsuda et al (2015)	0.20 (0.01, 4.46)	2.29
Subtotal (I-squared = 24.1%, p = 0.222)	1.27 (0.97, 1.68)	88.21
Overall (I-squared = 28.9%, p = 0.170)	1.20 (0.92, 1.56)	100.00

dCRT — Surgery

B

Study ID	OR (95% CI)	% Weight
RCT		
Sun (2006)	1.13 (0.68, 1.85)	13.69
Teoh (2013)	0.33 (0.13, 0.86)	8.85
Subtotal (I-squared = 79.8%, p = 0.028)	0.65 (0.20, 2.16)	22.54
nRCT		
CHAN (1999)	0.90 (0.44, 1.85)	11.31
HIRONAKA (2003)	1.26 (0.57, 2.80)	10.44
TOH (2006)	5.33 (1.55, 18.30)	8.75
Yamashita (2008)	1.20 (0.50, 2.90)	9.59
ARIGA (2009)	0.16 (0.02, 1.38)	3.00
Yamamoto (2011)	1.35 (0.62, 2.95)	10.63
Motoori (2012)	1.54 (0.78, 3.06)	11.62
Park (2014)	0.47 (0.16, 1.32)	8.17
Matsuda et al (2015)	0.26 (0.07, 1.00)	5.94
Subtotal (I-squared = 55.6%, p = 0.021)	1.03 (0.64, 1.67)	77.46
Overall (I-squared = 57.9%, p = 0.008)	0.95 (0.63, 1.43)	100.00
NOTE: Weights are from random effects analysis		

dCRT — Surgery

Fig. 2 Forest plot comparison of the ORs of the OS between the dCRT and surgery arms. **a** The OR of the 2-year OS was 1.199 (95% CI 0.922–1.560; $P = 0.177$). Publication bias test: $P = 0.640$ (Begg's test); $P = 0.240$ (Egger's test). Weights are from fixed-effects analyses. **b** The OR of the 5-year OS was 0.947 (95% CI 0.628–1.429; $P = 0.796$). Publication bias test: $P = 0.161$ (Begg's test), $P = 0.236$ (Egger's test). Weights are from random-effects analyses

Effect of dCRT and surgery on the OS of patients with ESCC

Nine studies [14, 15, 18, 20–26] were restricted to patients with ESCC. The pooled OR for the 5-year OS was not significantly different in patients with ESCC who were treated with dCRT compared with those who were treated with surgery (OR = 1.015, 95% CI 0.623–1.652; $P = 0.954$) (Fig. 3).

Subgroup analyses of the effects of dCRT and surgery in patients with different stages of esophageal cancer

Subgroup analyses of patients with stage I and stage II–III disease were performed, and none of the results demonstrated a significant difference between dCRT and surgery. The ORs for the 2-year OS of patients with stage I and stage II–III disease were 1.397 (95% CI 0.740–2.638; $P = 0.303$) and 0.418 (95% CI 0.022–7.833; $P = 0.560$), respectively (Fig. 4). An analysis of patients with stage I ESCC was also performed, and the OR of the 2-year OS was 1.021 (95% CI 0.488–2.134; $P = 0.957$) (Additional file 1: Figure S1).

Subgroup analyses of patients with and without lymph node metastasis

We identified two studies [14, 22] that included data from patients with and without positive lymph nodes. In these studies, all enrolled patients were diagnosed with ESCC. A trend towards improved survival was observed in patients with positive lymph nodes who were treated with dCRT; however, the difference was not statistically significant (OR = 0.226, 95% CI 0.044–1.169; $P = 0.076$). For patients without lymph node metastasis, no

significant difference was observed between the dCRT and surgery groups (OR = 1.419, 95% CI 0.613–3.289; $P = 0.414$) (Fig. 5). However, due to the small number of studies, heterogeneity was observed among patients with lymph node metastasis between the trials due to the small number of studies.

Subgroup analyses of patients from Asian and Western countries

We performed subgroup analyses to examine OS according to different regions. In this analysis, all patients from Asian countries were diagnosed with ESCC [14, 19–26], while Western studies included patients with esophageal adenocarcinoma (EAC) (56%) [17, 18]. The pooled results revealed no differences in terms of the 2-year OS of Asian patients who received dCRT compared with those who underwent surgery, while the estimated OR favoured surgery for patients from North America. The ORs for dCRT compared with that of surgery regarding the 2-year OS were 0.970 (95% CI 0.674–1.395; $P = 0.868$) and 1.522 (95% CI 1.035–2.238; $P = 0.033$) in Asian and Western patients, respectively (Fig. 6). We also performed an analysis on Asian patients with ESCC. The OR of the 2-year OS was 0.886 (95% CI 0.604–1.302; $P = 0.538$) (Additional file 2: Figure S2).

Effect of dCRT and surgery on PFS

Six studies [14, 15, 18, 23–25] reported the 5-year PFS. The results showed that dCRT is equivalent to surgery in terms of the 5-year PFS (OR = 1.06, 95% CI 0.79–1.42; $P = 0.70$) (Fig. 7). The 5-year PFS for ESCC patients between the dCRT and surgery arms was not significantly

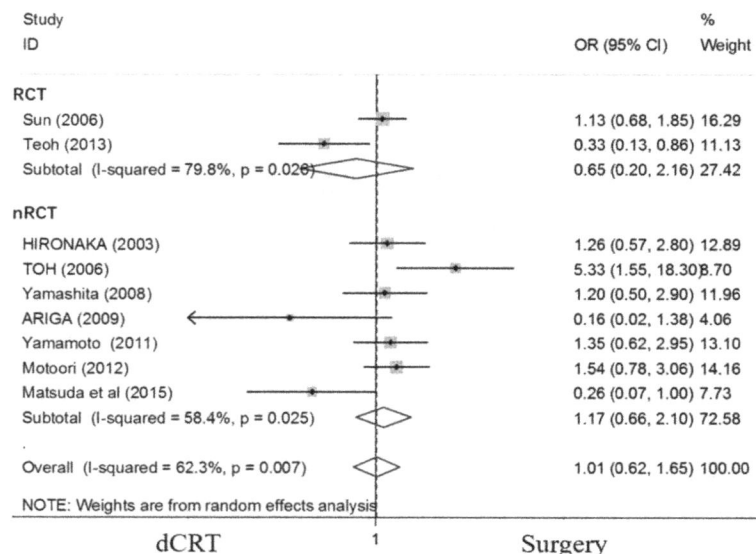

Study ID		OR (95% CI)	% Weight
RCT			
Sun (2006)		1.13 (0.68, 1.85)	16.29
Teoh (2013)		0.33 (0.13, 0.86)	11.13
Subtotal (I-squared = 79.8%, p = 0.026)		0.65 (0.20, 2.16)	27.42
nRCT			
HIRONAKA (2003)		1.26 (0.57, 2.80)	12.89
TOH (2006)		5.33 (1.55, 18.30)	3.70
Yamashita (2008)		1.20 (0.50, 2.90)	11.96
ARIGA (2009)		0.16 (0.02, 1.38)	4.06
Yamamoto (2011)		1.35 (0.62, 2.95)	13.10
Motoori (2012)		1.54 (0.78, 3.06)	14.16
Matsuda et al (2015)		0.26 (0.07, 1.00)	7.73
Subtotal (I-squared = 58.4%, p = 0.025)		1.17 (0.66, 2.10)	72.58
Overall (I-squared = 62.3%, p = 0.007)		1.01 (0.62, 1.65)	100.00
NOTE: Weights are from random effects analysis			

dCRT   1   Surgery

Fig. 3 Forest plot comparison of the ORs of the OS between the dCRT and surgery arms for patients with ESCC. The OR of the 5-year OS was 1.015 (95% CI 0.623–1.652; $P = 0.954$). Publication bias test: $P = 0.348$ (Begg's test), $P = 0.350$ (Egger's test). Weights are from random-effects analyses

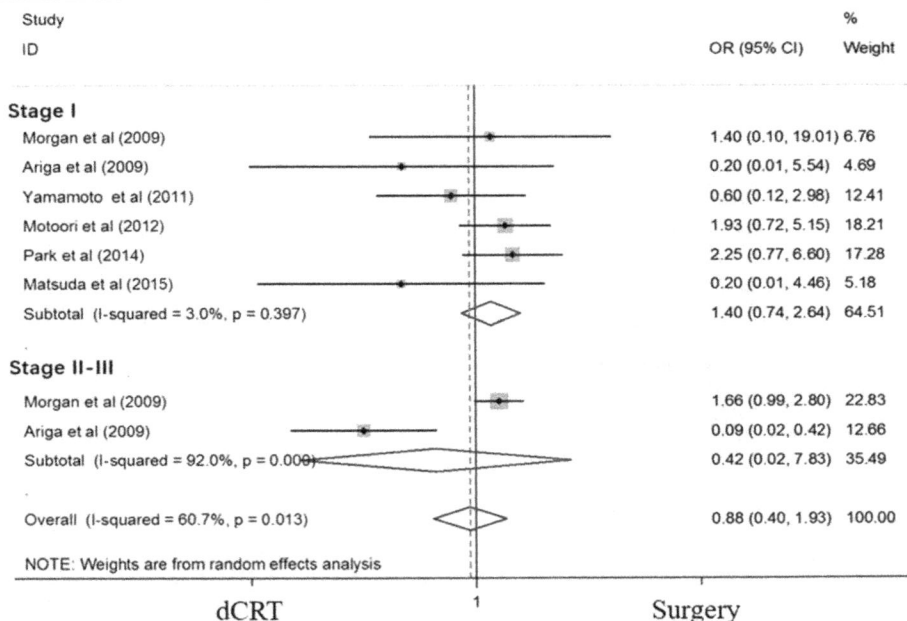

Fig. 4 Forest plot comparison of the ORs of the OS between the dCRT and surgery arms for patients with different stages of esophageal cancer. The OR of the 2-year OS for stage I esophageal cancer was 1.397 (95% CI 0.740–2.638; $P = 0.303$). Publication bias test: $P = 0.133$ (Begg's test), $P = 0.039$ (Egger's test). The OR of the 2-year OS for stage II–III esophageal cancer was 0.418 (95% CI 0.022–7.833; $P = 0.560$). Publication bias (not available due to lack of studies). Weights are from random-effects analyses

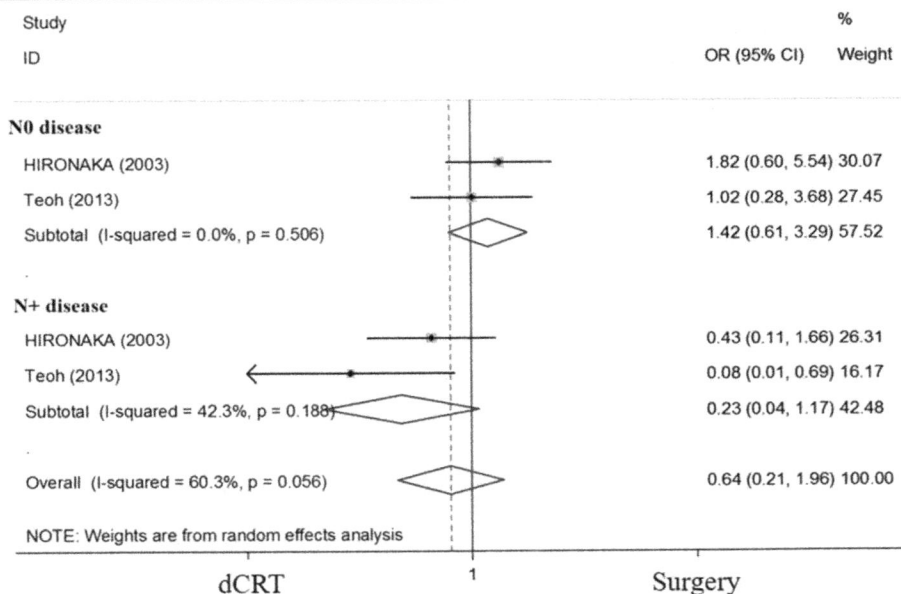

Fig. 5 Forest plot comparison of the ORs of the OS between the dCRT and surgery arms for patients with N0 disease and N+ diseases. The OR of the 5-year OS for N0 disease was 1.419 (95% CI 0.613–3.289; $P = 0.414$). Publication bias: not available due to lack of studies. The OR of the 5-year OS for N+ disease was 0.226 (95% CI 0.044–1.169; $P = 0.076$). Publication bias: not available due to lack of studies. Weights are from random-effects analyses

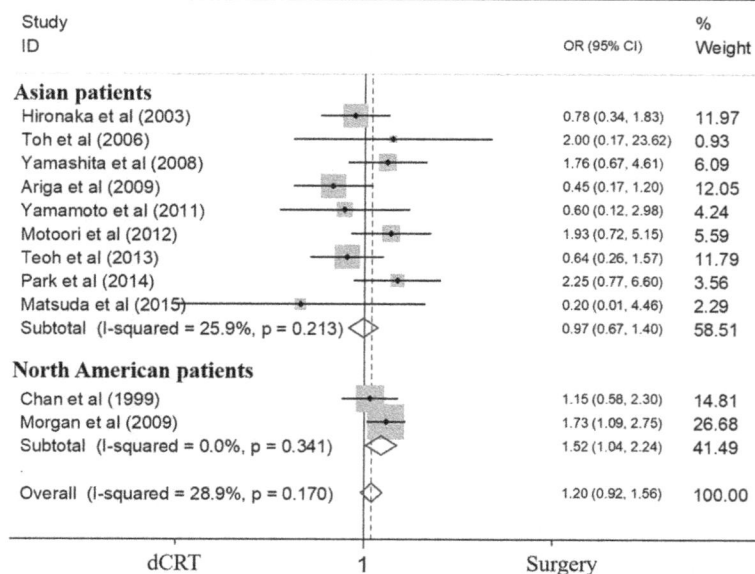

Fig. 6 Forest plot comparison of ORs of the OS between the dCRT and surgery arms for Asian patients and Western patients. The OR of the 2-year OS for Asian patients was 0.970 (95% CI 0.674–1.395; P = 0.868). Publication bias test: P = 0.835 (Begg's test); P = 0.807 (Egger's test). The OR of the 2-year OS for Western patients was 1.522 (95% CI 1.035–2.238; P = 0.033). Publication bias: not available due to lack of studies. Weights are from fixed-effects analyses

different. The OR of the 5-year PFS was 1.047 (95% CI 0.623–1.760; P = 0.862) (Additional file 3: Figure S3).

Discussion

In this meta-analysis, the outcomes between dCRT and surgery as initial treatments for resectable esophageal cancer across 13 RCTs and nRCTs were compared. No statistically significant differences were observed in either short- or long-term OS or PFS. Subgroup analyses showed a trend towards improved outcomes for patients with positive lymph nodes who were treated with dCRT; however, the difference was not statistically significant. Patients from Western countries who underwent surgery had a better 2-year OS than those who received dCRT.

The number of clinical stage I esophageal cancer patients has recently increased [27, 28]. The survival rate following surgery for submucosal tumours is high; however, the postoperative quality of life is often

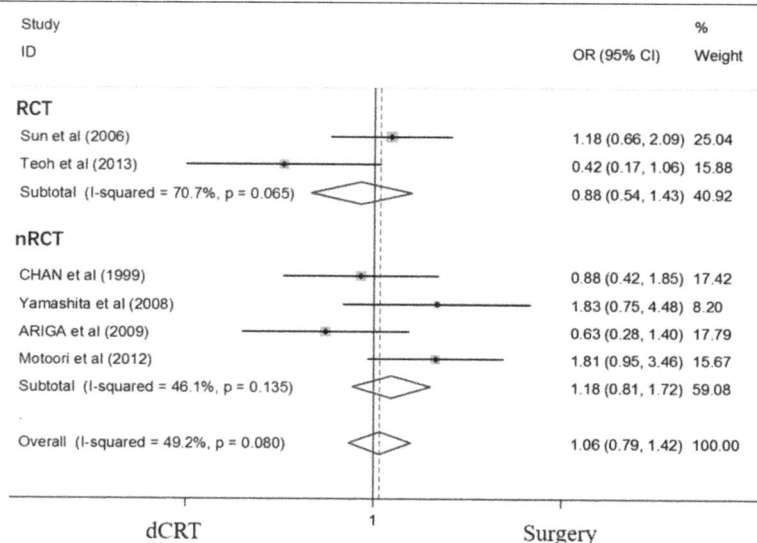

Fig. 7 Forest plot comparison of ORs of the PFS between the dCRT and surgery arms. The OR of the 5-year PFS was 1.060 (95% CI 0.789–1.424; P = 0.698). Publication bias test: P = 0.260 (Begg's test); P = 0.350 (Egger's test). Weights are from fixed-effects analyses

compromised. Some studies [29, 30] have demonstrated encouraging clinical results for dCRT in these patients. In this meta-analysis, the 2-year OS of patients with stage I esophageal cancer was comparable between the dCRT and esophagostomy groups. Therefore, dCRT may be considered a treatment modality in selected patients. The ongoing JCOG0502 study by the Japan Clinical Oncology Group is investigating the non-inferiority of dCRT compared with surgery for stage I esophageal cancer patients.

Esophageal cancer is characterised by a high rate of lymph node metastasis [31], which is the most reliable predictor of survival after surgery [32]. In addition, because its pattern of spread is not always predictable and since skip node metastases may also occur, lymph node dissections may be difficult to perform. As suggested by our subgroup analyses, dCRT was superior to surgery among patients with lymph node metastases.

The pathological types of esophageal cancer are characterised by obvious demographic variations. The incidence of ESCC is much higher in Asia than in Western countries, whereas EAC accounts for only 1–4% of cases in Asian countries [2]. In addition, the incidence of EAC in Western countries is increasing rapidly [33]. We extracted data from all patients with ESCC and found no difference between dCRT and surgery in terms of long-term OS. Moreover, the subgroup analysis of the geographic areas showed that the 2-year OS was comparable between Asian patients who received dCRT and those who received surgery. In Western patients, surgical treatment has obvious therapeutic benefits. Studies on preoperative chemoradiotherapy [4, 6, 34] have shown that the pathological complete response rate of patients with EAC was lower than that of patients with ESCC. In this meta-analysis, two studies enrolled patients with EAC from Western countries [17, 18] (proportion of EAC, 44.1% and 62.9%), whereas almost all patients from Asian countries had ESCC. In addition, these two studies, which were performed in Western countries, included a large proportion of patients with lower esophageal cancer (66.9% and 77.3%). Patients with lower esophageal cancer were more amenable to surgery.

The progression rate of esophageal cancer is usually high when treated with either dCRT or surgery alone [34–37]. For long-term PFS, dCRT is equivalent to surgery when used as the initial treatment modality. A multidisciplinary approach is the ideal strategy, especially for the treatment of esophageal cancer.

This meta-analysis has several limitations. First, retrospective studies were included; therefore, selection bias may exist. For example, patients treated with dCRT in these studies were diagnosed with more advanced disease than those treated with surgery. Second, individual results from each patient were not applied. Third, modest heterogeneity was observed in terms of the surgical methods that were used and the dosing schedules between studies. In addition, the number of studies in the subgroup analyses was limited, especially those that included patients with lymph node metastasis and those with Western ethnicity. Finally, the studies were limited to two languages, which may present another bias.

Conclusions

Our study demonstrates that dCRT is similar to surgery as an initial treatment for esophageal cancer with respect to the long-term survival of patients. Surgery may lead to a better OS in patients from Western countries, but further randomised trials are required to confirm these results.

Additional files

Additional file 1: Figure S1. Forest plot comparison of ORs of the OS between the dCRT and surgery arms for stage I ESCC patients. The OR of the 2-year OS was 1.021 (95% CI 0.488–2.134; $P = 0.957$). Publication bias test: $P = 0.308$ (Begg's test); $P = 0.042$ (Egger's test). Weights are from fixed-effects analyses.

Additional file 2: Figure S2. Forest plot comparison of ORs of the OS between the dCRT and surgery arms for Asian ESCC patients. The OR of the 2-year OS was 0.886 (95% CI 0.604–1.302; $P = 0.538$). Publication bias test: $P = 0.902$ (Begg's test); $P = 0.769$ (Egger's test). Weights are from fixed-effects analyses.

Additional file 3: Figure S3. Forest plot comparison of ORs of the PFS between the dCRT and surgery arms for ESCC patients. The OR of the 5-year PFS was 1.047 (95% CI 0.623–1.760; $P = 0.862$). Publication bias test: $P = 0.462$ (Begg's test); $P = 0.432$ (Egger's test). Weights are from random-effects analyses.

Abbreviations

5-FU: 5-Fluorouracil; CI: Confidence interval; dCRT: Definitive chemoradiotherapy; EAC: Esophageal adenocarcinoma; ESCC: Esophageal squamous cell carcinoma; LCAF: Late course accelerated fractionation; nRCT: Non-randomised clinical trial; OR: Odds ratio; OS: Overall survival; PF: Fluorouracil and cisplatin; PFS: Progression-free survival; PRISMA: Preferred Reporting Items for Reviews and Meta-Analyses; RCT: Randomised clinical trial; RT: Radiation therapy; U: Unavailable; XP: Cisplatin + capecitabine

Authors' contributions

MWM designed the study, analysed the data, and drafted the manuscript. XBG, MC, MX, and LL collected and verified the data. HY, MZ, and LL analysed and interpreted the data. LQC and XSG designed the study, interpreted the data, revised the manuscript, and made the decision to submit for publication. All authors read and approved the final manuscript.

Competing interests

The authors declare that they have no competing interests.

Author details
[1]Department of Radiation Oncology, Peking University First Hospital, No.7 Xishiku Street, Beijing 100034, People's Republic of China. [2]Department of Medical and Pharmaceutical Science and Technology Strategy Research, Institute of Medical Information, Chinese Academy of Medical Sciences, No. 3 Yabao Road, Beijing, China. [3]Department of Thoracic Surgery, West China School of Medicine/West China Hospital of Sichuan University, No. 37 Guoxue Alley, Chengdu 610041, Sichuan, People's Republic of China.

References
1. Mariette C, Piessen G, Triboulet JP. Therapeutic strategies in oesophageal carcinoma: role of surgery and other modalities. Lancet Oncol. 2007;8:545–53.
2. Hongo M, Nagasaki Y, Shoji T. Epidemiology of esophageal cancer: Orient to Occident. Effects of chronology, geography and ethnicity. J Gastroenterol Hepatol. 2009;24:729–35.
3. Sjoquist KM, Burmeister BH, Smithers BM, Zalcberg JR, Simes RJ, Barbour A, Gebski V. Survival after neoadjuvant chemotherapy or chemoradiotherapy for resectable oesophageal carcinoma: an updated meta-analysis. Lancet Oncol. 2011;12:681–92.
4. van Hagen P, Hulshof MC, van Lanschot JJ, Steyerberg EW, van Berge Henegouwen MI, Wijnhoven BP, Richel DJ, Nieuwenhuijzen GA, Hospers GA, Bonenkamp JJ, et al. Preoperative chemoradiotherapy for esophageal or junctional cancer. N Engl J Med. 2012;366:2074–84.
5. Bosset JF, Gignoux M, Triboulet JP, Tiret E, Mantion G, Elias D, Lozach P, Ollier JC, Pavy JJ, Mercier M, Sahmoud T. Chemoradiotherapy followed by surgery compared with surgery alone in squamous-cell cancer of the esophagus. N Engl J Med. 1997;337:161–7.
6. Urba SG, Orringer MB, Turrisi A, Iannettoni M, Forastiere A, Strawderman M. Randomized trial of preoperative chemoradiation versus surgery alone in patients with locoregional esophageal carcinoma. J Clin Oncol. 2001;19:305–13.
7. Nygaard K, Hagen S, Hansen HS, Hatlevoll R, Hultborn R, Jakobsen A, Mantyla M, Modig H, Munck-Wikland E, Rosengren B, et al. Pre-operative radiotherapy prolongs survival in operable esophageal carcinoma: a randomized, multicenter study of pre-operative radiotherapy and chemotherapy. The second Scandinavian trial in esophageal cancer. World J Surg. 1992;16:1104–9. discussion 1110
8. Walsh TN, Noonan N, Hollywood D, Kelly A, Keeling N, Hennessy TP. A comparison of multimodal therapy and surgery for esophageal adenocarcinoma. N Engl J Med. 1996;335:462–7.
9. Birkmeyer JD, Stukel TA, Siewers AE, Goodney PP, Wennberg DE, Lucas FL. Surgeon volume and operative mortality in the United States. N Engl J Med. 2003;349:2117–27.
10. Steyerberg EW, Neville BA, Koppert LB, Lemmens VE, Tilanus HW, Coebergh JW, Weeks JC, Earle CC. Surgical mortality in patients with esophageal cancer: development and validation of a simple risk score. J Clin Oncol. 2006;24:4277–84.
11. D'Journo XB, Thomas PA. Current management of esophageal cancer. J Thorac Dis. 2014;6(Suppl 2):S253–64.
12. Kato H, Sato A, Fukuda H, Kagami Y, Udagawa H, Togo A, Ando N, Tanaka O, Shinoda M, Yamana H, Ishikura S. A phase II trial of chemoradiotherapy for stage I esophageal squamous cell carcinoma: Japan Clinical Oncology Group Study (JCOG9708). Jpn J Clin Oncol. 2009;39:638–43.
13. Liberati A, Altman DG, Tetzlaff J, Mulrow C, Gotzsche PC, Ioannidis JP, Clarke M, Devereaux PJ, Kleijnen J, Moher D. The PRISMA statement for reporting systematic reviews and meta-analyses of studies that evaluate healthcare interventions: explanation and elaboration. BMJ. 2009;339:b2700.
14. Teoh AY, Chiu PW, Yeung WK, Liu SY, Wong SK, Ng EK. Long-term survival outcomes after definitive chemoradiation versus surgery in patients with resectable squamous carcinoma of the esophagus: results from a randomized controlled trial. Ann Oncol. 2013;24:165–71.
15. Sun XD, Yu JM, Fan XL, Ren RM, Li MH, Zhang GL. Randomized clinical study of surgery versus radiotherapy alone in the treatment of resectable esophageal cancer in the chest. Zhonghua Zhong Liu Za Zhi. 2006;28: 784–7.
16. Yamashita H, Okuma K, Seto Y, Mori K, Kobayashi S, Wakui R, Ohtomo K, Nakagawa K. A retrospective comparison of clinical outcomes and quality of life measures between definitive chemoradiation alone and radical surgery for clinical stage II-III esophageal carcinoma. J Surg Oncol. 2009;100:435–41.
17. Morgan MA, Lewis WG, Casbard A, Roberts SA, Adams R, Clark GW, Havard TJ, Crosby TD. Stage-for-stage comparison of definitive chemoradiotherapy, surgery alone and neoadjuvant chemotherapy for oesophageal carcinoma. Br J Surg. 2009;96:1300–7.
18. Chan A, Wong A. Is combined chemotherapy and radiation therapy equally effective as surgical resection in localized esophageal carcinoma? Int J Radiat Oncol Biol Phys. 1999;45:265–70.
19. Park I, Kim YH, Yoon DH, Park SR, Kim HR, Kim JH, Jung HY, Lee GH, Cho KJ, Kim SB. Non-surgical treatment versus radical esophagectomy for clinical T1N0M0 esophageal carcinoma: a single-center experience. Cancer Chemother Pharmacol. 2014;74:995–1003.
20. Matsuda S, Tsubosa Y, Niihara M, Sato H, Takebayashi K, Kawamorita K, Mori K, Tsushima T, Yokota T, Ogawa H, et al. Comparison of transthoracic esophagectomy with definitive chemoradiotherapy as initial treatment for patients with esophageal squamous cell carcinoma who could tolerate transthoracic esophagectomy. Ann Surg Oncol. 2015;22:1866–73.
21. Toh Y, Ohga T, Itoh S, Kabashima A, Yamamoto K, Adachi E, Sakaguchi Y, Okamura T, Hirata H. Treatment results of radical surgery and definitive chemoradiotherapy for patients with submucosal esophageal squamous cell cancinomas. Anticancer Res. 2006;26:2487–91.
22. Hironaka S, Ohtsu A, Boku N, Muto M, Nagashima F, Saito H, Yoshida S, Nishimura M, Haruno M, Ishikura S, et al. Nonrandomized comparison between definitive chemoradiotherapy and radical surgery in patients with T(2-3)N(any) M(0) squamous cell carcinoma of the esophagus. Int J Radiat Oncol Biol Phys. 2003;57:425–33.
23. Ariga H, Nemoto K, Miyazaki S, Yoshioka T, Ogawa Y, Sakayauchi T, Jingu K, Miyata G, Onodera K, Ichikawa H, et al. Prospective comparison of surgery alone and chemoradiotherapy with selective surgery in resectable squamous cell carcinoma of the esophagus. Int J Radiat Oncol Biol Phys. 2009;75:348–56.
24. Motoori M, Yano M, Ishihara R, Yamamoto S, Kawaguchi Y, Tanaka K, Kishi K, Miyashiro I, Fujiwara Y, Shingai T, et al. Comparison between radical esophagectomy and definitive chemoradiotherapy in patients with clinical T1bN0M0 esophageal cancer. Ann Surg Oncol. 2012;19:2135–41.
25. Yamashita H, Nakagawa K, Yamada K, Kaminishi M, Mafune K, Ohtomo K. A single institutional non-randomized retrospective comparison between definitive chemoradiotherapy and radical surgery in 82 Japanese patients with resectable esophageal squamous cell carcinoma. Dis Esophagus. 2008;21:430–6.
26. Yamamoto S, Ishihara R, Motoori M, Kawaguchi Y, Uedo N, Takeuchi Y, Higashino K, Yano M, Nakamura S, Iishi H. Comparison between definitive chemoradiotherapy and esophagectomy in patients with clinical stage I esophageal squamous cell carcinoma. Am J Gastroenterol. 2011;106: 1048–54.
27. Ozawa S. Comprehensive registry of esophageal cancer in Japan. In: bits 3rd annual world cancer congress-2012; 2012. p. 21–47.
28. Kodaira T, Fuwa N, Tachibana H, Nakamura T, Tomita N, Nakahara R, Inokuchi H, Mizoguchi N, Takada A. Retrospective analysis of definitive radiotherapy for patients with superficial esophageal carcinoma: consideration of the optimal treatment method with a focus on late morbidity. Radiother Oncol. 2010;95:234–9.
29. Yamada K, Murakami M, Okamoto Y, Okuno Y, Nakajima T, Kusumi F, Takakuwa H, Matsusue S. Treatment results of chemoradiotherapy for clinical stage I (T1N0M0) esophageal carcinoma. Int J Radiat Oncol Biol Phys. 2006;64:1106–11.
30. Nemoto K, Yamada S, Hareyama M, Nagakura H, Hirokawa Y. Radiation therapy for superficial esophageal cancer: a comparison of radiotherapy methods. Int J Radiat Oncol Biol Phys. 2001;50:639–44.
31. Akiyama H, Tsurumaru M, Udagawa H, Kajiyama Y. Radical lymph node dissection for cancer of the thoracic esophagus. Ann Surg. 1994;220:364–72. discussion 372-363
32. Zhu YM, Li MH, Kong L, Yu JM. Postoperative radiation in esophageal squamous cell carcinoma and target volume delineation. Oncotargets Therapy. 2016;9:4187–96.
33. Bollschweiler E, Wolfgarten E, Gutschow C, Holscher AH. Demographic variations in the rising incidence of esophageal adenocarcinoma in white males. Cancer. 2001;92:549–55.
34. Burmeister BH, Smithers BM, Gebski V, Fitzgerald L, Simes RJ, Devitt P, Ackland S, Gotley DC, Joseph D, Millar J, et al. Surgery alone versus chemoradiotherapy followed by surgery for resectable cancer of the oesophagus: a randomised controlled phase III trial. Lancet Oncol. 2005;6: 659–68.

35. Stahl M, Stuschke M, Lehmann N, Meyer HJ, Walz MK, Seeber S, Klump B, Budach W, Teichmann R, Schmitt M, et al. Chemoradiation with and without surgery in patients with locally advanced squamous cell carcinoma of the esophagus. J Clin Oncol. 2005;23:2310–7.

36. Minsky BD, Pajak TF, Ginsberg RJ, Pisansky TM, Martenson J, Komaki R, Okawara G, Rosenthal SA, Kelsen DP. INT 0123 (Radiation Therapy Oncology Group 94-05) phase III trial of combined-modality therapy for esophageal cancer: high-dose versus standard-dose radiation therapy. J Clin Oncol. 2002;20:1167–74.

37. Bedenne L, Michel P, Bouche O, Milan C, Mariette C, Conroy T, Pezet D, Roullet B, Seitz JF, Herr JP, et al. Chemoradiation followed by surgery compared with chemoradiation alone in squamous cancer of the esophagus: FFCD 9102. J Clin Oncol. 2007;25:1160–8.

13

The application of fibular free flap with flexor hallucis longus in maxilla or mandible extensive defect: a comparison study with conventional flap

Youkang Ni, Ping Lu, Zhi Yang, Wenlong Wang, Wei Dai, Zhong-zheng Qi, Weiyi Duan, Zhong-fei Xu, Chang-fu Sun and Fayu Liu*

Abstract

Background: The repair and reconstruction of maxillary and mandibular extensive defects have put huge challenges to surgeons. The fibular free flap (FFF) is one of the standard treatment choices for reconstruction. The conventional FFF has deficiencies, such as forming poor oral mucosa, limited flap tissue, and perforator vessel variation. To improve the use of FFF, we add the flexor hallucis longus (FHL) in the flap (FHL-FFF). In this paper, we described the advantage and indication of FHL-FFF and conducted a retrospective study to compare FHL-FFF and FFF without FHL.

Methods: Fifty-four patients who underwent FFF were enrolled and divided into two groups: nFHL group (using FFF without FHL, 38 patients) and FHL group (using FHL-FFF, 16 patients). The perioperative clinical data of patients was collected and analyzed.

Results: The flaps all survived in two groups. We mainly used FHL to fill dead space, and the donor-site morbidity was slight. In FHL group, flap harvesting time was shorter (118.63 ± 11.76 vs 125.74 ± 11.33 min, $P = 0.042$), the size of flap's skin paddle was smaller (16.5 (0–96) vs 21.0(10–104) cm^2, $P = 0.027$) than nFHL group. There were no significant differences ($P > 0.05$) in hospital days, hospitalization expense, rate of perioperative complications, etc. between the two groups. Compared with FFF without FHL, FHL-FFF will neither affect the use of flap nor bring more problems.

Conclusion: The FHL-FFF simplifies the flap harvesting operation. The FHL can form good mucosa and make FFF rely less on skin paddle. It can be used for adding flap tissue and dealing with perforator vessel variation in reconstruction of maxillary and mandibular extensive defects.

Keywords: Fibular free flap, Flexor hallucis longus, Maxillary and mandibular defect, Extensive defect, Reconstruction

Background

The maxillary and mandibular extensive defects are often caused by tumor surgery, trauma, etc. The defects can cause severe functional and cosmetic deformities and have harmful effects on the patients' quality of life. So, the patients have urgent desires to repair and reconstruct the defects.

Fibular free flap (FFF) was firstly described by Taylor in 1975 [1], and then Hidalgo [2] firstly introduced it for

mandibular reconstruction in 1989. In 1993, Sadove reported simultaneous maxillary and mandibular reconstruction with one fibular free osteocutaneous flap [3]. The advantages of FFF, such as sufficient osseous tissue, reliable blood supply, precise shaping, simple flap harvesting operation, and limited donor site morbidity, make it popularly used in the clinical work [4, 5, 6]. With the development of microsurgery, it has become one of the most common methods to repair and reconstruct the maxillary and mandibular defects [6].

In our department, the conventional FFF is mainly composed of fibula and skin paddle. The skin paddle can be used as a monitoring window for the flap's survival

* Correspondence: lfyhjk@126.com
Department of Oromaxillofacial-Head and Neck Surgery, School of Stomatology, China Medical University, No. 117 Nanjing North Street, Heping District, Shenyang 110002, Liaoning, People's Republic of China

[7]. In practice, we find that only fibula and skin paddle are not enough to repair extensive defect. In follow-up visits, the patients always complain about the skin paddle's discomfort in the oral cavity.

In spite of thorough presurgical planning, emergency situations that require prompt processing may arise during FFF surgeries, including perforator vessel variation and the limited flap tissue.

In 1994, Hidalgo mentioned the use of FHL in FFF for filling in the soft tissue defect in mandibular reconstruction [4]. But the indication of FHL-FFF and the comparison of FHL-FFF and FFF without FHL lack detailed description. Inspired by Hidalgo, and in order to resolve the deficiencies of the FFF and deal with the emergency during the surgery, we added flexor hallucis longus in FFF (FHL-FFF).

In this paper, we collected our FHL-FFF and FFF without FHL in the same time. We described the use of FHL in FFF and the indication of FHL-FFF. We compared FHL-FFF and FFF without FHL in patients' clinical data and analyzed the advantages and disadvantages of the two methods. In addition, we share two cases flexibly using FHL-FFF to repair the maxillary and mandibular extensive defects.

Methods
Patient
From Nov. 2013 to Apr. 2017, 60 patients underwent head and neck tumor resection and reconstruction with FFF at the Department of Oromaxillofacial-Head and Neck Surgery, School of Stomatology, China Medical University. The exclusion criteria are as follows: (1) the lower limb has a history of severe trauma, neuropathy, and diabetic foot; and (2) history of bone grafts more than one time. Finally, we excluded six patients and included 16 patients in FHL group, 38 patients in nFHL group (see Fig. 1).

All cases had detailed clinical records. The patient's preoperative data include demographics, smoking and drinking history, comorbidities, etc. The operation data include time of operation, operation method and data of the flap, etc. The postoperative data include hospital stay, hospitalization expenses, etc. Patient's informed consent was obtained, and approval was obtained from the ethics committee of the School of Stomatology, China Medical University.

Follow-up visit was conducted by telephone, Internet, and periodic review. The donor-site morbidity was observed.

Operative technique
The primary difference between two methods is whether the FHL is harvested in the flap. The operation is under an automatic tourniquet system (ATS-III) to reduce bleeding. First, we mark the design of the flap and skin paddle on the lower extremity. Then, we take the posterolateral approach of crus to harvest the flap. After cutting and separating skin, subcutaneous and fascia tissue, we seek one or two perforator vessels and confirm the vessels are from FHL. Then, we separate peroneus longus from the fibula and interrupt intermuscular septum and bone septum. Then, the fibula is fully revealed. We could conveniently cut off the fibula. Then, we harvest the skin paddle as needed. We continue to separate tissue and seek the spatium between FHL and soleus and use finger to separate the FHL from the fibula. Finally, we only need to ligate the vessels of superior and inferior fibula, then check the fibula flap's blooding (see Fig. 2). While in our conventional method, we need to dissect carefully the FHL from fibula and dissect peroneal artery and vein. It will prolong time of operation and increase risks of blood vessel and nerve injuries.

When we transplant the FHL-FFF to recipient site, we can use the FHL to fill the dead space after tumor resection and then use skin paddle to close defect. We can also cover the fibula with muscle and use the muscular fasciae of FHL to fill the intraoral defect.

Statistical methods
The statistical software SPSS version 18.0 was used to analyze the data. A P value < 0.05 was considered statistically significant.

Patient's age, weight, operation time, flap harvesting time, the length of harvested fibula, and hospitalization expenses obey normal distribution. To compare the differences of these items between the two groups, independent sample T test was used to analyze these data. Skin paddle size, total hospital days, and postoperative hospital days obey abnormal distribution. To compare the differences, Wilcoxon rank sum test was used to analyze these data. Chi-squared test was used to analyze the ratios, such as sex ratio and rate of smoking.

Results
Preoperative data
The FHL group had 16 patients, 15 males, and 1 female. The nFHL group had 38 patients, 18 males and 20 females. Male ratios of FHL group were significantly higher than that in nFHL group (93.75 vs 47.37%, $P = 0.001$). The mean age of FHL group was 46.44 ± 13.80 years old and nFHL group was 43.73 ± 13.66 years old. There was no significant difference in age ($P = 0.511$). The mean weight of FHL group was 66.22 ± 9.15 kg and nFHL group was 66.42 ± 13.45 kg. There was no significant difference ($P = 0.956$). The FHL group had 8 patients with smoking history and 4 patients with drinking history. The nFHL group had 9 patients with smoking history and 2 patients with drinking history.

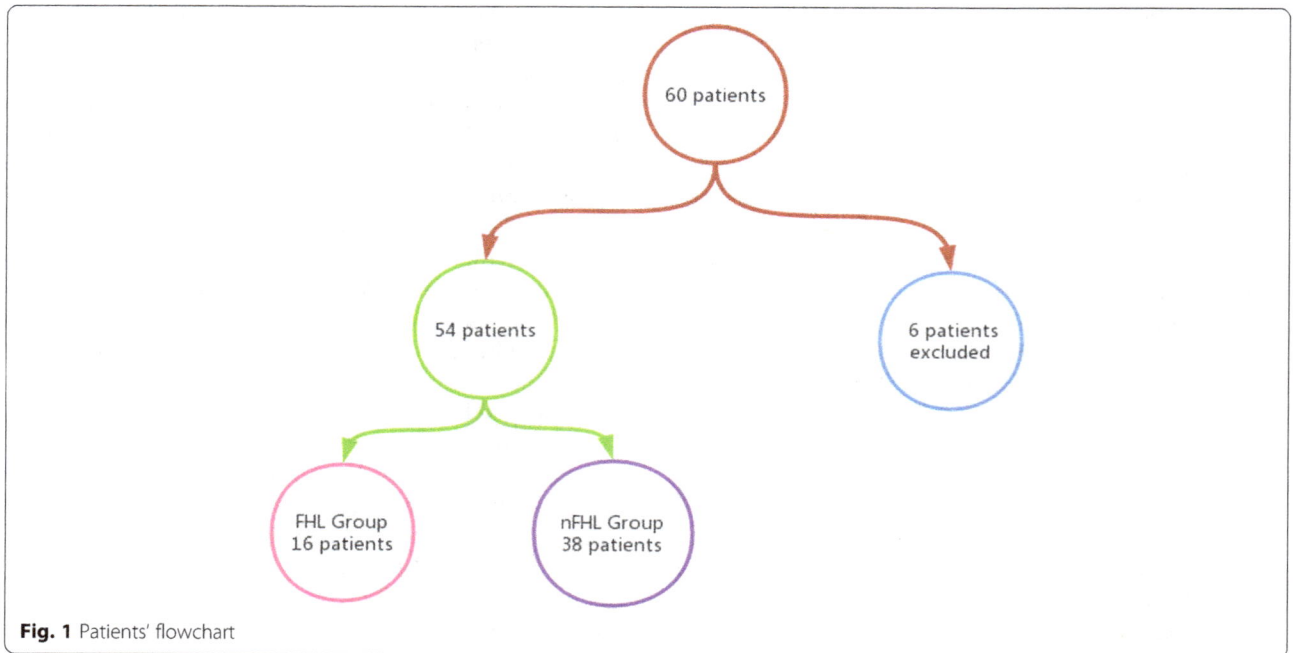

Fig. 1 Patients' flowchart

There were no significant differences in smoking and drinking rate (smoking% 50 vs 23.68%, $P = 0.106$; drinking% 25.00 vs 5.26%, $P = 0.102$). The major comorbidity was hypertension. The FHL group had 3 patients, and nFHL group had 8 patients. There was no significant difference (hypertension% 18.75 vs 21.05%, $P = 1.000$). The two groups had no history of chemoradiotherapy before the operation. In nature of tumor, the FHL group had 9 cases of benign tumor, including 8 cases of ameloblastoma and 1 case of odontogenic keratocyst; and 7 cases of malignant tumor, including 6 cases of squamous cell carcinoma and 1 case of adenoid cystic carcinoma. The nFHL group had 21 cases of benign tumor, including 16 cases of ameloblastoma, 3 cases of odontogenic myxoma, 1 case of odontogenic keratocyst, and 1 case of giant cell lesion; and 17 cases of malignant tumor,

including 11 cases of squamous cell carcinoma, 1 case of clear cell carcinoma, and 5 cases of osteosarcoma. The malignant tumor rates were 56.25 and 55.26%. There was no significant difference ($P = 0.947$). In malignant tumor, the rates of carcinoma were 43.75 and 31.58%; there was no significant difference ($P = 0.392$). The rates of sarcoma were 0 and 13.16%; there was no significant difference ($P = 0.313$) (see Table 1).

Table 1 Preoperative data

N	FHL group 16	nFHL group 38	P
Sex (n)			
Male%	93.75% (15)	47.37% (18)	0.001*
Female%	6.25% (1)	52.63% (20)	
Age (year)	46.44 ± 13.80	43.73 ± 13.66	0.511
Weight (kg)	66.22 ± 9.15	66.42 ± 13.45	0.956
Smoking%	50.00% (8)	23.68% (9)	0.106
Drinking%	25.00% (4)	5.26% (2)	0.102
Hypertension%	18.75% (3)	21.05% (8)	1.000
Nature			
Benign%	56.25% (9)	55.26% (21)	0.947
Malignant%	43.75% (7)	44.74% (17)	
Malignant			
Carcinoma%	43.75% (7)	31.58% (12)	0.392
Sarcoma%	0.00% (0)	13.16% (5)	0.313

*Statistically significant ($P < 0.05$)

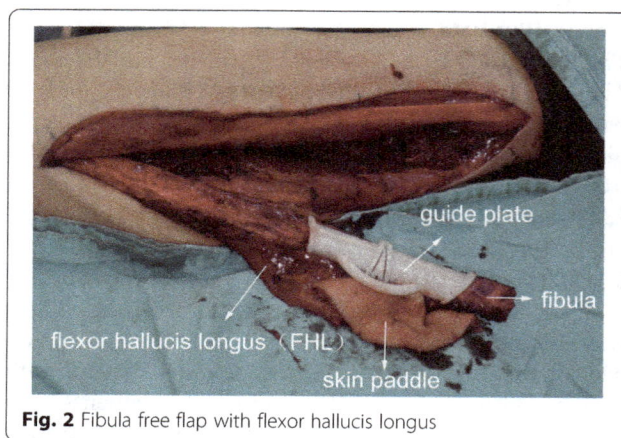

Fig. 2 Fibula free flap with flexor hallucis longus

The preoperative data of the two groups, including demographics, smoking and drinking history, comorbidities, nature of tumor, except for sex, have no significant differences, which make the two groups comparable.

Operation data

The FHL group had 16 patients. All the FHL were used to fill the dead space left by tumor resection. Fourteen patients of them used skin paddle to repair mucous defects. One case used FHL to repair mucous defect because of the unavailable skin paddle. One case used both FHL and skin paddle to repair mucous and skin defect. The nFHL group had 38 patients and used skin paddle to repair mucous defects.

The FHL group had 2 cases used for maxillary reconstruction and 14 cases for mandibular reconstruction. The nFHL group had 38 cases all for mandibular reconstruction. The rates of mandibular were 0.00 and 12.50%; there was no significant difference ($P = 0.152$). In neck dissection, the FHL group had 7 cases, 2 cases of which were bilateral neck dissection. The nFHL group had 13 cases, 2 cases of which were bilateral neck dissection. The neck dissection rates were 43.75 and 34.21%; there was no significant difference ($P = 0.507$). In donor site, the FHL group had 9 cases in the right, 7 cases in the left. The nFHL group had 8 cases in the right and 30 cases in the left. The rate of the left was 43.75 and 57.89%. The difference was significant ($P = 0.011$). The mean overall operation time was higher in the FHL group (11.90 ± 2.55 h vs 8.91 ± 1.29 h) than nFHL group. The difference was significant ($P = 0.000$). The mean flap harvesting time was 118.63 ± 11.76 min in the FHL group. It was shorter than nFHL group, 125.74 ± 11.33 min. The difference was significant ($P = 0.042$). The mean length of the fibula was 19.94 ± 2.67 cm in FHL group. The nFHL group was 19.8 ± 2.88 cm. There was no significant difference ($P = 0.935$). The median size of skin paddle is 16.5 (range 0–96) cm^2 in FHL group. It was smaller than the nFHL group, 21(range 10–104) cm^2. The difference was significant ($P = 0.027$). Two cases in FHL group received skin grafting and 3 cases in nFHL group (see Table 2).

Postoperative data

The median total hospital days of FHL group were 21.5 (range 18–37) days. The nFHL group was 25.5 (range 15–71) days. There was no significant difference ($P = 0.095$). The median postoperative hospital days of FHL group was 12 (range 8–27) days, nFHL group was 12.5 (range 6–27) days. There was no significant difference ($P = 0.696$). The mean hospitalization expenses of FHL group were 71.29 ± 18.37 thousand yuan; nFHL group was 72.50 ± 19.57 thousand yuan. There was no significant difference ($P = 0.833$). We observed the patients'

Table 2 Operation data

	FHL group	nFHL group	P
Site			
Maxilla%	12.50% (2)	0.00% (0)	0.152
Mandible%	87.50% (14)	100.00% (38)	
Neck dissection%	43.75% (7)	34.21% (13)	0.507
Bilateral ND%	12.5% (2)	7.89% (3)	0.985
Donor side			
Left%	43.75% (7)	78.95% (30)	0.011*
Right%	56.25% (9)	21.05% (8)	
Skin-grafting%	12.5% (2)	7.89% (3)	0.985
Operation time (hour)	11.90 ± 2.55	8.91 ± 1.29	0.000*
Flap harvesting time (min)	118.63 ± 11.76	125.74 ± 11.33	0.042*
Fibula length (cm)	19.94 ± 2.67	19.87 ± 2.88	0.935
Skin paddle size (cm²)	16.5 (0–96)	21.0 (10–104)	0.027*

*Statistically significant ($P < 0.05$)

recovery condition after operation. All the flaps survived completely with the overall success rate of 100%. No vascular crisis happened in FHL group, and one case of vascular crisis happened in nFHL group. All patients were satisfied with the treatment and esthetics effect. In terms of perioperative complications, the main complication was infection. There were 5 cases of infection in the FHL group and 8 cases in the nFHL group. The infection rates were 31.25 and 21.05%. There was no significant difference ($P = 0.651$) (see Table 3).

Donor-site morbidity

As for donor-site morbidity, we had observed the morbidity of the FHL group. And as a contrast, we chose 16 patients of the nFHL group, of which the operation date was close to the FHL group. We thought that the follow-up time of the two groups was accordant. Eleven patients in FHL group and 12 patients in nFHL group received follow-up. Five patients in FHL group and 4 patients in nFHL group lost to follow-up because of being out of touch. The median follow-up time was 20 months (range 3–42 months) in FHL group. And the nFHL group is 16 months (range 3–41 months). Among 11 patients in FHL group, 9 patients were satisfied with the recovery of the feet. Among 12 patients in nFHL group, 10 patients were satisfied with the recovery of the feet. In the FHL group, 3 cases had gait abnormality, 3

Table 3 Postoperative data

	FHL group	nFHL group	P
Hospital days (day)	21.5(18–37)	25.5(15–71)	0.095
Postoperative hospital days (day)	12.0(8–27)	12.5(6–27)	0.696
Hospitalization expense (yuan)	71.29 ± 18.37	72.50 ± 19.57	0.833
Infection%	31.25%(5)	21.05%(8)	0.651

cases had claw toe, 2 cases had chronic pain, 2 cases had edema, and 1 case had weakness. In nFHL the group, 7 cases had claw toe, 4 cases had sensory deficit, 1 case had chronic pain, 1 case had gait abnormality, and 1 case had edema.

Above all, comparing the two groups, there were significant differences in the operation time, flap harvesting time, and skin paddle size. There were no significant differences in hospital days, postoperative hospital days, hospitalization expense, and rate of perioperative complications.

Compared with FFF without FHL, FFF-FHL will neither affect the use of flap nor bring more time cost, economic burden, and perioperative complications. The donor-site morbidity was slight.

In the operation, some emergency situations may happen. Here are two cases using FHL-FFF to repair the maxillary and mandibular extensive defect when dealing with the emergency situations.

Case 1

Case 1 is a male, 65 years old, having squamous cell carcinoma of upper gingiva.

The emergency situation in flap harvesting was the perforator vessel variation. When seeking perforator, we found that the perforator was not from the peroneal artery. It resulted in the unavailability of the skin paddle. The patient had both bone defect and soft tissue defect. We had to abandon the unavailable skin paddle and seek substitution to replace it. The operator flexibly used the FHL to close the intraoral defect (Fig. 3). The FFF was without skin paddle. To accelerate the intraoral mucosa forming, we used an artificial biological membrane to cover the myofascial surface of FHL and used an iodoform cotton wrapping for pressing. The skin paddle was sutured in situ. One week later, when we removed the iodoform cotton wrapping, the intraoral mucosa recovered well. (Fig. 4a–d) And the fibular flap survived and

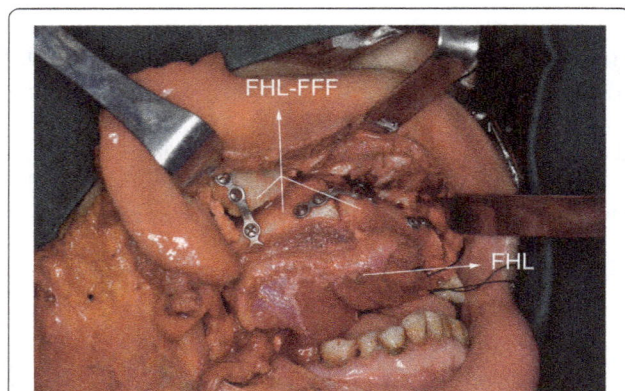

Fig. 3 FHL-FFF in repairing maxillary extensive defect: the FHL for intraoral defect

had no infection and necrosis. The patient was satisfied with the appearance and oral functional recovery.

Case 2

Case 2 is a male, 67 years old, having squamous cell carcinoma of lower gingiva.

The emergency situation in flap harvesting was not enough flap tissue volume. Beyond our expectation, the tumor violated the facial skin. When we removed the violated facial skin, the skin paddle could not meet the intraoral defect and facial defect simultaneously. The operator flexibly used skin paddle repair facial defect and used it as a extraoral "window" that made it convenient to observe flap survival (Figs. 5 and 6). The FHL was used to repair the intraoral defect. And in case 1, we used an artificial biological membrane and an iodoform cotton wrapping. Ten days later, the intraoral mucosa recovered well (Fig. 7a–c). And the fibular flap survived and had no infection and necrosis. The patient was satisfied with the appearance and oral functional recovery.

Discussion

The maxillary and mandibular extensive defects bring huge challenge in the reconstruction. Some epithelial benign tumors, such as ameloblastoma, will sometimes leave extensive osseous and soft tissue defects after tumor excision. The epithelial malignant tumors will accompany more extensive defects. The conventional FFF, consisting of fibula and skin paddle cannot fully fill the dead space after tumorectomy. In order to repair the extensive defects, we need to increase the size of skin paddle. When the size is more than 4 to 6 cm, it is difficult to suture the incision. It will increase the risks of wound dehiscence and compartment syndrome if we try to suture the incision [8, 9]. In 1986, Hidalgo mentioned that the FHL muscle can help fill the dead space and repair the defects [10].

The conventional FFF relies on skin paddle to repair soft tissue defect. The perforator vessel variation limits the use of skin paddle. Some skin paddles may be unavailable because of the miss of perforator vessel. Although FFF in the contralateral leg can be harvested, it will increase the damage and operation time. In our department, there was once a patient had to undergo another FFF because of the perforator of one leg was not found. In our study, we used a FHL-FFF without skin paddle to deal with perforator vessel variation.

The skin paddle has hair follicle and subcutaneous fat. Some patients feel annoyed because of the hair growing. The hair and wrinkled skin make it hard to stay clean in oral. The heavy subcutaneous fat has a poor influence on chewing and try-in of denture base and dental implant. The volume of skin paddle often needs to be

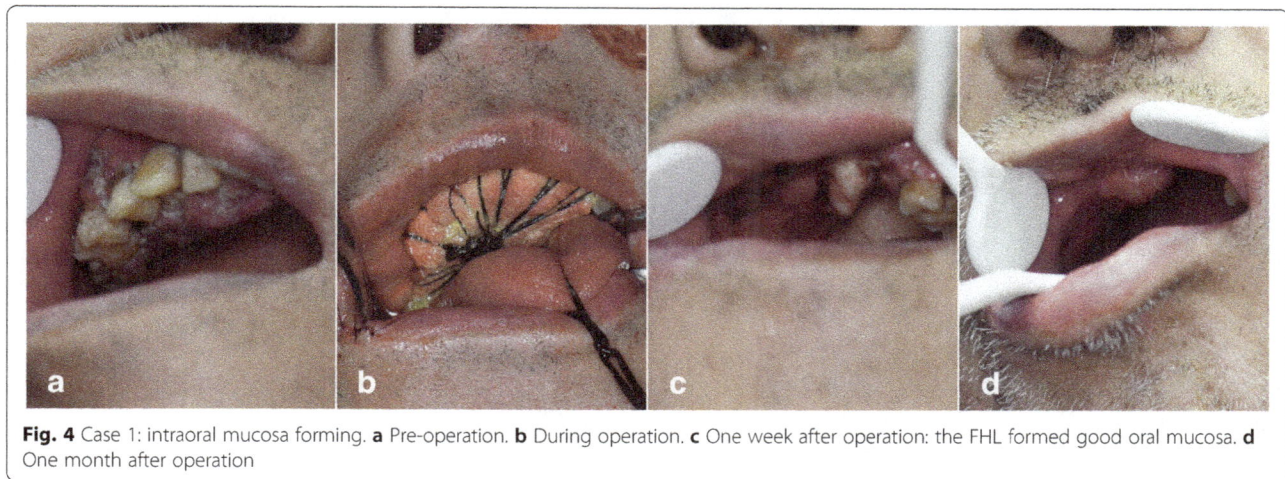

Fig. 4 Case 1: intraoral mucosa forming. **a** Pre-operation. **b** During operation. **c** One week after operation: the FHL formed good oral mucosa. **d** One month after operation

reduced to make denture and implant try-in smoothly [9]. In dental implant, the establishment and maintenance of a soft tissue seal around the transmucosal part of an implant is vital for implant treatment's success [11]. The skin paddle does not provide an appropriate peri-implant environment [11, 12]. It results in peri-implant mucositis and peri-implantitis and reduces lifetime of dental implant [11]. In our study, we used FHL to form good oral mucosa.

Summarized above conventional FFF's deficiencies, we find that the not enough flap tissue volume, perforator vessel variation, and poor oral mucous epithelization are the top three problems. To resolve these problems, we add the FHL in FFF.

To cope with the not enough flap tissue volume, we can harvest a FHL-FFF in advance for the preparation. In case 2, we harvested the FHL-FFF before the tumor resection. Owing to the FHL-FFF, we could repair the intraoral and extraoral defect simultaneously. To resolve the not enough tissue volume, some researchers raised the double and triple skin paddle FFF to reconstruct

defects [13–15]. The multi-skin paddle FFF may be a good solution for multi-defect of jaw. But it may increase operation time and the difficulty of operation. The harder close of donor site's incision and the uncertain perforators also limit the use of multi-skin paddle FFF.

To cope with the perforator vessel variation, we can seek perforators firstly. If the perforators cannot be used, we can immediately change the operation plan and turn to harvest a FHL-FFF. In case 1, if we did not have any preparation, the flap harvesting may fail because of perforator vessel variation. It proved that FHL-fibula flap could be survived without a skin paddle. A FFF without skin paddle can no doubt avoid the shortcoming of a skin paddle, while it loses the function of observation window of the skin paddle.

The two cases have formed good mucosa. It suggests that the FHL-FFF can resolve the problem of poor oral mucous epithelization. The use of artificial biological membrane is to protect the FHL from being exposed and accelerate mucous epithelization. The good mucosa is also helpful for the dental implant. When using the

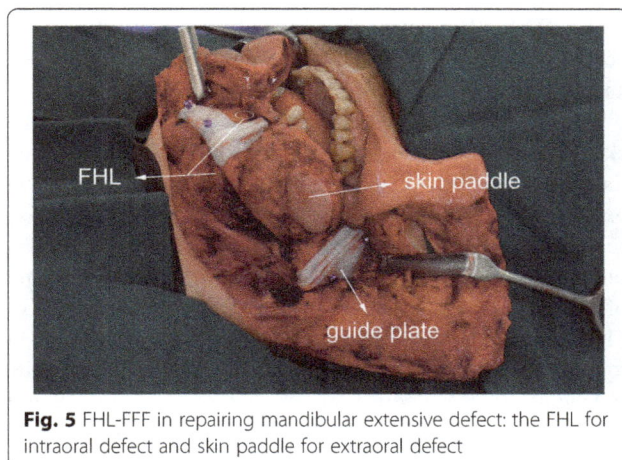

Fig. 5 FHL-FFF in repairing mandibular extensive defect: the FHL for intraoral defect and skin paddle for extraoral defect

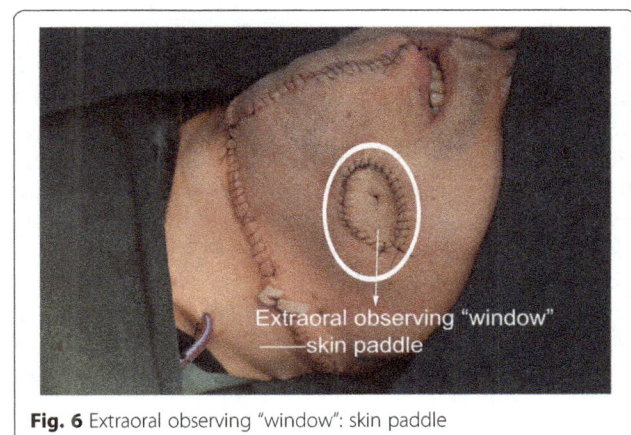

Fig. 6 Extraoral observing "window": skin paddle

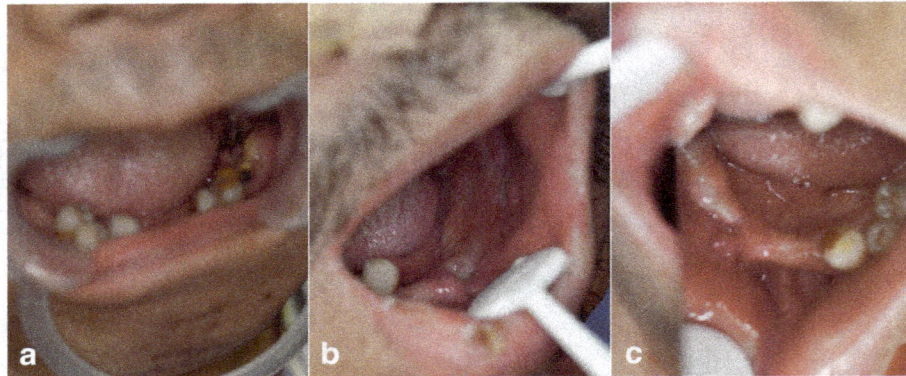

Fig. 7 Case 2: intraoral mucosa forming. **a** Pre-operation. **b** Two weeks after operation: the oral mucosa recovered well. **c** Three weeks after operation

FHL for good mucosa, the FHL covers on the fibula and muscular fasciae of FHL repair the mucosal defect. If we want to implant, we may need to reduce the muscle thickness. It needs further study cooperating with Oral Implantology Center.

The FFF with FHL has been reported since early time. In 1992, Schusterman et al. recommended that a cuff of soleus and flexor hallucis longus be incorporated into the flap to help ensure flap viability in using the osteocutaneous fibula flap [16]. In 1994, Hidalgo introduced that flexor hallucis longus muscle lay conveniently under the fibula to fill in the soft tissue defect in mandible reconstruction [4]. And in 1995, Hidalgo mentioned that flexor hallucis longus muscle was anatomically convenient for obliterating dead space in a review of 60 consecutive fibula free flap mandible reconstruction [10]. In 1997, Ruch et al. used the fibula-flexor hallucis longus osteomuscular flap to reconstruct a massive defect in limb salvage [17]. These were the early application of FHL-FFF. In 2001, Cho et al. studied the blood supply of osteocutaneous free fibula flap and found that it was recommended that a soleus and flexor hallucis longus muscle cuff be included to incorporate these perforators when designing an osteocutaneous free fibula flap 10 to 20 cm from the fibular head [18]. From Schusterman et al. and Cho et al.'s research, we can learn that the FHL incorporated into the flap can help raise the reliability of perforators. In 2002, Schoeller reported that they applied the reinnervated fibula-flexor hallucis longus free flap in the functional recovering and reconstruction after the Ewing sarcoma excision [19]. The function of upper limb recovered well. It proves that FHL-FFF has become a popular source of vascularized bone and skin for limb reconstructions. In 2003 and 2011, Peng and Mao et al. reported the use of free fibula-flexor hallucis longus myofascial flap in maxillary reconstruction [9, 20]. They found that the flexor hallucis longus myofascial flap could replace the skin paddle and improve the shortage

of the skin paddle. In their research, they used the flexor hallucis longus myofascial flap to repair the intraoral defect and the mucosa totally formed after 3 month. In our study, FHL has been proved to be able to repair the intraoral defect and the use of artificial biological membrane can accelerate the myofascial flap's mucosa forming. About 10 days after surgery, it can be found the mucosa totally forms. Through enough time to observe, the mucosa of FHL's surface is steady and safe (see Figs. 3a–d and 6a–c).

To review our control study, the carcinoma rate of FHL group was higher than nFHL group. Although the difference was not significant, in some degree, it suggests that the FHL-FFF may be better for large carcinoma. The overall operation time depends on multi factors, such as neck dissection. Although it is higher significantly in FHL group, in the flap harvesting time, it is shorter significantly in FHL group. The proportion of neck dissection, especially bilateral neck dissection, in FHL group was higher, which also suggests the FHL-FFF is better for large carcinoma. It suggests that the FHL-FFF can reduce the flap harvesting time. The reason is that we do not need to dissect the peroneal artery and FHL. So, the harvesting procedure is simplified. The size of skin paddle in FHL group was smaller significantly. It suggests that the FHL-FFF can reduce the dependency of skin paddle and reduce the loss of the leg skin. There were no significant differences in total hospital days, postoperative hospital days, and hospitalization expenses. It suggests that the FHL-FFF does not increase time cost and economic burden compared with FFF (without FHL). There was no significant difference in the rate of perioperative complications. It suggests that the FHL-FFF does not lead to more perioperative complications. As for the long-term complications, such as donor-site morbidity, it needs more follow-up study. In our present study, the donor-site morbidity is slight. Most patients were satisfied with the recovery of the feet. The more reliable results about morbidity depend on more patients and longer follow-up time.

The advantages of FHL-FFF are as follows: FHL can increase the volume of soft tissue and help fill the dead space and repair the defects. The FHL-FFF can simplify the flap harvesting operation and save time. The FHL can make FFF rely less on skin paddle and replace the skin paddle in some cases. The FHL incorporated into the flap can help raise the reliability of perforators. The FHL-FFF can form good mucosa.

The indication of FHL-FFF is an extensive bone defect with moderate soft tissue defect if we only use the FHL to fill dead space. If we want to use the muscular fasciae of FHL to repair the intraoral defect and form oral mucosa, the indication is more strict: an extensive bone defect with moderate soft tissue defect as well as limited mucosa defect. The reason is that the movability of FHL is poor because of the blood supply. For this reason, the FHL-FFF is not suitable for folding. The folding will have a bad influence on the blood supply of FHL and increase the risk of necrosis.

The influence of removing FHL on donor-site function still needs further study. The FHL helps curve the ankle joint and hallux. The removing of FHL may have some influence on FHL function. Sassu said that nerve injury to the FHL muscle is unlikely during fibula flap harvest [21]. In 2014, van den Heuvel reported that free fibula flap donor site morbidity in terms of hallux function is independent of the inclusion or exclusion of the FHL muscle in the flap [22]. Another prospective study about the influence on patients' quality of life with/without FHL in the flap has been performed by us. The data at present suggests that the FHL-FFF has not brought more functional loss and more complication. We believe more reliable conclusions will be reached soon.

Overall, the retrospective study weakens the strength of this study. The limits of this study are obvious. The population is too small. The follow-up study is barely satisfactory. The case of maxillary defect is too small. In our further study, we will add more patients and raise reliability of the study.

Conclusions

FHL-FFF can be flexibly used in the reconstruction of the maxillary and mandibular extensive defect. FHL-FFF can provide more tissue volume and be used in larger carcinoma and emergency situation for perforator vessel variation as well as forming good mucosa. Furthermore, the simple and convenient flap harvesting makes it fitter for younger surgeons to conduct.

Acknowledgements
Thanks to all who have contributed and all the patients in our research.

Funding
This research was supported by grants from the National Natural Science Foundation of China grant (No.81372877), Excellent Talent Fund Project of Higher Education Liaoning province (LJQ2014087), Doctoral Scientific Research Launching Fund Project of Liaoning province (No. 201501002), Scientific project of Shenyang City (No. 17-230-9-12), Basic scientific research projects of colleges of Liaoning Province (No. LQNK201725), Key research and development guidance program in Liaoning Province (No. 2017225037), and Youth Science and Technology Innovation Plan of Shenyang city (RC170489).

Authors' contributions
YN collected the data and wrote the paper. PL, ZY, and WW collected the data. WDai, Z-zQ, WDuan, Z-fX, and C-fS modified the paper. FL contributed to the concept design and guided in writing. All authors read and approved the final manuscript.

Competing interests
The authors declare that they have no competing interests.

References
1. Taylor GI, Miller GD, Ham FJ. The free vascularized bone graft. A clinical extension of microvascular techniques. Plast Reconstr Surg. 1975;55:533.
2. Hidalgo DA. Fibula free flap: a new method of mandible reconstruction. Plast Reconstr Surg. 1989;84:71.
3. Sadove RC, Powell LA. Simultaneous maxillary and mandibular reconstruction with one free osteocutaneous flap. Plast Reconstr Surg. 1993;92:141.
4. Hidalgo DA. Fibula free flap mandible reconstruction. Microsurgery. 1994;15:238.
5. Coghlan BA, Townsend PL. The morbidity of the free vascularised fibula flap. Br J Plast Surg. 1993;46:466.
6. Xu ZF, Bai S, Zhang ZQ, Duan WY, Wang ZQ, Sun CF. A critical assessment of the fibula flap donor site. Head Neck. 2017;39:279.
7. Al QMM, Boyd JB. "Mini paddle" for monitoring the fibular free flap in mandibular reconstruction. Microsurgery. 1994;15:153.
8. Berzofsky C, Shin E, Mashkevich G. Leg compartment syndrome after fibula free flap. Otolaryngol Head Neck Surg. 2013;148:172.
9. Mao C, Peng X, Yu GY, Guo CB, Huang MX. A preliminary study of maxillary reconstruction using free fibula-flexor hallucis longus myofascial flap. Zhonghua Kou Qiang Yi Xue Za Zhi. 2003;38:401.
10. Hidalgo DA, Rekow A. A review of 60 consecutive fibula free flap mandible reconstructions. Plast Reconstr Surg. 1995;96:585.
11. Carbiner R, Jerjes W, Shakib K, Giannoudis PV, Hopper C. Analysis of the compatibility of dental implant systems in fibula free flap reconstruction. Head Neck Oncol. 2012;4:37.
12. Raoul G, Ruhin B, Briki S, et al. Microsurgical reconstruction of the jaw with fibular grafts and implants. J Craniofac Surg. 2009;20:2105.
13. Chang EI, Yu P. Prospective series of reconstruction of complex composite mandibulectomy defects with double island free fibula flap. J Surg Oncol. 2017;116:258.
14. Jones NF, Vögelin E, Markowitz BL, Watson JP. Reconstruction of composite through-and-through mandibular defects with a double-skin paddle fibular osteocutaneous flap. Plast Reconstr Surg. 2003;112:758.
15. Maciejewski A, Szymczyk C, Wierzgoń J. Triple skin island fibula free flap: a good choice for combined mandibular and tongue defect reconstruction. J Reconstr Microsurg. 2008;24:461.
16. Schusterman MA, Reece GP, Miller MJ, Harris S. The osteocutaneous free fibula flap: is the skin paddle reliable. Plast Reconstr Surg. 1992;90:787.
17. Ruch DS, Koman LA. The fibula-flexor hallucis longus osteomuscular flap. J Bone Joint Surg Br. 1997;79:964.
18. Cho BC, Kim SY, Park JW, Baik BS. Blood supply to osteocutaneous free fibula flap and peroneus longus muscle: prospective anatomic study and clinical applications. Plast Reconstr Surg. 2001;108:1963.
19. Schoeller T, Wechselberger G, Meirer R, Bauer T, Piza-Katzer H, Ninković M. Functional osteomuscular free-tissue transfer: the reinnervated fibula-flexor hallucis longus free flap. Plast Reconstr Surg. 2002;109:253.
20. Peng X, Mao C, Yu GY, et al. Functional maxillary reconstruction with free composite fibula flap. Beijing Da Xue Xue Bao. 2011;43:18.

14

Differences in gene mutations according to gender among patients with colorectal cancer

Yi-Jian Tsai[1], Sheng-Chieh Huang[1,2], Hung-Hsin Lin[1,2], Chun-Chi Lin[1,2], Yuan-Tzu Lan[1,2], Huann-Sheng Wang[1,2], Shung-Haur Yang[1,2], Jeng-Kai Jiang[1,2], Wei-Shone Chen[1,2], Tzu-chen Lin[1,2], Jen-Kou Lin[1] and Shih-Ching Chang[1,2]* (iD)

Abstract

Background: The incidence, site distribution, and mortality rates of patients with colorectal cancer differ according to gender. We investigated gene mutations in colorectal patients and wanted to examine gender-specific differences.

Methods: A total of 1505 patients who underwent surgical intervention for colorectal cancer were recruited from March 2000 to January 2010 at Taipei Veterans' General Hospital and investigated for gene mutations in K-ras, N-ras, H-ras, BRAF, loss of 18q, APC, p53, SMAD4, TGF-β, PIK3CA, PTEN, FBXW7, AKT1, and MSI.

Results: There were significant differences between male and female patients in terms of tumor location ($p < 0.0001$) and pathological stage ($p = 0.011$). The female patients had significantly more gene mutations in BRAF (6.4 vs. 3.3%, OR 1.985, $p = 0.006$), TGF-β (4.7 vs. 2.5%, OR 1.887, $p = 0.027$), and revealed a MSI-high status (14.0 vs. 8.3%, OR 1.800, $p = 0.001$) than male patients. Male patients had significantly more gene mutations in N-ras (5.1 vs. 2.3%, OR 2.227, $p = 0.012$); however, the significance was maintained only for mutations in BRAF (OR 2.104, $p = 0.038$), MSI-high status (OR 2.003 $p = 0.001$), and N-ras (OR 3.000, $p = 0.010$) after the groups were divided by tumor site.

Conclusion: Gene mutations in BRAF, MSI-high status, and N-ras differ according to gender among patients with colorectal cancer.

Keywords: Colorectal cancer, Gender, Gene mutation

Background

Although the colorectal mucosa and colorectal cancer are morphologically identical in genders, gender-specific differences in incidence, site distribution, and mortality rates of colorectal cancer are evident. These differences were thought to be related with hormonal factors, e.g., estrogen level, or behavioral factors, e.g. nutritional habits, physical activity, and alcohol consumption [1, 2]. Previous studies revealed postmenopausal women treated with estrogen replacement therapy have a significant reduction in both risk and rate of developing colon cancer, [3] and estrogen

* Correspondence: changsc@vghtpe.gov.tw
[1]Division of Colon and Rectal Surgery, Department of Surgery, Taipei-Veterans General Hospital, No 201,Sec 2, Shih-Pai Rd, 11217 Taipei, Taiwan
[2]Department of Surgery, Faculty of Medicine, National Yang-Ming University, Taipei, Taiwan

exposure is a protective factor against microsatellites instability (MSI), while the lack of estrogen in older women increased the risk of MSI-high colon cancer [4]. Alcohol consumption may affect the risk of colorectal cancer and rectal cancer, particularly in men [5].

A recent review on the clinical and molecular characteristics of colon cancer revealed a higher incidence of right-sided colon cancer in women than in men [6, 7]. In addition, high status MSI, CpG island methylator phenotype (CIMP), and BRAF mutations are often observed in right-sided colon cancer [1, 2]. On the other hand, chromosomal instability, which is associated with 60 to 70% cases of colorectal cancer, is more often observed in left sided colon cancer and defective genes include adenomatous polyposis coli (APC), K-ras, deleted in colorectal cancer (DCC), and p53 [8]. Our goal was to identify gender-specific molecular differences, especially current known colorectal-cancer-related gene mutation, in colorectal cancer, and determine its association with the side of tumor distribution.

Methods

Study setting and population

This was a retrospective cohort study. Cases were retrieved from the database of the Division of Colorectal Surgery, Taipei Veterans General Hospital. Patients with adenocarcinoma of the colon and rectum, undergoing curative resections, were retrieved. Clinical information that had been prospectively obtained and stored in the database included age, gender, TNM stage, differentiation, location of tumor, pathological prognostic features, personal and family medical history, and follow-up conditions. The right-sided colon was defined as the colon between the cecum and the splenic flexure of the colon. The left sided colon was defined as the colon from the splenic flexure to rectum. Patients who had undergone preoperative chemo-radiotherapy, emergent operations, or who were dead within 30 days of surgery were excluded. In addition, definite germline mutations of MMR genes were noted in 30 patients, and they were also excluded.

Collection of tumor tissue

All patients gave their informed consent for inclusion before tissue collection before the operation and sample collection. The study was conducted in accordance with the Declaration of Helsinki, and the protocol was approved by the Ethic Committee of Institutional Review Board of Taipei Veterans General Hospital in Taiwan.(no. 2013–04-042B) Tumors were dissected and collected from different quadrants of the tumors and were then snap frozen in liquid nitrogen. Samples were stored at the Taipei Veterans' General Hospital Biobank.

DNA isolation and quantification

Samples were obtained from the Biobank for the study. DNA was extracted from the sample using the QIAamp DNA Tissue Kit (Qiagen, Valencia, CA, USA) according to the manufacturer's protocol. The purity and quantity of DNA were confirmed using Nanodrop ND-1000 Spectrophotometer (Thermo Scientific, Wilmington, DE, USA).

MassArray-based mutation characterization

According to hotspots found in previous studies and the Catalogue of Somatic Mutations in Cancer (COSMIC) database, The MassDetect colorectal cancer (CRC) panel (v2.0) was designed, enabling the identification of 139 mutations in 12 genes. The primers of polymerase chain reaction (PCR) and extension for the mutations were made with the MassArray Assay Design 3.1 software (Sequenom, San Diego, CA, USA). Multiplexed reactions were spotted onto SpectroCHIP II arrays, DNA fragments were resolved electrophoretically on MassArray Analyzer 4 System (Sequenom, USA), and the spectrum was analyzed (Typer 4.0 software (Sequenom, USA)) to detect mutations.

We defined a putative mutation as one with a 5% abnormal signal and then filtered it by manual review. Sanger sequencing was performed to confirm any detected mutation in BRAF, KRAS, and NRAS. The concordance was 99.1% using MassArray and Sanger sequencing.

MSI analysis

As international criteria, we used D5S345, D2S123, BAT25, BAT26, and D17S250 as reference microsatellite markers for the determination of MSI, and obtained the primer sequences for these genes from GenBank [9] The detection of MSI was done as previously described. We defined high status MSI as samples with more than or equal to 2 MSI markers, and microsatellite stability as those with 1 or without an MSI marker.

Statistical analysis

Patient baseline characteristics, including age, gender, tumor site, tumor staging were collected. The patients were divided according to gender. Then, each gene mutation was tested by Pearson's chi-square test to find the difference between the two groups. All p values are two-sided and are considered significant if they are less than .05. The demographic data between two the groups were checked with Pearson chi-square test to identify any possible confounding factors. Data management was done using SPSS software, version 22. (IBM Corp. Armonk, NY, USA).

Results

From March 2000 to January 2010, 1505 patients were recruited from the database. The demographic data of patients are presented in Table 1.

Most of our patients were men (65.8%), and the median age at diagnosis was 72.17 years. The tumors were most often located on left side of the colon and rectum (73.4%), and only 6% of patients had a poorly differentiated histopathological grade. Most patients were at pathological TNM stages II (37.5%) and III (31.4%). The stage IV patients accounted for 17% of all patients. There were significant differences between male and female patients in terms of tumor location ($p < 0.0001$) and pathological stage ($p = 0.011$). For example, the female group had more right-sided tumors, more stage III patients, and less stage II patients. The female patients had significantly higher number of BRAF gene mutations (6.4 vs. 3.3%, OR 1.985, $p = 0.006$), TGF-β mutations (4.7 vs. 2.5%, OR 1.887, $p = 0.027$), and revealed a higher MSI status (14.0 vs. 8.3%, OR 1.800, $p = 0.001$) than male patients. (Table 2).

Table 1 Demographic data of patients

			Men	Women
Gender				
Men	990	65.8%		
Women	515	34.2%		
Age (years)				$p < 0.001$
Median(range)	72.17	28~107	73.95 (28~107)	67.20 (31~95)
≤ 70 years	646	42.9%	355 (35.9%)	291 (56.5%)
> 70 years	859	57.1%	635 (64.1%)	224 (43.5%)
Pathological staging				$p = 0.011$
I	212	14.1%	132 (13.3%)	80 (15.5%)
II	564	37.5%	399 (40.3%)	165 (32.0%)
III	473	31.4%	291 (29.4%)	182 (35.3%)
IV	256	17.0%	168 (17.0%)	88 (17.1%)
Tumor localization				$p < 0.0001$
Right colon	400	26.6%	232 (23.4%)	168 (32.6%)
Left colon and rectum	1105	73.4%	758 (76.6%)	347 (67.4%)
Histopathology grade				$p = 0.368$
Well and moderately differentiated	1417	94.2%	936 (94.5%)	481 (93.4%)
Poorly differentiated	88	5.8%	54 (5.5%)	34 (6.6%)

Male patients had significantly higher gene mutations in N-ras (5.1 vs. 2.3%, OR 2.227, $p = 0.012$) than female patients. (Table 3).

We then separated the patients according to tumor sides and performed the same statistical analysis. The female patients still had a high number of gene mutations in BRAF (OR 2.104, $p = 0.038$), MSI-high status (OR 2.003 $p = 0.001$) at right side colon, (Table 4), and the male still had a high number of gene mutations in N-ras (OR 3.000, $p = 0.010$) (Table 5).

Discussion

Several studies have revealed that certain genetic and epigenetic differences between sexes may determine colorectal cancer risk. A recent systemic review reported that the proportion of women presenting with right-sided colon cancer, which is often at a more advanced stage at diagnosis, was higher than men [7]. Hendifar et al. reported that in patients with metastatic colorectal cancer, women were more likely to have right-sided or proximal lesion [10]. In our study, the female group was more likely to have right-sided

colon cancer and more female patients were at stage III at diagnosis. This is consistent with previous studies.

Our study revealed that there is a gender-specific difference in patients with colorectal cancer regarding gene mutations of BRAF, N-ras, and high status MSI. Sporadic MSI/MMR-deficient (dMMR) colorectal cancer is associated with the BRAF V600E mutation, though its association with CIMP (CpG island methylator phenotype) [11] has been reported. In addition, an earlier study reported that female patients were 8.8 times more likely than male patients to have methylation-positive cancers [12], and previously published studies suggested that [13–15] sporadic MSI/dMMR metastatic colorectal cancer occurred more in female patients. Our study revealed that females had significantly more gene mutations than males in terms of high status MSI and BRAF which has been suggested in previous reports. Breivik et al. reported MSI tumors were more common among old women and younger men [16]. Lindblom reviewed previous study and concluded that estrogen may have a protective effect for MSI cancer in women and a possible mechanism could be an increased methylation. We have also performed further analysis toward gender, age, and MSI status in our study, no significant statistical difference was found in patients below 70 years for MSI

Table 2 Genes with higher mutation rate in female patients

Gene mutation	F vs. M	OR	CI 95%	p value
BRAF	6.4 vs. 3.3%	1.985	1.211~3.256	0.006
TGF-β	4.7 vs. 2.5%	1.887	1.066~3.338	0.027
MSI-high status	14.0 vs. 8.3%	1.800	1.286~2.519	0.001

F female, *M* male, *OR* odds ratio, *CI* confidence interval

Table 3 Genes with higher mutation rate in male patients

Gene mutation	M vs. F	OR	CI 95%	p value
N-ras	5.1 vs. 2.3%	2.227	1.176~4.219	0.012

M male, *F* female, *OR* odds ratio, *CI* confidence interval

Table 4 Genes with higher mutation rate in female patients after divided by tumor side

Gene mutation	Right side			Left side		
	OR	CI 95%	p value	OR	CI 95%	p value
BRAF	2.104	1.030~4.298	0.038	1.514	0.739~3.101	0.254
TGF-β	1.897	0.895~4.020	0.091	1.280	0.500~3.280	0.606
MSI-high status	2.003	1.212~3.311	0.006	1.349	0.835~2.179	0.220

OR odds ratio, *CI* confidence interval

tumor by genders.(p = 0.334) And the female older than 70 years had 2.45 times risk for MSI tumors than men. ($p < 0.001$).

The approximate frequency of N-ras mutations in colorectal adenocarcinoma is 2 to 8% [17–21]. The frequency in our study was 4.1%, which is consistent with previous studies; however, the significance between genders was not seen in previous reports. While some gender-specific differences were noted in our study, no other chromosomal instability-related genes demonstrated gender-specific differences.

Besides, for the interests in early-onset colorectal cancer (EOCRC) patients, we have done subgroup analysis for EOCRC. EOCRCs are disproportionately located in the distal colon, and there is a longer interval between symptoms and diagnosis [22]. In our study, 63 patients (4.2%) are below 50 years old. Distal distribution was noted (left colon, including rectum, 77%; rectum, 41%), and there was a trend that increased incidence rectal cancer in more men than in women, but there is no statistical significance (p = 0.124).

Due to retrospective design and single center data, the study has its inherited limitation. Our databases did not query menopausal status, history of hormone replacement therapy, or contraceptive use; therefore, this limited our ability to investigate its interaction with our findings.

Conclusions

Gene mutations in high status MSI, BRAF, and N-ras differ according to gender among patients with colorectal cancer. No other chromosomal instability-related genes demonstrated gender-specific differences. Hormone status may play role in the development and pathogenesis of colorectal cancer and warrant further studies to determine it.

Table 5 Genes with higher mutation rate in male patients after divided by tumor side

Gene mutation	Right side			Left side		
	OR	CI 95%	p value	OR	CI 95%	p value
N-ras	1.472	0.541~4.000	0.446	3.000	1.256~7.142	0.010

OR odds ratio, *CI* confidence interval

Abbreviations
APC: Adenomatous polyposis coli; CI: Confidence interval; CIMP: CpG island methylator phenotype; CRC: Colorectal cancer; DCC: Deleted in colorectal cancer; MSI: Microsatellite instability; PCR: Polymerase chain reaction; PI3K: Phosphoinositol-3-kinase; TGF-β: Transforming growth factor beta; TNM: Tumor-node-metastasis

Funding
This research was funded by grants from the Taipei Veterans General Hospital, (V101E2–005) Department of Health, Taipei City Government (10401-62-031; 10601-62-059), and Ministry of Science and Technology, Taiwan (105-2314-B-075-010 -MY2).

Authors' contributions
Y-JT analyzed the data and drafted the manuscript. S-CH, H-HL, C-CL, Y-TL, H-SW, S-HY, W-SC, J-KJ, T-cL, and J-KL carried out collecting patients' records and samples. S-CC conceived and designed the experiments and completed the manuscript. All authors read and approved the final manuscript.

Competing interests
The authors declare that they have no competing interests.

References
1. DeCosse JJ, Ngoi SS, Jacobson JS, Cennerazzo WJ. Gender and colorectal cancer. Eur J Cancer Prev. 1993;2:105–15.
2. Kim SE, Paik HY, Yoon H, Lee JE, Kim N, Sung MK. Sex- and gender-specific disparities in colorectal cancer risk. World J Gastroenterol. 2015;21:5167–75.
3. Rossouw JE, Anderson GL, Prentice RL, LaCroix AZ, Kooperberg C, Stefanick ML, Jackson RD, Beresford SA, Howard BV, Johnson KC, et al. Risks and benefits of estrogen plus progestin in healthy postmenopausal women: principal results from the Women's Health Initiative randomized controlled trial. JAMA. 2002;288:321–33.
4. Slattery ML, Potter JD, Curtin K, Edwards S, Ma KN, Anderson K, Schaffer D, Samowitz WS. Estrogens reduce and withdrawal of estrogens increase risk of microsatellite instability-positive colon cancer. Cancer Res. 2001;61:126–30.
5. Longnecker MP. A case-control study of alcoholic beverage consumption in relation to risk of cancer of the right colon and rectum in men. Cancer Causes Control. 1990;1:5–14.
6. Benedix F, Kube R, Meyer F, Schmidt U, Gastinger I, Lippert H, Colon/rectum carcinomas study G. Comparison of 17,641 patients with right- and left-sided colon cancer: differences in epidemiology, perioperative course, histology, and survival. Dis Colon Rectum. 2010;53:57–64.
7. Hansen IO, Jess P. Possible better long-term survival in left versus right-sided colon cancer - a systematic review. Dan Med J. 2012;59:A4444.
8. Missiaglia E, Jacobs B, D'Ario G, Di Narzo AF, Soneson C, Budinska E, Popovici V, Vecchione L, Gerster S, Yan P, et al. Distal and proximal colon cancers differ in terms of molecular, pathological, and clinical features. Ann Oncol. 2014;25:1995–2001.
9. Genbank. https://blast.ncbi.nlm.nih.gov/Blast.cgi, accessed on 24 June 2014.
10. Hendifar A, Yang D, Lenz F, Lurje G, Pohl A, Lenz C, Ning Y, Zhang W, Lenz HJ. Gender disparities in metastatic colorectal cancer survival. Clin Cancer Res. 2009;15:6391–7.
11. Colle R, Cohen R, Cochereau D, Duval A, Lascols O, Lopez-Trabada D, Afchain P, Trouilloud I, Parc Y, Lefevre JH, et al. Immunotherapy and patients treated for cancer with microsatellite instability. Bull Cancer. 2017; 104:42–51.

12. Wiencke JK, Zheng S, Lafuente A, Lafuente MJ, Grudzen C, Wrensch MR, Miike R, Ballesta A, Trias M. Aberrant methylation of p16INK4a in anatomic and gender-specific subtypes of sporadic colorectal cancer. Cancer Epidemiol Biomark Prev. 1999;8:501–6.

13. Cohen R, Buhard O, Cervera P, Hain E, Dumont S, Bardier A, Bachet JB, Gornet JM, Lopez-Trabada D, Dumont S, et al. Clinical and molecular characterisation of hereditary and sporadic metastatic colorectal cancers harbouring microsatellite instability/DNA mismatch repair deficiency. Eur J Cancer. 2017;86:266–74.

14. Tran B, Kopetz S, Tie J, Gibbs P, Jiang ZQ, Lieu CH, Agarwal A, Maru DM, Sieber O, Desai J. Impact of BRAF mutation and microsatellite instability on the pattern of metastatic spread and prognosis in metastatic colorectal cancer. Cancer. 2011;117:4623–32.

15. French AJ, Sargent DJ, Burgart LJ, Foster NR, Kabat BF, Goldberg R, Shepherd L, Windschitl HE, Thibodeau SN. Prognostic significance of defective mismatch repair and BRAF V600E in patients with colon cancer. Clin Cancer Res. 2008;14:3408–15.

16. Breivik J, Lothe RA, Meling GI, Rognum TO, Borresen-Dale AL, Gaudernack G. Different genetic pathways to proximal and distal colorectal cancer influenced by sex-related factors. Int J Cancer. 1997;74:664–9.

17. Cercek A, Braghiroli MI, Chou JF, Hechtman JF, Kemeny N, Saltz L, Capanu M, Yaeger R. Clinical features and outcomes of patients with colorectal cancers harboring NRAS mutations. Clin Cancer Res. 2017;23:4753–60.

18. Scott AJ, Lieu CH, Messersmith WA. Therapeutic approaches to RAS mutation. Cancer J. 2016;22:165–74.

19. Schirripa M, Cremolini C, Loupakis F, Morvillo M, Bergamo F, Zoratto F, Salvatore L, Antoniotti C, Marmorino F, Sensi E, et al. Role of NRAS mutations as prognostic and predictive markers in metastatic colorectal cancer. Int J Cancer. 2015;136:83–90.

20. Vaughn CP, Zobell SD, Furtado LV, Baker CL, Samowitz WS. Frequency of KRAS, BRAF, and NRAS mutations in colorectal cancer. Genes Chromosomes Cancer. 2011;50:307–12.

21. Irahara N, Baba Y, Nosho K, Shima K, Yan L, Dias-Santagata D, Iafrate AJ, Fuchs CS, Haigis KM, Ogino S. NRAS mutations are rare in colorectal cancer. Diagn Mol Pathol. 2010;19:157–63.

22. Patel SG, Ahnen DJ. Colorectal Cancer in the Young. Curr Gastroenterol Rep. 2018;20:15. https://doi.org/10.1007/s11894-018-0618-9.

15

Patient Blood Management improves outcome in oncologic surgery

Vivienne Keding[1], Kai Zacharowski[2], Wolf O. Bechstein[1], Patrick Meybohm[2†] and Andreas A. Schnitzbauer[1*†]

Abstract

Background: Patient Blood Management (PBM) is a systematic quality improving clinical model to reduce anemia and avoid transfusions in all kinds of clinical settings. Here, we investigated the potential of PBM in oncologic surgery and hypothesized that PBM improves 2-year overall survival (OS).

Methods: Retrospective analysis of patients 2 years before and after PBM implementation. The primary endpoint was OS at 2 years after surgery. We identified a sample size of 824 to detect a 10% improvement in survival in the PBM group.

Results: The analysis comprised of 836 patients that underwent oncologic surgery, 389 before and 447 after PBM, was implemented. Patients in the PBM+ presented significantly more frequent with normal hemoglobin values before surgery than PBM− (56.6 vs. 35.7%; $p < 0.001$). The number of transfusions was significantly reduced from 5.5 ± 11.1 to 3.0 ± 6.9 units/patient ($p < 0.001$); moreover, the percentage of patients being transfused during the clinic stay was significantly reduced from 62.4 to 40.9% ($p < 0.001$). Two-year OS was significantly better in the PBM+ and increased from 67.0 to 80.1% ($p = 0.001$). A normal hemoglobin value (> 12 g/dl in female and > 13 g/dl in male) before surgery (HR 0.43, 95% CI 0.29–0.65, $p < 0.001$) was the only independent predictive factor positively affecting survival.

Conclusions: PBM is a quality improvement tool that is associated with better mid-term surgical oncologic outcome. The root cause for improvement is the increase of patients entering surgery with normal hemoglobin values.

Keywords: Patient Blood Management, Oncologic surgery, Transfusion

Background

The discussion of whether a liberal or restrictive transfusion regimen adversely or positively affects the patient outcome is long lasting in medicine. In 1999, Hébert et al. published one of the first randomized controlled trials showing that a restrictive strategy of red-cell transfusion is at least as effective as a liberal transfusion strategy in critically ill patients [1]. Other authors confirmed these findings for different indications, e.g., septic shock and large cohorts detected the application of already 1 unit of blood as an independent risk factor for increased morbidity and mortality [2, 3]. Recently, a large national initiative was launched in Germany: the so-called Patient Blood Management project to increase patient safety. In a first prospective analysis in surgical patients, it was shown that more careful handling of red blood cells with adjusted and strict triggers for transfusion did not increase morbidity and mortality. Moreover, an algorithmic approach to minimize anemia before surgery in patients scheduled for elective surgery was established. All these measures together led to a significant reduction in the application of blood products, resulting in a relevant potential for economization [4–6]. Specifically, Meybohm et al. and other authors showed that the use of 1 unit of blood during general surgical procedures already led to an increase in morbidity and mortality of patients [7].

Besides the clinical and economic evidence of PBM, transfusions may also have immunologic effects that increase morbidity and mortality, e.g., an enhanced recurrence rate after tumor resection [8]. Dixon et al. named the RBC transfusion rate as a neglected potential quality parameter of outcome in oncologic surgery

* Correspondence: andreas.schnitzbauer@kgu.de
†Patrick Meybohm and Andreas A. Schnitzbauer contributed equally to this work.
[1]Clinic for General and Visceral Surgery, University Hospital Frankfurt, Goethe University Frankfurt/Main, Theodor-Stern-Kai 7, 60590 Frankfurt/Main, Germany
Full list of author information is available at the end of the article

[9]. Nevertheless, there is no clinical evidence that a structured program of PBM may lead to an improved long-term outcome in oncologic surgery [10]. Therefore, we analyzed all patients undergoing elective surgery for oncologic indications. We hypothesized that there is a consistent improvement in 2 years overall survival of at least 10% after PBM implementation.

Methods

Patient selection, the period of evaluation and data-collection, endpoints

All consecutive inpatients (aged ≥ 18 years) undergoing abdominal oncologic surgery were included in the analysis, 24 months before and after implementation of PBM at University Hospital Frankfurt [4]. The cutoff date for the implementation of PBM was on July 1, 2013.

ICD-10- and OPS-codes had to refer to malignant disease. If a patient had multiple hospital admissions during the study period, only the first hospital stay was included to avoid overlap. Surgical procedures were classified according to the German surgery and procedure classification, based on the International Classification of Procedures in Medicine.

Data collected were age, gender, indications for resection (hepatobiliary, colorectal liver metastases, pancreatic, gastric, intestinal, esophagus, primary other and metastasis other), history of concomitant disease in accordance with ICD10 coding (cardiovascular I00-I99, pulmonic J00-J99, endocrine E00-E35, gastrointestinal K00-K93, renal N00-N29, hematologic D50-D90, malignant other C00-C97, infection A00-B99), hemoglobin prior to and post surgery, percentage of patients with a normal hemoglobin value prior to and post surgery, number of RBC units transfused until hospital discharge, percentage of patients receiving at least 1 RBC unit, the complication rate in accordance with the classification of Dindo and Clavien as well as 30-day, 90-day, and overall survival rates. The ethics review board (Ethikkommission des Fachbereichs Medizin) granted permission for analysis (number 218/17, dated July 17, 2017).

The primary endpoint was 2-year overall survival. Secondary endpoints were 30-day and 90-day survival, the percentage of patients with anemia, number of RBC units transfused, the percentage of patients with RBC transfusion, and complication rates following the classification of Dindo and Clavien [11].

Intervention––Patient Blood Management

Patient Blood Management is a clinical quality program. The implementation of a structured Patient Blood Management included six bundles. As a first bundle, dedicated project management with involvement of crucial PBM stakeholders was founded. Education included undergraduate and post graduate teaching as well as the establishment of local standards and protocols. Moreover, bundle 2 consisted of specific diagnosis and treatment of anemia. Bundle 3 focused on management of coagulopathy during surgery. Bundles 4 and 5 mainly yielded at the reduction of diagnostic-associated blood loss and reduction of surgery associated blood loss. Finally, outcome measures were defined in bundle 6 including the endpoints targeted in this study. Exact information can be obtained in the English version of https://www.patientbloodmanagement.de/en/pbm-bundles/ and was published by the group elsewhere [12]. The PBM program focused on preoperative optimization of hemoglobin levels, blood-sparing techniques, standardization of transfusion practice, and regular education sessions. Compliance with guideline-based transfusion triggers was supervised by electronic-based checklists, in which the indication of each RBC transfusion had to be documented in the patient's record.

In brief, if a patient has a hemoglobin value of < 12 (f) or < 13 (m) g/dl and the transfusion probability is > 10%, iron status is measured. In case iron deficiency as the leading course for anemia was present, iron i.v. was supplemented. Intraoperative and postoperative thresholds for transfusion were adjusted to hemoglobin < 6 g/dl in the absence of other triggers like shock or dyspnea and 6 to 8 g/dl in case a patient has specific risk factors or signs for hypoxia. These bundles applied for the indication of every single transfused RBC. The exact algorithm is displayed in the Additional file 1: Figures S1 and S2.

Data management and statistical analysis

Data were extracted from the electronic patient charts. For survival data, the University Cancer Center database was used to identify patient follow-up and status. In case a patient was lost to follow up, the date of the last known and documented status was used. To estimate the power, sample size calculations for the validity of the findings were made based on 2-year overall survival data. We estimated that the average 2-year overall survival probability was 70% for all surgical oncologic procedures. Considering a 10% benefit in patients with PBM, a two-sided alpha-value of 0.05, and a beta-value of 0.20 reflecting the power of 80%, overall 824 patients were necessary for analysis.

Differences in demographics were detected using paired t tests, Fisher's exact test, and the Pearson X^2 test. Demographic data are given as means with standard deviation or distribution in percentage between the groups. Kaplan-Meier-estimations were used to detect differences in 2-year, 30-day, and 90-day overall survival between the groups. Patients dying within 2 years after surgery were censored for death; patients lost to follow up were censored alive on the day of the last follow-up. Univariate and multivariate analysis were performed using COX regression analysis with stepwise backward

Results

Patients and baseline demographics

Between July 1, 2011, and July 1, 2015, a total of 7041 cases were treated in the Clinic for Abdominal and Visceral Surgery at University Hospital Frankfurt. A total of 6662 surgeries were coded and performed. Of those, 836 patients were treated for malignant diagnosis and underwent oncological surgery with a curative approach. Of the 836 patients included, 389 were included in the pre-PBM cohort (PBM−) and 447 in the PBM cohort (PBM+). Indications are displayed in Table 1 and were equally distributed between groups.

Overall survival of patients

Mean overall follow-up was 43.6 ± 1.5 months in PBM− and 34.1 ± 0.8 months in PBM+ associated with significant differences in overall survival of 61.6 and 78.6% ($p < 0.001$).

Two-year overall survival was 73.9% in all patients, 66.8% in PBM−, and 80.1% in PBM+ ($p = 0.001$). In total, 129 patients died in PBM− and 89 patients in PBM+ within 2 years after surgery (Fig. 1). Notably, 30-day and 90-day mortality rates were not different between the investigated groups (92.8 vs. 91.9%; $p = 0.595$ and 85.7 vs. 87.7%; $p = 0.444$). Patients that were transfused had a significantly better 2-year overall survival (87.5 vs. 61.0%, $p < 0.001$). The trend was consistent in both the PBM-era (90.7 vs. 64.7%, $p < 0.001$) and in the non-PBM-era (81.6 vs. 58.2%, $p < 0.001$) (Fig. 2). However, there was a large transfusion sparing effect of more than 20% after the PBM program was introduced.

Secondary endpoints

There was a definite trend towards higher hemoglobin levels in the PBM+ group before surgery, which is an effect of the structured quality program. The number of patients with normal hemoglobin was significantly higher in PBM+ (56.6 vs. 35.7%, $p < 0.001$). The number of transfused RBCs/patient was significantly lower in the PBM+ group (5.5 ± 11.1 vs. 3.0 ± 6.9; $p < 0.001$), and the number

Table 1 Demographic data, indications, concomitant disease, pre-surgical anemia, and numbers of RBC transfusions

	Cumulative N = 836		PBM− N = 389		PBM+ N = 447		p value
Age (years)			64.8 ± 13.6		66.9 ± 12.4		0.019
Gender (m/f) (%)	508 (63.1%)	328 (39.2%)	216 (55.5%	173 (44.5%)	292 (65.3%)	155 (34.6%)	0.004
Indication							
Hepatobiliary	212 (25.7%)		92 (23.7%)		120 (26.8%)		0.06
Pancreatic	80 (9.5%)		48 (12.3%)		32 (7.1%)		0.09
CRLM	273 (32.6%)		136 (35.0%)		137 (30.6%)		1.00
Upper GI	99 (11.8%)		54 (13.9%)		45 (10.0%)		0.42
Intestinal	112 (13.4%)		38 (9.8%)		74 (16.6%)		0.001
Primary other	22 (2.6%)		14 (3.6%)		8 (1.8%)		0.29
Metastases other	38 (4.5%)		7 (1.8%)		31 (6.8%)		< 0.001
Concomitant disease							
Cardiovascular	437 (52.6%)		212 (54.5%)		225 (51.0%)		0.229
Pulmonic	86 (10.1%)		48 (12.3%)		38 (8.3%)		0.068
Endocrine	232 (27.6%)		97 (25.1%)		135 (29.8%)		0.090
Gastrointestinal	319 (38.1%)		178 (45.8%)		141 (31.5%)		< 0.001
Renal	71 (8.4%)		24 (6.1%)		47 (10.3%)		0.034
Hematologic	50 (6.0%)		27 (7.2%)		23 (5.0%)		0.246
Infection	84 (10.3%)		38 (9.7%)		46 (10.7%)		0.802
Hemoglobin prior to surgery (g/dl)			11.9 ± 2.2		12.5 ± 1.9		< 0.001
Hemoglobin before surgery normal			139 (35.7%)		253 (56.6%)		< 0.001
RBCs transfused per patient			5.5 ± 11.1		3.0 ± 6.9		< 0.001
Patients receiving at least 1 RBC			242 (62.4%)		180 (40.9%)		< 0.001
Complications DC > 3a (major)	142 (16.9%)		70 (17.9%)		72 (16.0%)		0.463

PBM Patient Blood Management, *CRLM* colorectal liver metastases, *GI* gastrointestinal, *RBC* red blood cells, *DC* Dindo-Clavien

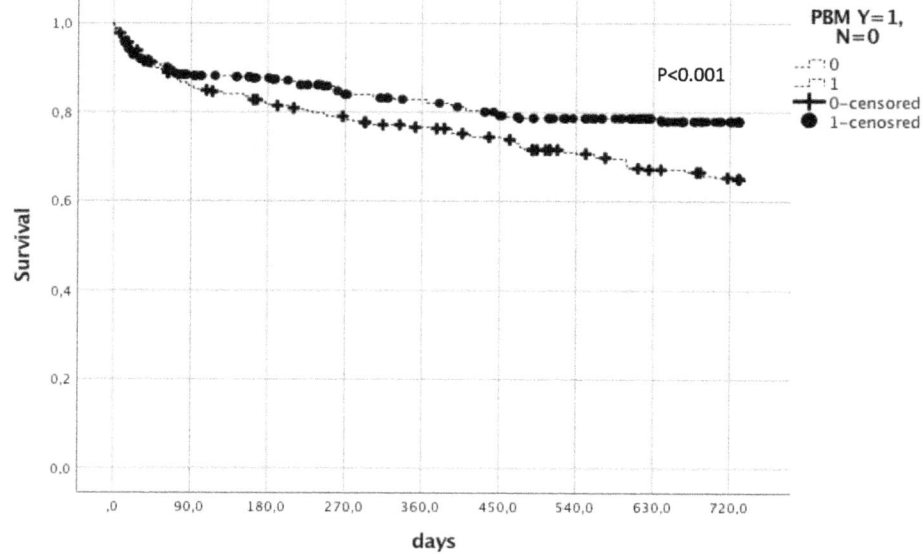

Fig. 1 Two-year overall survival comparing patients with and without Patient Blood Management

of transfused patients was also significantly lower (62.4 to 40.9%; $p < 0.001$). Complications (Dindo-Clavien>IIIa) were not different between the groups.

Age, gastrointestinal concomitant disease, normal hemoglobin before surgery, complications, and the number of transfused RBCs are independent predictors for 2-year overall survival

Univariate analysis identified 11 factors that were associated with outcome. Factors being significant were included in a multivariate analysis, which revealed

increasing age (HR 1.02, 95% CI 1.00–1.04, $p = 0.008$), the presence of gastrointestinal concomitant disease (HR 1.86, 95% CI 1.26–2.76, $p = 0.002$), the number of transfusions/patient (HR 1.03, 95% CI 1.00–1.05, $p = 0.023$), and the presence of major surgical complications (HR 7.52, 95% CI 4.50–12.57, $p < 0.001$) as independent risk factors for death; a normal hemoglobin value before surgery (HR 0.43, 95% CI 0.29–0.65, $p < 0.001$) was associated with improved overall survival (Table 2). A ROC analysis revealed an AUC-ROC of 0.595 for age and 0.729 for the number of transfused RBC units. For the number of units

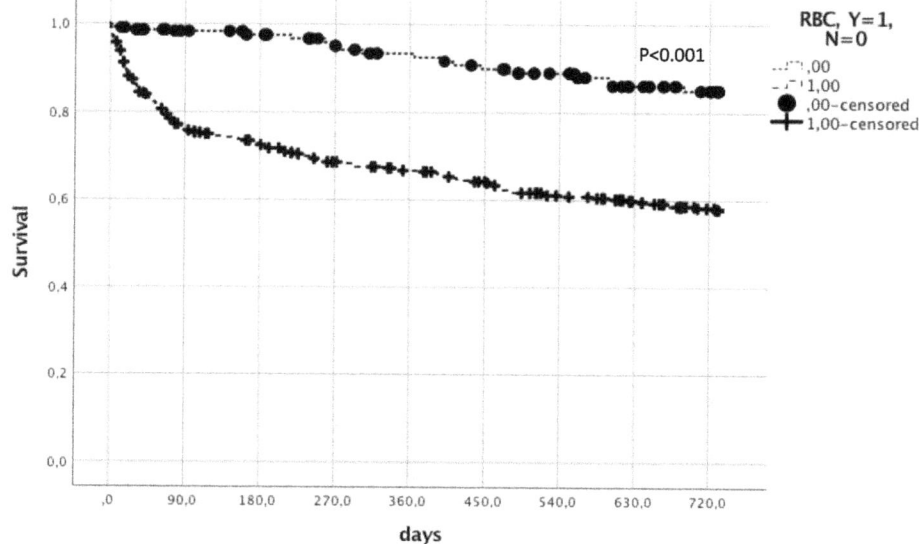

Fig. 2 Two-year overall survival comparing patients with and without transfusion. PBM Patient Blood Management, Y yes, N no, RBC red blood cells

Table 2 COX regression analysis of univariate and multivariate factors influencing 2-year overall survival

Parameter	Univariate analysis				Multivariate analysis			
	HR	95% CI lower	95% CI upper	p value	HR	95% CI lower	95% CI upper	p value
Age (years)	1.03	1.015	1.039	< 0.001	1.02	1.00	1.04	0.02
Gender	0.94	0.71	1.25	0.68				
Transfusion of RBC	3.53	2.55	4.87	< 0.001	0.77	0.39	1.54	0.46
Endocrine concomitant disease	0.98	0.71	1.33	0.87				
GI concomitant disease	2.07	1.56	2.73	< 0.001	1.68	1.1	2.57	0.016
Hematologic concomitant disease	1.21	0.67	2.17	0.53				
Infection concomitant disease	0.95	0.60	1.49	0.81				
Cardiovascular concomitant disease	0.94	0.71	1.25	0.68				
Renal concomitant disease	1.61	1.01	2.56	0.04	1.32	0.68	2.57	0.42
Pulmonic concomitant disease	0.80	0.49	1.30	0.37				
Malignancy concomitant disease	1.63	1.24	2.16	0.001	0.88	0.52	1.48	0.62
PBM yes	0.66	0.50	0.90	0.006	0.89	0.48	1.65	0.71
Hemoglobin prior surgery	0.83	0.74	0.93	0.001	0.98	0.80	1.19	0.80
Hemoglobin post surgery	0.66	0.57	0.76	< 0.001	0.94	0.80	1.12	0.50
Hemoglobin prior surgery normal	0.49	0.32	0.75	0.001	0.48	0.31	0.74	0.001
Hb post surgery normal	1.40	0.70	2.78	0.34				
Complications > DC IIIA without V	8.90	6.69	11.85	< 0.001	12.39	7.88	19.48	< 0.001
Total number of RBCs	1.1	1.04	1.06	< 0.001	1.02	0.99	1.04	0.21

HR hazard ratio, *CI* confidence interval, *GI* gastrointestinal, *PBM* Patient Blood Management

transfused, a cutoff of 1 unit of transfusion was identified as a threshold for impaired survival reflecting a sensitivity of 75% and a specificity of 61%.

Subgroup analysis
Patients with minor complications may profit most from PBM
In total, 705 (84.3%) patients experienced minor complications (<Dindo-Clavien IIIb), (384 in PBM+ and 321 in PBM−). Two hundred ninety-seven patients in the minor-complication group (42%) were transfused, whereas 408 (58%) did not receive an RBC. Patients with minor complications had better oncologic outcome in the PBM+ (88.3 vs. 75.7%; $p < 0.001$) and without being transfused (88.7 vs. 74.1%; $p < 0.001$).

Notably, 142 patients (16.9%) experienced major complications (>Dindo-Clavien IIIa), of which 134 (94%) received at least one transfusion. Major complications were present in 70 patients in PBM− and 73 in PBM+. When patients experienced major complications, overall survival decreased, independently from RBC transfusion (33.3 vs. 32.1%; $p = 0.669$) or PBM−/PBM+ (37.0 vs. 27.1%; $p = 0.850$).

PBM improved 2-year overall survival for the majority of indications
Regarding indications, there was an improvement in survival after 2 years for mostly all indications after PBM

($p = 0.001$). Liver diseases without colorectal liver metastases (CRLM) improved from 63.0 to 69.2% and CRLM from 71.3 to 85.4%. Overall survival for pancreatic malignancies improved from 56.3 to 68.8%, for upper-GI-indications from 71.7 to 84.8% for gastric cancer, and from 37.5 to 58.3% for esophageal cancer. Intestinal and colorectal cancer indications improved from 68.4 to 91.9%. Results for other cancers (78.6 to 87.5%) and other metastases (71.4 to 83.9%) were also improved.

Discussion
In this retrospective analysis of > 800 patients undergoing oncologic surgery, the implementation of a structured PBM program led to a significant reduction in RBC transfusion requirements. This reduced need for transfusions was associated with a significantly improved 2-year survival by 15%, while short-term surgical outcomes were not affected. Transfusion thus may be an early determinant on late outcome. The number of patients receiving RBC could be significantly reduced (20%) after PBM implementation, and the number of patients starting with normal hemoglobin was significantly higher in the PBM cohort, which reduced the risk for 2-year mortality by 50%. In patients with minor complications, the benefit of PBM could also be proven. Uncritical transfusion practice in these patients, however, was associated with adverse outcome.

In contrast, patients with significant complications had a dramatically decreased survival rate of about 30–35%. Almost all patients received at least one transfusion. In most patients, transfusion was necessary in case of a life-threatening condition, e.g., massive bleeding. Not surprisingly, major complications were associated with adverse outcome, while PBM and transfusion practice had no additional impact on survival.

In the literature, transfusions were associated with increased morbidity and mortality. Sutton et al. described an adverse outcome in pancreatic cancer (overall survival: 14 vs. 21 months) [13]. Other authors confirmed this for various indications: Martin et al. (CRLM: odds ratio (OR) 4.18, 95% CI 2.18–8.02) and mortality (OR 14.5, 95% CI 3.08–67.8) [14], Schiergens et al. (reduced recurrence-free survival (32 vs. 72 months in CRLM) [15], and Reim et al. (gastric cancer: hazard ratio (HR) 1.31, 95% CI 1.01–1.69) [16]. However, these findings were based on dichotomization of data and not on the introduction of a structured program to reduce transfusions, which is the crucial difference to our work. Our investigation concentrated on a real-life scenario of an era with Patient Blood Management that aims at minimization of perioperative transfusions and compares it with an era where this program has not been present in our clinic. Data in the non-transfusion group thus may even be better. However, the systematic introduction of PBM (still including patients with transfusions, but reduced by 20%) naturally reached similar results than cohorts with no transfusion at all, by avoiding transfusions in patients that have an increased risk instead of benefit from sometimes––necessary blood supplementation in daily clinical practice.

This is reflected by beneficial survival data for individual indications, which were also in good agreement with data in the literature: Jarnagin et al. (intrahepatic and perihilar cholangiocarcinoma, 63 and 69% [17]; Zaydfudim et al. (hepatocellular carcinoma, 6059 [18]; Schiergens et al. and Margonis et al. (CRLM 68% with transfusion and 82% without transfusion) [15, 19]; esophageal cancer (40% with transfusion vs. 60% without transfusion) [20]; gastric cancer (82 vs. 60%) [16]; and pancreatic cancer (50 to 60% vs. 20%) [13, 21]. Last not least, Mörner et al. showed that anemia and transfusions were associated with adverse outcome [22]. Moreover, Mörner and also Wilson stress that pre-surgical normal hemoglobin is an essential reducer for the risk of death after surgery, which is also in perfect agreement with our data [22, 23].

Nonetheless, there are some limitations to the study, like its retrospective nature in however without selection for indications or concomitant disease. Positively, the sample size calculation aimed at analysis of 845 patients to be able to detect a significant difference of at least

10% in overall survival. Therefore, this retrospective single-center cohort is a good indicator of the potential of PBM. Undoubtedly, the awareness for a responsive transfusion practice has sustainably been established. Where other studies describe a benefit of restricted transfusion regimens more as a coincidental finding, this is the first report in which a complete system in a clinic was changed, and results of this change by otherwise stable conditions can be shown.

From a clinical perspective, our policy is that every surgical procedure has to be at least assisted by a board-certified surgeon and that steps of every operation have to be assisted whenever possible. Data from various analysis of the American NSQIP database show that outcomes are not influenced by resident involvement [24]. Moreover, every patient requires presentation in a multidisciplinary tumor board. As we are one of two German University Clinics that are certified for every abdominal tumor by the German Cancer Society, our pre-therapeutic discussion rate in multidisciplinary boards is close to 100%. Post procedural multidisciplinary boards and annual audits by the German Cancer Society for recertification do not show personnel or oncologic indication-specific variations.

Unfortunately, the mechanisms that lead to the improved outcome in the oncologic surgical cohort after PBM remain unclear and speculative. In general, the assumed immunologic effects of long-term improvement are unclear and not backed-up by refined translational clinical trials of the mechanisms leading to tumor growth, tethering and dissemination caused by transfusion, or a complicated clinical course. Goubran et al. therefore called for substantial retrospective data analysis and well-designed prospective translational trials to clarify the yet unclear mechanisms of transfusion-tumor interaction on an immunologic level [25].

Conclusion

In conclusion, this retrospective analysis shows that a complex PBM program focusing on normal hemoglobin before surgery, multimodal blood-sparing techniques, and a rationale transfusion regimen improve outcome after oncologic surgery. Presumed that evidence will be further increased, PBM may be a future key element of long-term patient safety and outcome in a multidisciplinary setting of oncologic surgery.

Authors' contributions
VK collected data, performed data analysis, wrote the manuscript, and interpreted the data. KZ and WOB gave significant input in the discussion of the data. PM gave significant input in the discussion of data and wrote the manuscript. AAS performed data analysis, wrote the manuscript, and generated the idea of analysis. All authors read and approved the final manuscript.

Competing interests
The authors declare that they have no competing interests.

Author details
[1]Clinic for General and Visceral Surgery, University Hospital Frankfurt, Goethe University Frankfurt/Main, Theodor-Stern-Kai 7, 60590 Frankfurt/Main, Germany. [2]Department of Anesthesiology, Intensive Care Medicine, and Pain Therapy, University Hospital Frankfurt, Goethe University Frankfurt, Frankfurt/Main, Germany.

References

1. Hébert PC, Wells G, Blajchman MA, Marshall J, Martin C, Pagliarello G, et al. A multicenter, randomized, controlled clinical trial of transfusion requirements in critical care. Transfusion Requirements in Critical Care Investigators. Canadian Critical Care Trials Group N Engl J Med. 1999;340:409–17.

2. Holst LB, Haase N, Wetterslev J, Wernerman J, Guttormsen AB, Karlsson S, et al. Lower versus higher hemoglobin threshold for transfusion in septic shock. N Engl J Med. 2014;371:1381–91.

3. Whitlock EL, Kim H, Auerbach AD. Harms associated with single unit perioperative transfusion: retrospective population-based analysis. BMJ. 2015;350:h3037.

4. Meybohm P, Fischer DP, Geisen C, Müller MM, Weber CF, Herrmann E, et al. Safety and effectiveness of a Patient Blood Management (PBM) program in surgical patients—the study design for a multi-center prospective epidemiologic non-inferiority trial. BMC Health Serv Res. 2014;14:576.

5. Meybohm P, Herrmann E, Steinbicker AU, Wittmann M, Gruenewald M, Fischer D, et al. Patient Blood Management is associated with a substantial reduction of red blood cell utilization and safe for patient's outcome: a prospective, multicenter cohort study with a noninferiority design. Ann Surg. 2016;264:203–11.

6. Meybohm P, Fischer D, Schnitzbauer A, Zierer A, Schmitz-Rixen T, Bartsch G, et al. Patient blood management: current state of the literature. Chir Z Alle Geb Oper Medizen. 2016;87:40–6.

7. Bernard AC, Davenport DL, Chang PK, Vaughan TB, Zwischenberger JB. Intraoperative transfusion of 1 U to 2 U packed red blood cells is associated with increased 30-day mortality, surgical-site infection, pneumonia, and sepsis in general surgery patients. J Am Coll Surg. 2009;208:931–7. 937-2-939

8. Acheson AG, Brookes MJ, Spahn DR. Effects of allogeneic red blood cell transfusions on clinical outcomes in patients undergoing colorectal cancer surgery: a systematic review and meta-analysis. Ann Surg. 2012;256:235–44.

9. Dixon E, Datta I, Sutherland FR, Vauthey J-N. Blood loss in surgical oncology: neglected quality indicator? J Surg Oncol. 2009;99:508–12.

10. Ecker BL, Simmons KD, Zaheer S, Poe S-LC, Bartlett EK, Drebin JA, et al. Blood transfusion in major abdominal surgery for malignant tumors: a trend analysis using the National Surgical Quality Improvement Program. JAMA Surg. 2016;151:518–25.

11. Dindo D, Demartines N, Clavien P-A. Classification of surgical complications: a new proposal with evaluation in a cohort of 6336 patients and results of a survey. Ann Surg. 2004;240:205–13.

12. Meybohm P, Richards T, Isbister J, Hofmann A, Shander A, Goodnough LT, et al. Patient Blood Management bundles to facilitate implementation. Transfus Med Rev. 2017;31:62–71.

13. Sutton JM, Kooby DA, Wilson GC, Squires MH, Hanseman DJ, Maithel SK, et al. Perioperative blood transfusion is associated with decreased survival in patients undergoing pancreaticoduodenectomy for pancreatic adenocarcinoma: a multi-institutional study. J Gastrointest Surg Off J Soc Surg Aliment Tract. 2014;18:1575–87.

14. Martin AN, Kerwin MJ, Turrentine FE, Bauer TW, Adams RB, Stukenborg GJ, et al. Blood transfusion is an independent predictor of morbidity and mortality after hepatectomy. J Surg Res. 2016;206:106–12.

15. Schiergens TS, Rentsch M, Kasparek MS, Frenes K, Jauch K-W, Thasler WE. Impact of perioperative allogeneic red blood cell transfusion on recurrence and overall survival after resection of colorectal liver metastases. Dis Colon Rectum. 2015;58:74–82.

16. Reim D, Strobl AN, Buchner C, Schirren R, Mueller W, Luppa P, et al. Perioperative transfusion of leukocyte depleted blood products in gastric cancer patients negatively influences the oncologic outcome: a retrospective propensity score weighted analysis on 610 curatively resected gastric cancer patients. Medicine (Baltimore). 2016;95:e4322.

17. Jarnagin WR, Shoup M. Surgical management of cholangiocarcinoma. Semin Liver Dis. 2004;24:189–99.

18. Zaydfudim VM, McMurry TL, Harrigan AM, Friel CM, Stukenborg GJ, Bauer TW, Adams RB, Hedrick TL. Improving treatment and survival: a population-based study of current outcomes after a hepatic resection in patients with metastatic colorectal cancer. HPB (Oxford). 2015;17(11):1019–24.

19. Margonis GA, Kim Y, Samaha M, Buettner S, Sasaki K, Gani F, et al. Blood loss and outcomes after resection of colorectal liver metastases. J Surg Res. 2016;202:473–80.

20. Reeh M, Ghadban T, Dedow J, Vettorazzi E, Uzunoglu FG, Nentwich M, et al. Allogenic blood transfusion is associated with poor perioperative and long-term outcome in esophageal cancer. World J Surg. 2017;41:208–15.

21. Hwang HK, Jung MJ, Lee SH, Kang CM, Lee WJ. Adverse oncologic effects of intraoperative transfusion during pancreatectomy for left-sided pancreatic cancer: the need for strict transfusion policy. J Hepato-Biliary-Pancreat Sci. 2016;23:497–507.

22. Mörner MEM, Edgren G, Martling A, Gunnarsson U, Egenvall M. Preoperative anaemia and perioperative red blood cell transfusion as prognostic factors for recurrence and mortality in colorectal cancer—a Swedish cohort study. Int J Color Dis. 2017;32:223–32.

23. Wilson MJ, van Haaren M, Harlaar JJ, Park HC, Bonjer HJ, Jeekel J, et al. Long-term prognostic value of preoperative anemia in patients with colorectal cancer: a systematic review and meta-analysis. Surg Oncol. 2017;26:96–104.

24. Saliba AN, Taher AT, Tamim H, Harb AR, Mailhac A, Radwan A, et al. Impact of Resident Involvement in Surgery (IRIS-NSQIP): looking at the bigger picture based on the American College of Surgeons-NSQIP database. J Am Coll Surg. 2016;222:30–40.

25. Goubran HA, Elemary M, Radosevich M, Seghatchian J, El-Ekiaby M, Burnouf T. Impact of transfusion on cancer growth and outcome. Cancer Growth Metastasis. 2016;9:1–8.

16

Diffusion-weighted imaging in monitoring the pathological response to neoadjuvant chemotherapy in patients with breast cancer

Wen Gao[1], Ning Guo[2] and Ting Dong[3*] [iD]

Abstract

Background: Diffusion-weighted imaging (DWI) is suggested as an non-invasive and non-radioactive imaging modality in the identification of pathological complete response (pCR) in breast cancer patients receiving neoadjuvant chemotherapy (NACT). A growing number of trials have been investigating in this aspect and some studies found a superior performance of DWI compared with conventional imaging techniques. However, the efficiency of DWI is still in dispute. This meta-analysis aims at evaluating the accuracy of DWI in the detection of pCR to NACT in patients with breast cancer.

Methods: Pooled sensitivity, specificity, and diagnostic odds ratio (DOR) were drawn to estimate the diagnostic effect of DWI to NACT. Summary receiver operating characteristic curve (SROC), the area under the SROC curve (AUC), and Youden index (*Q) were also calculated. The possible sources of heterogeneity among the included studies were explored using single-factor meta-regression analyses. Publication bias and quality assessment were assessed using Deek's funnel plot and QUADAS-2 form respectively.

Results: Twenty studies incorporated 1490 participants were enrolled in our analysis. Pooled estimates revealed a sensitivity of 0.89 (95% CI, 0.86–0.91), a specificity of 0.72 (95% CI, 0.68–0.75), and a DOR of 27.00 (95% CI, 15.60–46.73). The AUC of SROC curve and *Q index were 0.9088 and 0.8408, respectively. The results of meta-regression analyses showed that pCR rate, time duration of study population, and study design were not the sources of heterogeneity.

Conclusion: A relatively high sensitivity and specificity of DWI in diagnosing pCP for patients with breast cancer underwent NACT treatment was found in our meta-analysis. This finding indicated that the use of DWI might provide an accurate and precise assessment of pCR to NACT.

Keywords: Neoadjuvant chemotherapy, Breast cancer, Diffusion-weighted imaging, Pathological response, Meta-analysis

Background

Neoadjuvant chemotherapy (NACT), since its first appearance until nowadays, has become a standard therapy for patients with breast cancer. It is suggested to have beneficial effect especially on locally advanced or inflammatory breast cancer [1]. The major benefit of NACT is to reduce the tumor size and to downstage the tumor burden, which may lead to the successful performance of breast-conserving surgery instead of mastectomy [2]. In addition, assessing the treatment responses to NACT can also help to determine the right time to perform the operation or to adjust the therapy regimen in case of an unfavorable tumor response at an early stage [3]. It is well-established in some previous studies that the response to NACT is correlated with long-term outcomes for breast cancer patients. Studies also reveal that pathological complete response (pCR) patients may have a superior chance to achieved disease-free survival and overall survival [4–6]. Nevertheless, only a minority of patients were featured with pCR due to the heterogeneity of breast cancer. We could not accurately

* Correspondence: tingdong666@126.com
[3]Department of Cardiovascular Medicine, Guizhou Provincial People's Hospital, No. 83 Zhongshandong Road, Guiyang City 550002, Guizhou, China
Full list of author information is available at the end of the article

observe the pCR until the definitive breast surgery was completed, which always led to inappropriate surgery decision-making for patients [7, 8]. Therefore, it is crucial to find an effective method to separate the patients who have achieved pCR from pathological non-responders (pNR) before surgery.

Mammography, ultrasonography, positron emission tomography-computed tomography (PET/CT) and magnetic resonance imaging (MRI) are the most commonly applied conventional imaging techniques for the detection of NACT responses. Previous studies found that MRI was superior to mammography or ultrasonography in evaluating therapeutic response of NACT in breast cancer [9, 10]. A meta-analysis demonstrated a higher sensitivity in PET/CT and a higher specificity in MRI for the assessment of pCR [11]. Currently, contrast-enhanced magnetic resonance imaging (DCE-MRI) is frequently and commonly used for tumor response evaluation after NACT. However, the information provided by DCE-MRI regarding blood flow and vessel permeability might cause difficulty in differentiating viable residual cancer form surrounding scar, necrosis, fibrosis, or reactive inflammation resulting from NACT response. Thus, DCE-MRI has deficiencies for the examination of pathological response to NACT [12].

Diffusion-weighted imaging (DWI), with its unique tissue contrast mechanism, is regarded as a potential modality to overcome the limitations of traditional DCE-MRI evaluation [13]. DWI reveals the thermally driven motion of water molecules in the target tissue. It offers information concerning the integrity of cell membranes and cancer cellularity. The apparent diffusion coefficient (ADC), which can be quantified and measured on DWI, represents the complex diffusion of water in tissues [14]. With those characteristics, DWI can be sensitive in detecting the changes in the intratumor induced by NACT [15].

The accuracy of conventional imaging modality including MRI, PET/CT, mammography, and ultrasonography in the assessment of the pCR to NACT has been investigated by several recent meta-analyses [16–19]. However, no previous study has focused on analyzing the performance of DWI in detecting the pCR in breast cancer to NACT systematically. In researches providing DWI evaluation, the data were limited. They only involved a small amount of studies which might weaken the statistic power of the analysis. By combining all available data, the present meta-analysis intended to evaluate the diagnostic role of DWI in monitoring pCR in breast cancer to NACT.

Method
Literature search
Databases PubMed and EMBASE were systematically searched from database inception to August 2017 for all the potential publications. Articles in regard to DWI assessing tumor response in patients with breast cancer underwent NACT treatment were retrieved using the following search terms: "diffusion-weighted imaging" or "DW-MRI" or "DWI," "breast cancer" or "breast tumor" or "breast," "response" or "prediction," "neoadjuvant chemotherapy" or "chemotherapy" or "NACT," "diagnosis" or "accuracy" or "performance." One reviewer screened all the titles and abstracts for eligibility. The remaining studies after removing the duplications and non-related articles were examined in full text by a second reviewer. Reference list of the enrolled studies and other meta-analyses were searched manually for any additional publication that was not included in the original search. Articles published in English and Chinese were eligible for inclusion.

Eligibility criteria
Studies were considered as usable if they met the following criteria: (1) patients were diagnosed with breast cancer and received NACT treatment; (2) DWI scan should be performed before and during (after) NACT; (3) studies provided available data of true positive (TP), true negative (TN), false positive (FP), false negative (FN), sensitivity and specificity findings, either directly or indirectly; (4) studies that with different additional surgery or other adjunctive treatment were all considered available. We excluded studies with inseparable combined data of different diagnostic methods, duplicated articles, reviews, case reports, and other non-related studies.

Data extraction
The following information were extracted in the process of full-text review of the eligible studies: first author, region where the study took place, year of publication, patients' demographic (sample size, gender, age) and clinical characteristics (disease stages, histologic subtype), chemotherapeutic regimens used in NACT, cycles of NACT, image interpretation (blinded or not), magnet strength of DWI, timing of DWI evaluation, applied surgery after NACT, reference standard of pathologic response, definition of pCR, and number of complete responders and non-responders. The number of TP, TN, FP, and FN was obtained from the pathological results of the DWI scan. Two independent reviewers carried out the data extraction process, and discrepancies were solved by discussion till consensus was reached.

Quality assessment
The updated version of quality assessment of diagnosis accuracy study form (QUADAS-2) was used in the assessment of methodological quality of the enrolled studies. This appliance was specifically developed for systematic review and meta-analysis of diagnostic accuracy studies [20]. The QUADAS-2 test contains four aspects of questions: patients' selection, index text, reference standard, and flow and timing. Risk of bias was assessed in all fields,

and the concerns regarding applicability was evaluated in the first three domains. The signaling questions of each key domain can help in judging studies as having high, low, or unclear risk.

Statistical analysis

A 2-by-2 contingency table separating patients into TP, TN, FP, and FN groups was constructed for each enrolled study. Based on this table, sensitivity and specificity were calculated. Diagnostic odds ratio (DOR) was measured to estimate the effectiveness of DWI by calculating the odds of achieving pCR in patients with a positive test result to patients with a negative test result. The area under the curve (AUC) of the summary receiver operating characteristic curve (SROC) was calculated to measure the performance of DWI. An AUC close to 1 indicates a favorable diagnostic performance, whereas a close to 0.5 AUC implies a poor test result. The Youden index (*Q), which is used in conjunction with SROC analysis and recognized as a preferred statistic to reflect the diagnostic value, were also assessed. A *Q index of 1 indicates a perfect test result. All data analyses were carried out using statistical software package Meta-DiSc 1.4 and Stata version 15.0.

The heterogeneity among studies was evaluated with chi-squared test and I^2 statistics. A random effects model was used for outcome estimation if $I^2 < 50\%$, and a fixed effects model was chosen if $I^2 > 50\%$. Threshold effect was one of the important sources of heterogeneity in diagnostic accuracy test. The Spearman correlation coefficients can determine the existence of threshold effect. It indicated no threshold effects among studies if P value > 0.05. Then, the bivariate mixed-effect models were used to draw the forest plot and SROC. In addition, heterogeneity caused by non-threshold effect was also explored utilizing single-factor meta-regression analyses. We separated the studies into different subgroups, in terms of pCR rate (mean = 21%), the duration of the study population (midpoint = 2009), and whether the image interpretation was blinded. Variances were considered as sources of heterogeneity if their regression coefficients reached statistical significance ($P < 0.05$). Publication bias was analyzed using Deeks' funnel plot and an asymmetry test. The absence of a non-zero slope coefficient ($P > 0.05$) indicates no publication bias exists among the included studies.

Results

Study selection

The systematic search and manual cross-checking of references yielded 648 articles in total from PubMed and EMBASE database initially. After excluding the obviously irrelevant articles according to titles and abstracts, 190 remained as potential candidates for inclusion. One hundred fifty-four articles were further ruled out as they disagreed with our inclusion criteria. An additional of 16

articles were excluded after careful full-text review. The reasons for exclusion were as follows: studies lacked of raw data ($n = 4$); the provided data were not sufficient to construct or calculate the contingency table ($n = 7$); studies presented repetitive data from author with additional studies ($n = 5$). Eventually, 20 studies were enrolled in the analysis. Figure 1 presented the procedure of literature search and study selection.

Study description

The included 20 studies consisted a total of 1490 patients [7, 12, 21–38]. The sample size ranged from 28 to 225 (median 75) patients. Thirteen of the enrolled studies used a 1.5 T magnet strength and 6 used 3 T for measurement. The study of Mani et al. [30] did not provide information about the applied magnet strength. In more than a half of the studies, radiologists were blinded to the pathological data. The basic information of each included trail were described in Table 1. The classifications used to identify pathologic response after NACT were varied from study to study. Three studies utilized Miller-Payne grading system, another three studies applied Mandard's tumor regression grade (TRG) criteria, one study used a Japanese Breast Cancer Society criteria, and one used the Chevalier-Sataloff classifications. The remaining articles applied a standard set by the researchers. Therefore, the definition of pCR after NACT of each study was not identical. Patients who reached Miller-Payne grade V, TRG 1, Japanese Breast Cancer Society grade 3, and Chevalier class 1, Sataloff A were classified as pCR in studies using the above criteria. Of the other 12 studies, 5 of them considered patients with no residual invasive cancer in the breast or lymph nodes as achieving pCR. Five studies defined pCR as the absence of invasive cancer and two studies defined pCR as the disappearance of recognizable invasive tumor cells but ductal carcinoma in situ (DCIS) may have been present. Breast-conserving surgery or mastectomy was performed in nine studies and lumpectomy or mastectomy was conducted in two studies. Four studies declared that patients received surgery after NACT treatment, but they did not clarify the type of surgery. The final five studies did not mention surgery after NACT. As for NACT regimens, patients in the same study or in different studies received diverse chemotherapy. The detailed information of NACT treatment of the enrolled literature were presented in Table 2.

Quality assessment

The result of the QUADAS-2 form revealed that the included studies contained satisfying and eligible qualities. The detailed information and the distribution results of each enrolled study were displayed in Fig. 2.

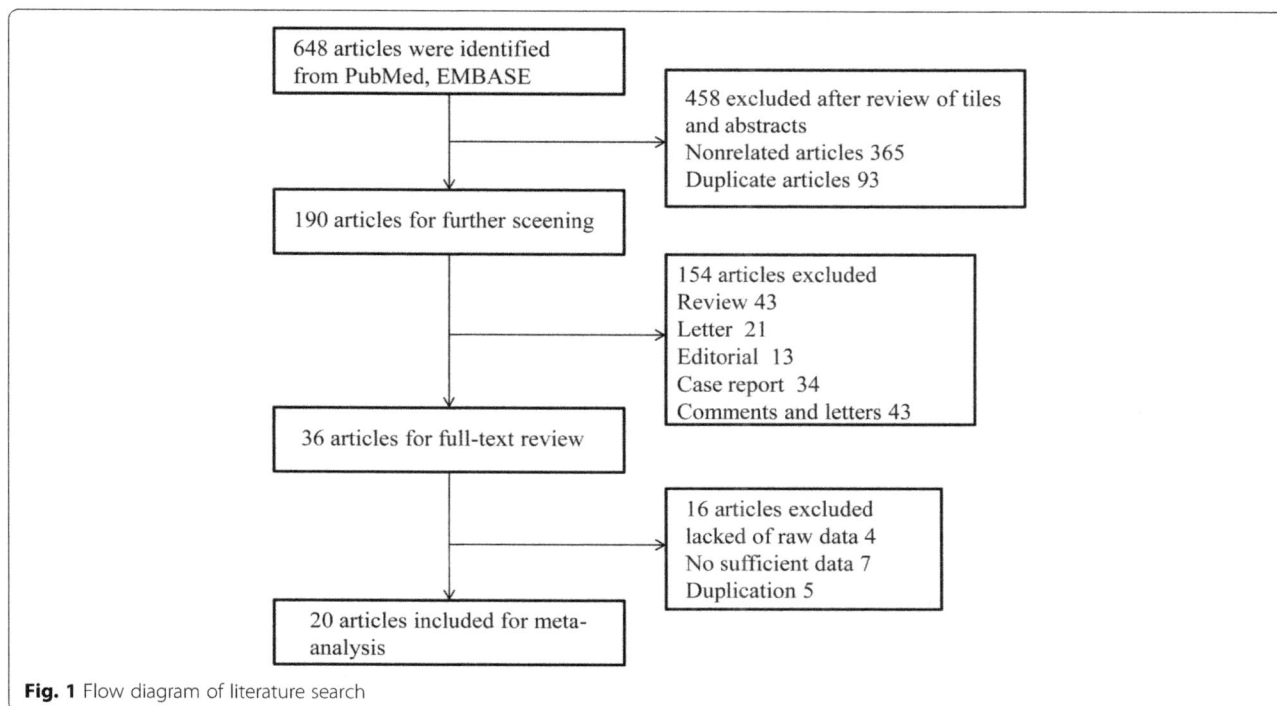

Fig. 1 Flow diagram of literature search

Performance of DWI

The sensitivity and specificity of all 20 selected studies ranged from 0.68 (95% CI, 0.43–0.87) to 1.00 (95% CI, 0.59–1.00), and from 0.38 (95% CI, 0.28–0.49) to 0.95 (95% CI, 0.90–0.98), respectively. The pooled estimate of 20 studies demonstrated a sensitivity of 0.89 (95% CI, 0.86–0.91) (Fig. 3), a specificity of 0.72 (95% CI, 0.68–0.75) (Fig. 4), and a DOR of 27.00 (95% CI, 15.60–46.73) (Fig. 5). Figure 6 presented the AUC value, which represented the overall diagnostic accuracy of DWI, was 0.9088 ± 0.0230, and the *Q index was 0.8408 ± 0.0254. The outcomes of the analyses suggested that DWI modality was provided with eligible diagnostic performance in the differentiation of NACT responders and non-responders. The publication bias was shown in Fig. 7. Confirming by the Deeks' funnel plot asymmetry test, no significant publication bias ($P = 0.51$) existed in the present study.

Heterogeneity text

The statistical results confirmed that there was heterogeneity of DWI both in sensitivity ($I^2 = 62.7\%$) and in specificity ($I^2 = 84.9\%$). The Spearman correlation coefficients' P values (0.565, $P > 0.05$) disclosed the absence of threshold effect in the DWI evaluation.

Single-factor meta-regression analyses were also performed to assess the non-threshold effect. Three subgroups, regarding different pCR rate, treatment duration of patients and whether the researchers were blinded to patients' therapeutic responses to NACT and pathological findings, were analyzed. Table 3 listed the results of meta-regression analyses. The results demonstrated no statistically significant differences among each subgroup, which indicated that pCR rate, treatment duration, and study design (blinded or not) were not strongly associated with DWI accuracy.

Discussion

DWI, with its rapid, non-invasive, and without the use of contrast agent characteristic, has emerged as a practical mean to overcome the limitation of DCE-MRI [23, 39]. However, to our knowledge, no previous meta-analysis focused on evaluating the diagnostic performance of DWI in detecting patients' complete response to NACT in breast cancer. Thus, we designed the current meta-analysis specific for this purpose. By combining data from 20 studies, we detected a 0.89 sensitivity and a 0.72 specificity for DWI, which indicated that DWI could be a valuable imaging method for assessing pCR to NACT in breast cancer. An approximately 0.91 AUC value, which was close to 1 (the perfect test result), also indicated an ideal diagnostic performance. The DOR of a test can serve as a single summary measure since it obtains from combining different sensitivity and specificity. It is defined as the ratio of the odds of positivity in disease relative subjects to the odds of positivity in the non-diseased [40]. The DOR value display in a wide range from 0 to infinity. A higher DOR value represents a better ability for the discrimination of the test performance. The outcome of our study has shown that the DOR estimated for DWI was 27.00 (95% CI, 15.60–46.73). This benign high-DOR value indicated that DWI could monitor pCR in NACT accurately.

Table 1 Basic characteristics of included studies

Study	Year	Study design	No. of cases	Age (mean range)	Disease stages	Histologic subtype	Magnet strenth (T)	Duration of the patients (years, month)	Blind	Timing of evaluation
Agarwal	2017	NR	38	44.2(19–65)	LABC, stage II/III	IDC/DCIS	1.5 T	NR		Pre-NAC and after 1.3 cycles
Atuegwu	2013	NR	28	44.9 (28–67)	Stage II/III	NR	3.0 T	NR		Pre-NAC and after 1 cycle, and post-NAC
Belli	2011	Pro	51	48.4 (26–66)	NR	IDC/ILC	1.5 T	2007.01–2009.01	Blind	Pre-NAC and post-NAC within 4 weeks
Bufi	2014	Retro	225	47 (26–67)	Stage II/III	IDC/ILC	1.5 T	2007–2012	Blind	Pre-NAC and post-NAC within 4 weeks
Bufi	2015	Retro	225	47 (26–67)	LABC, stage II/III/IV	IDC/ILC	1.5 T	2007–2012	Blind	Pre-NAC and post-NAC within 4 weeks
Che	2016	NR	36	50.9 (27–75)	LABC	IDC/ILC	3.0 T	2014.03–2015.05	Blind	Pre-NAC and after 2 cycles
Fangberget	2010	Pro	31	50.7 (37–72)	Stage II/III/IV	IDC/ILC	1.5 T	2007.04–2008.10	Blind	Pre-NAC and after 4 cycles, and post-NAC
Fujimoto	2013	NR	56	50.9(27–70)	Stage II/III	IDC	1.5 T	2006.02–2009.12	Blind	Pre-NAC and post-NAC within 3 weeks
Li	2011	Pro	32	46 (25–63)	LABC	NR	1.5 T	2007.07–2010.07		Pre-NAC and after 1 cycle
Li	2015	Pro	42	46.8 (28–67)	Stage II/III	NR	3.0 T	NR		Pre-NAC and after 1 cycle, post-NAC
Luo	2014	Retro	71	46.1 (29–72)	NR	IDC	3.0 T	2010.03–2012.12	Blind	Pre-NAC, after 2 cycles and post-NAC
Mani	2013	NR	28	45 (28–67)	Stage II/III	NR	NR	NR		Pre-NAC, after 1 cycle and post-NAC
Study	Year	Study design	No. of cases	Age (mean range)	Disease stages	Histologic subtype	Magnet strenth(T)	Duration of the patients (year, months)	Blind	Timing of evaluation
Park	2010	Retro	53	43.7 (24–65)	Stage II/III	IDC/ILC	1.5 T	2007.03–2008.05	Blind	Pre-NAC and after 3 cycles
Park	2011	Retro	34	44 (27–60)	LABC	IDC/ILC	1.5 T	2007.04–2008.05	Blind	Pre-NAC and after 3–6 cycles
Richard	2013	Retro	118	53.2 (23–83)	LABC, stage II/III/IV	IDC/ILC	1.5 T	2008.07–2011.05	Blind	Pre-NAC and post-NAC less than 2 weeks
Sharma	2009	Retro	56	48.5 (25–75)	LABC	IDC	1.5 T	2003.12–2006.12		Pre-NAC and after 1, 2, 3 cycles
Shin	2012	Retro	90	46 (24–68)	Stage I/II/III	IDC/ILC	1.5 T	2009.01–2011.05		Pre-NAC and post-NAC
Weis	2015	Retro	33	46 (28–67)	Stage II/III	NR	3.0 T	NR		Pre-NAC, after 1 cycle and post-NAC
Woodhams	2010	NR	69	NR	NR	IDC/ILC	1.5 T	2005.01–2008.10	Blind	Pre-NAC, after 4 cycles the post-NAC
Xu	2017	NR	174	45.7 (28–64)	LABC, stage II/III	IDC/ILC	3.0 T	2011.09–2014.12	Blind	Pre-NAC, after 1 cycle and post-NAC

LABC locally advanced breast cancer; *IDL* invasive ductal carcinoma; *ILC* invasive lobular carcinoma; *Pro* prospective; *Retro* retrospective; *NR* not reported

Although the pooled statistic of our study implied that DWI might accurately detect pCR for breast cancer to NACT, significant heterogeneity in sensitivity ($I^2 =$ 62.7%) and specificity ($I^2 = 84.9\%$) were also noticed. The Spearman correlation coefficients of DWI (0.565, $P >$ 0.05) already eliminated the threshold effect had on DWI evaluation. However, the considerable heterogeneity might be attributed to many other factors, such as variations in definition to separate responders from non-responders, variations in the duration of the study population, or differences in pathologic complete response rate or study designs. To reduce the influence induced by these diversities, we carried out several subgroups analyses concerning pCR rate, time duration of study population, and study design. Meta-regression analyses revealed no significant difference among the

Table 2 Characteristics of included studies for neoadjuvant chemotherapy

Study	Year	No. of cases	Classification of pathologic response	Definition of pCR	NACT regimens	Surgery after NACT
Agarwal	2017	38	Miller-Payne	Miller-Payne grade V	CEF, CAF, CEF + DE, DE, DC + Herceptin, DEC	Modified radical mastectomy or wide local excision
Atuegwu	2013	28	–	No residual invasive cancer in the breast or lymph nodes	AC + taxol, Taxotere, Taxol + cisplatin ± everolimus, Trastuzumab +carboplatin + ixabepilone, Trastuzumab, and lapatinib	NR
Belli	2011	51	Mandard's TRG criteria	TRG 1	FEC, AT, TAC, and TC ± carboplatinum or trastuzumab	Surgery
Bufi	2014	225	Mandard's TRG criteria	TRG 1	Doxorubicin and cyclophosphamide, and taxanes-based regimens	Breast-conserving and nipple sparing surgery; Surgical excision
Bufi	2015	225	Mandard's TRG criteria	TRG 1	Doxorubicin, taxane, and cyclophosphamide-based regimens	Breast-conserving and nipple sparing surgery; Surgical excision
Che	2016	36	Miller-Payne	Miller-Payne grade V	Paclitaxel with epirubicin or paclitaxel with carboplatin	Breast-conserving surgery with axillary nodal clearance or modified radical mastectomy.
Fangberget	2010	31	–	Absence of invasive cancer	5-fluoro-uracil, epirubicin and cyclophosphamide	Surgery
Fujimoto	2013	56	Japanese Breast Cancer Society criteria	Necrosis or disappearance of all tumor cells	Adriamycin and cyclophosphamide, paclitaxel, 5-fluorouracil, epirubicin, and cyclophosphamide, paclitaxel	Lumpectomy or mastectomy
Li	2011	32	–	Absence of invasive cancer on breast tumor and lymph nodes	Docetaxel and epirubicin	Breast-conserving surgery or modified radical mastectomy
Li	2015	42		No invasive tumor in the breast	DOX + Cyc + Tax, Cis/Tax±RAD001, Tra + Car, Tra/Car/Her, Tax	Mastectomy or lumpectomy
Luo	2014	71	Miller-Payne	Miller-Payne grade V	NR	NR
Mani	2013	28	–	No residual tumor in the breast or lymph nodes	Adriamycin/cytoxan, taxol/trastuzumab; docetaxel, carboplatin, and trastuzumab; or lapatinib and trastuzumab	Surgery
Park	2010	53	–	Absence of recognizable invasive tumor cells (DCIS may have been present)	Docetaxel and doxorubicin with granulocyte colony–stimulating factor	Modified radical mastectomy or breast-conserving surgery
Park	2011	34	–	No residual malignancy and no sign of cancer cells; no residual invasive cancer and DCIS present	Doxorubicin and docetaxel; paclitaxel, gemcitabine and trastuzumab	Modified radical mastectomy or breast-conserving surgery
Richard	2013	118	Chevalier-Sataloff classifications	Chevalier class 1, Sataloff A	Epirubicin and cyclophosphamide, docetaxel; epirubicin and cyclophosphamide, trastuzumab	Mastectomy or breast-conservative surgery
Sharma	2009	56	–	No residual tumor	CEF; PpE	NR
Shin	2012	90	–	No residual tumor or absence of invasive cancer, but presence of DCIS	Doxorubicin and cyclophosphamide; cyclophosphamide and docetaxel; adriamycin plus docetaxel; 5-fluorouracil, epirubicin and cyclophos-phamide; trastuzumab plus paclitaxel	Surgery
Weis	2015	33	–	No residual tumor in the breast or nodes	Paclitaxel, carboplatin, and trastuzumab; doxorubicin and cyclophosphamide, paclitaxel; cisplatin and paclitaxel ± everolimus	NR
Woodhams	2010	69	–	No residual disease or no invasive cancer or DCIS present	Anthracycline and cyclophosphamide, paclitaxel	Quadrantectomy or mastectomy
Xu	2017	174	–	No residual tumor in the breast or nodes	Cyclophosphamide + epirubicin and tatotere	NR

Miller-Payne grade V, showed complete disappearance of malignant cells at the site of tumor with only vascular fibroelastotic stroma seen with macrophages; *TRG 1*, complete regression, absence of residual tumor cells; *Chevalier class 1*, disappearance of all tumors on either macroscopic or microscopic assessment; *Sataloff A*, total or near total therapeutic effect; *CEF*, cyclophosphamide epirubicin 5-Fluorouracil; *CAF* cyclophosphamide adriamycin 5-fluorouracil; *DE*, docetaxel epirubicin; *DC*, docetaxel cisplatin; *DEC*, docetaxel epirubicin cisplatin; *FEC*, fluorouracil + epirubicin + cyclophosphamide; *AT*, doxorubicin + taxanes; *TAC*, taxanes + doxorubicin + cyclophosphamide; *TC*, taxanes + cyclophosphamide; *Dox*, doxorubicin; *Cyc*, cyclophosphamide; *Cis*, cisplatin; *PpE*, paclitaxel and epirubicin; *NR*, not reported

	Risk of Bias				Applicability Concerns		
	Patient Selection	Index Test	Reference Standard	Flow and Timing	Patient Selection	Index Test	Reference Standard
agarwal2017	+	?	?	?	+	+	+
atuegwu2013	+	?	−	−	+	+	+
belli2011	+	+	+	+	+	+	+
Bufi2014	+	+	+	+	+	+	+
Bufi2015	+	+	+	+	+	+	+
che2016	+	+	+	+	+	+	+
fangberget2010	?	−	+	−	+	+	+
fujimoto2013	?	?	?	?	+	+	+
li2011	+	−	−	+	+	+	+
li2015	+	−	+	+	+	+	+
Luo2014	?	?	?	?	+	+	+
mani2013	+	−	?	+	+	+	+
park2010	+	−	+	?	+	+	+
park2011	+	?	+	+	+	+	+
richard2013	+	+	+	+	+	+	+
sharma2009	?	−	?	?	+	+	+
shin2012	+	−	+	+	+	+	+
weis2015	+	−	+	+	+	+	+
woodhams2010	+	+	+	+	+	+	+
Xu2017	+	?	+	+	+	+	+

− High   ? Unclear   + Low

Fig. 2 Methodological quality summary of 20 included studies

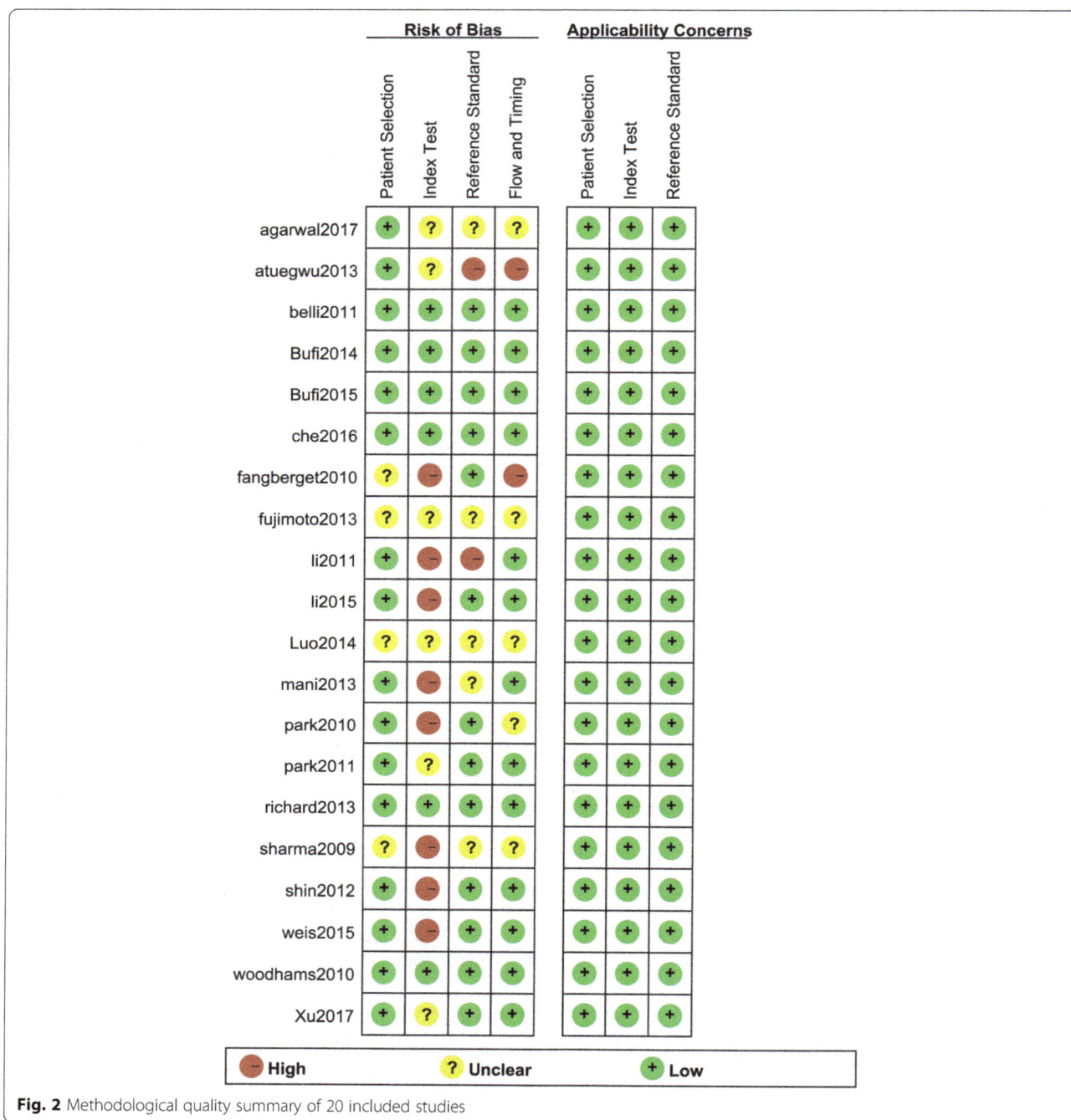

three subgroups. This finding implied that, although heterogeneity might exist between different studies, results across studies were still comparable with little or no differences outcomes.

Abundant studies have been conducted to evaluate the efficiency of DCE-MRI in diagnosing pathologic response to NACT for patients with breast cancer. Yet, only a few has investigated the DWI diagnostic accuracy for predicting pCR to NACT. Gu et al. [11] suggested that the sensitivity and specificity of DWI were 93 and 85%, respectively. Another meta-analysis, Wu et al. [41] reported a 93% sensitivity and a 82% specificity for DWI evaluation. It seems that both studies have a slightly higher sensitivity and a much higher specificity than our research. However, the two previous analyses only included a small amount of studies which provided DWI data. Gu et al. enrolled eight studies, and Wu et al. had six. Our study analyzed up to 20 groups of DWI data, and this might be the reason causing

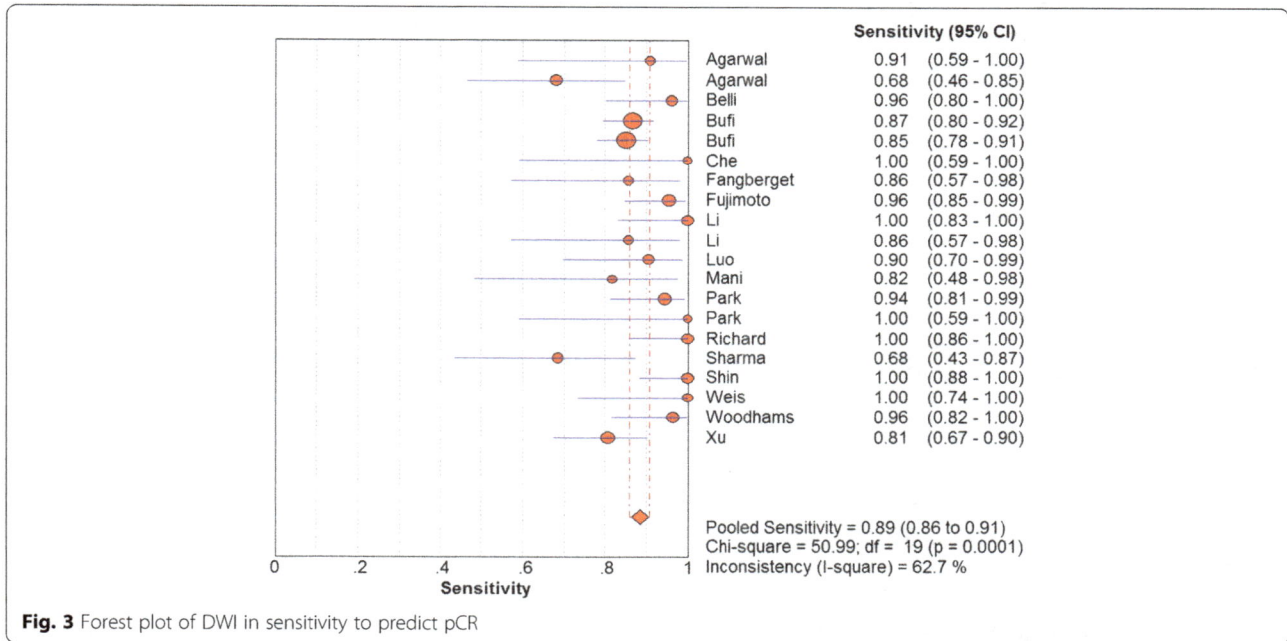

Fig. 3 Forest plot of DWI in sensitivity to predict pCR

discrepancy in our result. Interestingly, we can observe in all three studies that the sensitivity of DWI is higher than the specificity. This finding might further prove the hypothesis that DWI could accurately assess pCR in sensitivity. However, it might lack specificity.

Generally, by predicting the outcome and identifying the pCR to NACT treatment, breast cancer patients can avoid inappropriate chemotherapy at early stage as well as additional toxic therapies, and hold a better chance to achieve pCR [42, 43]. Therefore, some researchers argue that it is crucial to find a specific time for DWI evaluation.

However, the previous studies and our analysis all failed to find an exact time to perform DWI. The timing of DWI assessment in our research was varied from study to study. Many studies conducted DWI at several time points. Five studies performed DWI after 1 cycle of therapy, three conducted after 2 cycles, and four studies assessed after 3 cycles. The available data were limited and hampered us to perform subgroup analysis. Nevertheless, a pattern can still be observed from the included studies. It seems that the first 3 cycles might be the preferable timing for DWI assessment. This hypothesis needs further approval.

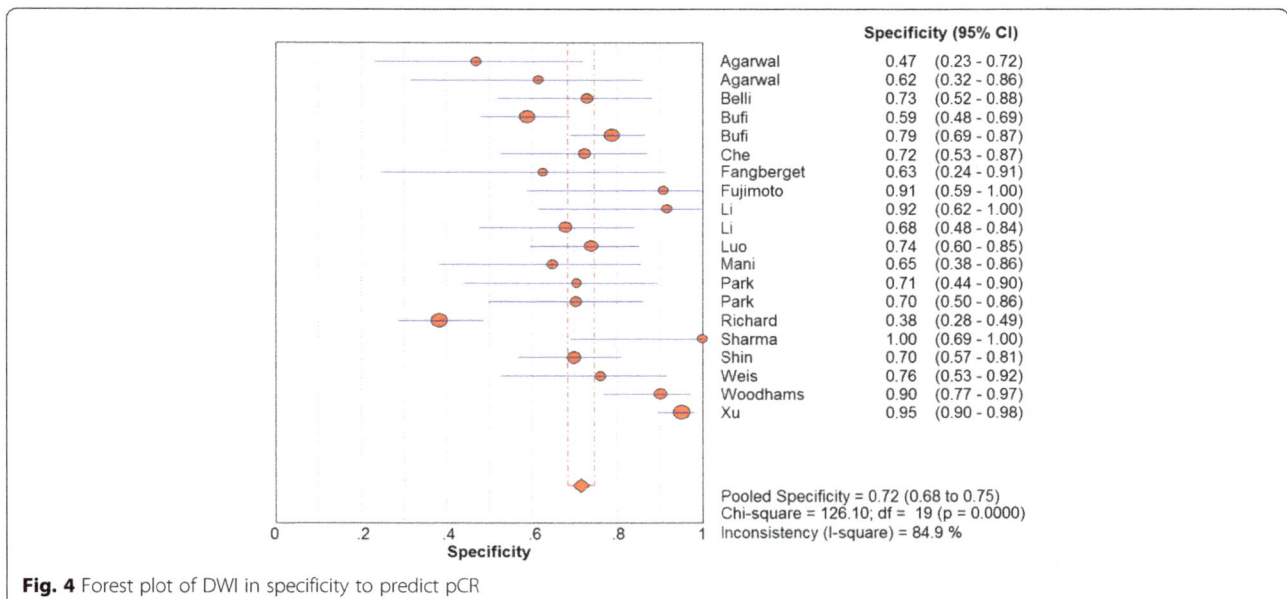

Fig. 4 Forest plot of DWI in specificity to predict pCR

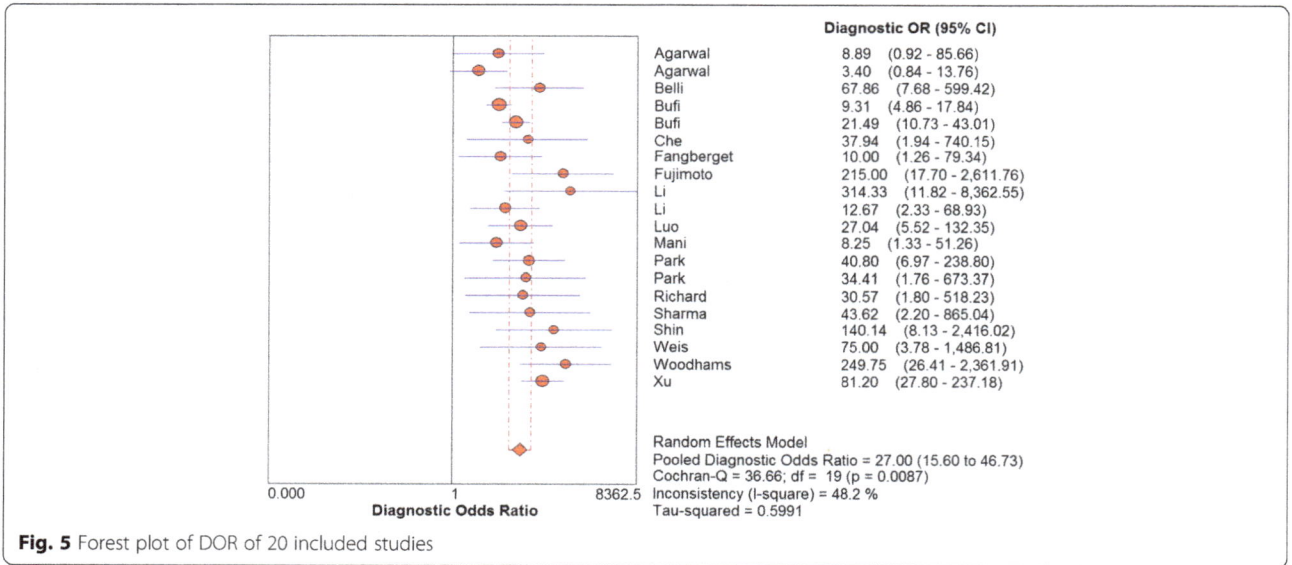

Fig. 5 Forest plot of DOR of 20 included studies

Some limitations should be taken into account in our analysis. First, a majority of the included studies contained a relatively small patients' population which might weaken the statistical power of the study and might bring about inconclusive and imprecise results. Although quality assessment and publication bias test confirmed that the included studies were eligible, the effect brought by different sample size still could not be neglected. Second, patients with different breast cancer subtypes would be assigned with different treatment regimens which might eventually lead to different pathological responses [24, 25, 33]. Bufi et al. remarked that DWI might achieve a better diagnostic performance in luminal and hybrid tumor subtypes [24]. Another study by Bufi et al. reported that pretreatment ADC was capable of detecting pCR in Triple negative and HER2$^+$ tumors [25]. Richard et al. found that luminal A and B subtypes had a lower pretreatment ADC than triple-negative tumors which indicated a superior performance of DWI in the prediction of pCR to NACT in triple-negative tumors [33]. Thus, subgroup analysis based on tumor phenotypes is desirable. However, the limited information, which only three studies had provided data of breast cancer subtypes, prevented us to conduct subgroup analysis on this aspect. Moreover, the definition of pCR could be a reason affecting the diagnostic accuracy test.

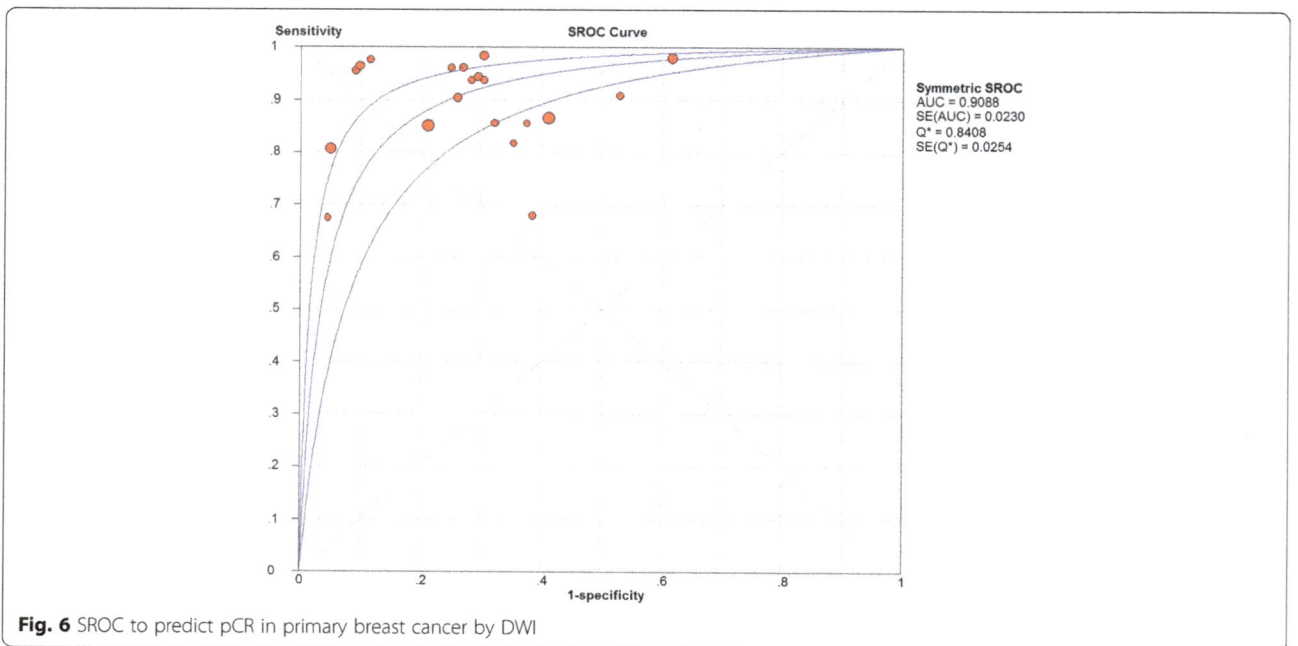

Fig. 6 SROC to predict pCR in primary breast cancer by DWI

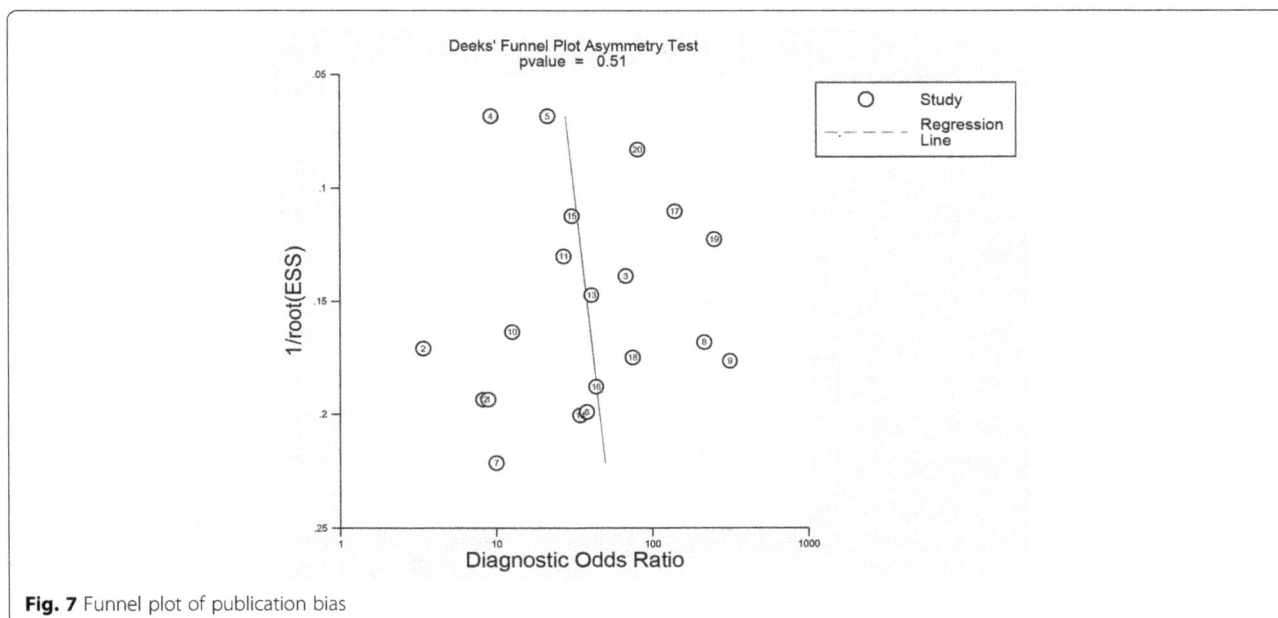

Fig. 7 Funnel plot of publication bias

Since too many various pCR definitions were applied in the included studies, such as Miller-Payne grading system, Mandard's TRG criteria, Japanese Breast Cancer Society criteria, Chevalier-Sataloff classifications and classification by user-defined, subgroup comparison could not be performed in our study. Yet, although subgroups and threshold effect evaluation has diminished the influence of heterogeneity, the effect of heterogeneity still cannot be eliminated completely. Several variables, regarding treatment regiments of NACT, timing of pCR evaluation, standards and pattern of DWI measurement, and the optimal cut-off values of diagnosis, should be taken into consideration. However, the information retrieved from the included studies were limited and inconsistent regarding the above factors, making it impossible to conduct subgroup analyses to eliminate their effect.

Conclusion

Despite some limitations, the findings of our study indicate that DWI modality holds a relatively high sensitivity and specificity for the evaluation and prediction of pCR of breast cancer to NACT. The result of our analysis suggests that the application of DWI in combination with other imaging modality may yield greater precision and accuracy in assessing the pCR after NACT.

Abbreviations
ADC: Apparent diffusion coefficient; AUC: Area under the curve; DCE-MRI: Contrast-enhanced magnetic resonance imaging; DOR: Diagnostic odds ratio; DWI: Diffusion-weighted imaging; FN: False negative; FP: False positive; MRI: Magnetic resonance imaging; NACT: Neoadjuvant chemotherapy; pCR: Pathological complete response; PET/CT: Positron emission tomography-computed tomography; pNR: Pathological non-responders; SROC: Summary receiver operating characteristic curve; TN: True negative; TP: True positive

Authors' contributions
WG and TD conceived and designed the study. WG, NG, and TD co-wrote the manuscript. WG, NG, and TD reviewed all the included publications, extracted the participants' data, and performed the statistical analysis. All authors read and approved the final manuscript.

Competing interests
The authors declare that they have no competing interests.

Author details
 Department of Trauma Surgery, Tianjin Fourth Central Hospital, No.1 Zhongshan Road, Hebei District, Tianjin 300010, China. ²Department of Breast Surgery, Tianjin Fourth Central Hospital, No.1 Zhongshan Road, Hebei District, Tianjin 300010, China. ³Department of Cardiovascular Medicine, Guizhou Provincial People's Hospital, No. 83 Zhongshandong Road, Guiyang City 550002, Guizhou, China.

Table 3 Results of regression meta-analysis

	Pathologic complete response rate	The duration of the patients	Blind
Coefficient	− 0.314	− 0.365	0.243
Standard error	0.7153	0.7715	0.7349
P value	0.6673	0.6427	0.7457
RDOR	0.73	0.69	1.27
[95% CI]	(0.16 to 3.36)	(0.13 to 3.59)	(0.27 to 6.11)

References
1. Liu SV, Melstrom L, Yao K, Russell CA, Sener SF. Neoadjuvant therapy for breast cancer. J Surg Oncol. 2010;101:283–91.
2. Avril N, Sassen S, Roylance R. Response to therapy in breast cancer. Journal of Nuclear Medicine Official Publication Society of Nuclear Medicine. 2009; 50(Suppl 1):55S.
3. Groheux D, Giacchetti S, Espié M, Rubello D, Moretti JL, Hindié E. Early monitoring of response to neoadjuvant chemotherapy in breast cancer with 18F-FDG PET/CT: defining a clinical aim. Eur J Nucl Med Mol Imaging. 2011;38:419–25.
4. Rastogi P, Anderson SJ, Bear HD, Geyer CE, Kahlenberg MS, Robidoux A, Margolese RG, Hoehn JL, Vogel VG, Dakhil SR. Preoperative chemotherapy: updates of National Surgical Adjuvant Breast and Bowel Project Protocols B-

18 and B-27. Journal of Clinical Oncology Official Journal of the. Proc Am Soc Clin Oncol. 2008;26:778.

5. Esserman LJ, Berry DA, Cheang MCU, Yau C, Perou CM, Carey L, Demichele A, Gray JW, Conway-Dorsey K, Lenburg ME. Chemotherapy response and recurrence-free survival in neoadjuvant breast cancer depends on biomarker profiles: results from the I-SPY 1 TRIAL (CALGB 150007/150012; ACRIN 6657). Breast Cancer Res Treat. 2012;132:1049–62.

6. Minckwitz GV, Untch M, Blohmer JU, Costa SD, Eidtmann H, Fasching PA, Gerber B, Eiermann W, Hilfrich J, Definition HJ. Impact of pathologic complete response on prognosis after neoadjuvant chemotherapy in various intrinsic breast cancer subtypes. Journal of Clinical Oncology Official Journal of the. Proc Am Soc Clin Oncol. 2012;30:1796.

7. Che S, Zhao X, Ou Y, Li J, Wang M, Wu B, Zhou C. Role of the intravoxel incoherent motion diffusion weighted imaging in the pre-treatment prediction and early response monitoring to neoadjuvant chemotherapy in locally advanced breast cancer. Medicine. 2016;95:e2420.

8. Ahmed MI, Lennard TWJ. Breast cancer: role of neoadjuvant therapy. Int J Surg. 2009;7:416–20.

9. Hylton NM, Blume JD, Bernreuter WK, Pisano ED, Rosen MA, Morris EA, Weatherall PT, Lehman CD, Newstead GM, Polin S. Locally advanced breast cancer: MR imaging for prediction of response to neoadjuvant chemotherapy–results from ACRIN 6657/I-SPY TRIAL. Breast Diseases A Year Book Quarterly. 2012;263:663–72.

10. Londero V, Bazzocchi M, Frate CD, Puglisi F, Loreto CD, Francescutti G, Zuiani C. Locally advanced breast cancer: comparison of mammography, sonography and MR imaging in evaluation of residual disease in women receiving neoadjuvant chemotherapy. Eur Radiol. 2004;14:1371–9.

11. Gu YL, Pan SM, Ren J, Yang ZX, Jiang GQ. The role of magnetic resonance imaging in detection of pathological complete remission in breast cancer patients treated with neoadjuvant chemotherapy: a meta-analysis. Clin Breast Cancer. 2017;17(4):245–255.

12. Fujimoto H, Kazama T, Nagashima T, Sakakibara M, Suzuki TH, Okubo Y, Shiina N, Fujisaki K, Ota S, Miyazaki M. Diffusion-weighted imaging reflects pathological therapeutic response and relapse in breast cancer. Breast Cancer. 2014;21:724–31.

13. Le BD, Breton E, Lallemand D, Grenier P, Cabanis E, Lavaljeantet M. MR imaging of intravoxel incoherent motions: application to diffusion and perfusion in neurologic disorders. Radiol. 1986;161:401.

14. Le BD. Diffusion, perfusion and functional magnetic resonance imaging. J Mal Vasc. 1995;20:203–14.

15. Padhani AR, Liu G, Koh DM, Chenevert TL, Thoeny HC, Takahara T, Dzik-Jurasz A, Ross BD, Van CM, Collins D. Diffusion-weighted magnetic resonance imaging as a cancer biomarker: consensus and recommendations. Neoplasia. 2009;11:102.

16. ML M, N H, P M, F S, L I, EP M, vM G. ME B and S C. Meta-analysis of magnetic resonance imaging in detecting residual breast Cancer after neoadjuvant therapy. J Natl Cancer Inst. 2013;105:321–33.

17. Yuan Y, Chen XS, Liu SY, Shen KW. Accuracy of MRI in prediction of pathologic complete remission in breast cancer after preoperative therapy: a meta-analysis. AJR Am J Roentgenol. 2010;195:260–8.

18. Mghanga FP, Lan X, Bakari KH, Li C, Zhang Y. Fluorine-18 Fluorodeoxyglucose positron emission tomography–computed tomography in monitoring the response of breast Cancer to neoadjuvant chemotherapy: a meta–analysis. Clin Breast Cancer. 2013;13:271.

19. Liu Q, Wang C, Li P, Liu J, Huang G, Song S. The role of 18F-FDG PET/CT and MRI in assessing pathological complete response to neoadjuvant chemotherapy in patients with breast cancer: a systematic review and meta-analysis. Biomed Res Int. 2016;2016:1235429.

20. Whiting PF, Rutjes AW, Westwood ME, Mallett S, Deeks JJ, Reitsma JB, Leeflang MM, Sterne JA, Bossuyt PM, Group Q. QUADAS-2: a revised tool for the quality assessment of diagnostic accuracy studies. Ann Intern Med. 2011;155:529–36.

21. Agarwal K, Sharma U, Sah RG, Mathur S, Hari S, Seenu V, Parshad R, Jagannathan NR. Pre-operative assessment of residual disease in locally advanced breast cancer patients: a sequential study by quantitative diffusion weighted MRI as a function of therapy. Magn Reson Imaging. 2017;42:88–94.

22. Atuegwu NC, Arlinghaus LR, Li X, Chakravarthy AB, Abramson VG, Sanders ME, Yankeelov TE. Parameterizing the logistic model of tumor growth by DW-MRI and DCE-MRI data to predict treatment response and changes in breast cancer cellularity during neoadjuvant chemotherapy. Transl Oncol. 2013;6:256.

23. Belli P, Costantini M, Ierardi C, Bufi E, Amato D, Mule' A, Nardone L, Terribile D, Bonomo L. Diffusion-weighted imaging in evaluating the response to neoadjuvant breast cancer treatment. Breast Journal. 2011;17:610.

24. Bufi E, Belli P, Matteo MD, Terribile D, Franceschini G, Nardone L, Petrone G, Bonomo L. Effect of breast cancer phenotype on diagnostic performance of MRI in the prediction to response to neoadjuvant treatment. Eur J Radiol. 2014;83:1631.

25. Bufi E, Belli P, Costantini M, Cipriani A, Di MM, Bonatesta A, Franceschini G, Terribile D, Mulé A, Nardone L. Role of the apparent diffusion coefficient in the prediction of response to neoadjuvant chemotherapy in patients with locally advanced breast cancer. Clin Breast Cancer. 2015;15:370.

26. Fangberget A, Nilsen LB, Hole KH, Holmen MM, Engebraaten O, Naume B, H.-J S, Olsen DR, Seierstad T. Neoadjuvant chemotherapy in breast cancer-response evaluation and prediction of response to treatment using dynamic contrast-enhanced and diffusion-weighted MR imaging. Int J Med Radiol. 2011;21(6):1188–99.

27. Li XR, Cheng LQ, Liu M, Zhang YJ, Wang JD, Zhang AL, Song X, Li J, Zheng YQ, Liu L. DW-MRI ADC values can predict treatment response in patients with locally advanced breast cancer undergoing neoadjuvant chemotherapy. Med Oncol. 2012;29:425–31.

28. Li X, Abramson RG, Arlinghaus LR, Kang H, Chakravarthy AB, Abramson VG, Farley J, Mayer IA, Kelley MC, Meszoely IM. Multiparametric magnetic resonance imaging for predicting pathological response after the first cycle of neoadjuvant chemotherapy in breast cancer. Investig Radiol. 2015;50:195.

29. Luo Y, Yu J, Xu Z, Zeng H, Chen H. Evaluation of pathologic response of breast cancer to neoadjuvant chemotherapy with magnetic resonance diffusion weighted imaging. Sheng wu yi xue gong cheng xue za zhi = J Biomed Eng = Shengwu yixue gongchengxue zazhi. 2014;31:1336.

30. Mani S, Chen Y, Li X, Arlinghaus L, Chakravarthy AB, Abramson V, Bhave SR, Levy MA. Xu H and Yankeelov TE. Machine learning for predicting the response of breast cancer to neoadjuvant chemotherapy. Journal of the American Medical Informatics Association. Jamia. 2013;20:688.

31. Park SH, Moon WK, Cho N, Chang JM, Im SA, Park IA, Kang KW, Han W, Noh DY. Comparison of diffusion-weighted MR imaging and FDG PET/CT to predict pathological complete response to neoadjuvant chemotherapy in patients with breast cancer. Eur Radiol. 2012;22:18–25.

32. Sang HP, Moon WK, Cho N, Song IC, Chang JM, Park IA, Han W, Noh DY. Diffusion-weighted MR imaging: pretreatment prediction of response to neoadjuvant chemotherapy in patients with breast cancer1. Radiol. 2010;257:56.

33. Richard R, Thomassin I, Chapellier M, Scemama A, Cremoux PD, Varna M, Giacchetti S, Espié M, Kerviler ED, Bazelaire CD. Diffusion-weighted MRI in pretreatment prediction of response to neoadjuvant chemotherapy in patients with breast cancer. Eur Radiol. 2013;23:2420–31.

34. Sharma U, Danishad KKA, Seenu V, Jagannathan NR. Longitudinal study of the assessment by MRI and diffusion-weighted imaging of tumor response in patients with locally advanced breast cancer undergoing neoadjuvant chemotherapy. NMR Biomed. 2009;22:104–13.

35. Shin HJ, Baek HM, Ahn JH, Baek S, Kim H, Cha JH, Kim HH. Prediction of pathologic response to neoadjuvant chemotherapy in patients with breast cancer using diffusion-weighted imaging and MRS. NMR Biomed. 2012;25:1349.

36. Weis JA, Miga MI, Arlinghaus LR, Li X, Abramson V, Chakravarthy AB, Pendyala P, Yankeelov TE. Predicting the response of breast Cancer to neoadjuvant therapy using a mechanically coupled reaction-diffusion model. Cancer Res. 2015;75:4697.

37. Woodhams R, Kakita S, Hata H, Iwabuchi K, Kuranami M, Gautam S, Hatabu H, Kan S, Mountford C. Identification of residual breast carcinoma following neoadjuvant chemotherapy: diffusion-weighted imaging—comparison with contrast-enhanced MR imaging and pathologic findings. Radiol. 2010;254:357–66.

38. Xu HD, Zhang YQ. Evaluation of the efficacy of neoadjuvant chemotherapy for breast cancer using diffusion-weighted imaging and dynamic contrast-enhanced magnetic resonance imaging. Neoplasma. 2017;64(3):430–436.

39. Peters NH, Borel Rinkes IH, Zuithoff NP, Mali WP, Moons KG, Peeters PH. Meta-analysis of MR imaging in the diagnosis of breast lesions. Radiology. 2008;246:116.

40. Glas AS, Lijmer JG, Prins MH, Bonsel GJ, Bossuyt PM. The diagnostic odds ratio: a single indicator of test performance. J Clin Epidemiol. 2003;56:1129.

41. Wu LM, Hu JN, Gu HY, Hua J, Chen J, Xu JR. Can diffusion-weighted MR imaging and contrast-enhanced MR imaging precisely evaluate and predict pathological response to neoadjuvant chemotherapy in patients with breast cancer? Breast Cancer Res Treat. 2012;135:17–28.

17

Prediction of key genes and pathways involved in trastuzumab-resistant gastric cancer

Chaoran Yu[1,2], Pei Xue[1,2], Luyang Zhang[1,2], Ruijun Pan[1,2], Zhenhao Cai[1,2], Zirui He[1,2], Jing Sun[1,2]* and Minhua Zheng[1,2]*

Abstract

Background: Trastuzumab has been prevailingly accepted as a beneficial treatment for gastric cancer (GC) by targeting human epidermal growth factor receptor 2 (HER2)-positive. However, the therapeutic resistance of trastuzumab remains a major obstacle, restricting the therapeutic efficacy. Therefore, identifying potential key genes and pathways is crucial to maximize the overall clinical benefits.

Methods: The gene expression profile GSE77346 was retrieved to identify the differentially expressed genes (DEGs) associated with the trastuzumab resistance in GC. Next, the DEGs were annotated by the gene ontology (GO) and Kyoto Encyclopedia of Genes and Genomes (KEGG) pathways. The DEGs-coded protein-protein interaction (PPI) networks and the prognostic values of the 20 hub genes were determined. Correlation of the hub genes were analyzed in The Cancer Genome Atlas. The prognostic values of hub genes were further validated by Kaplan-Meier (KM) plotter.

Results: A total of 849 DEGs were identified, with 374 in upregulation and 475 in downregulation. Epithelium development was the most significantly enriched term in biological processes while membrane-bounded vesicle was in cellular compartments and cell adhesion molecular binding was in molecular functions. Pathways in cancer and ECM-receptor interaction were the most significantly enriched for all DEGs. Among the PPI networks, 20 hub genes were defined, including CD44 molecule (CD44), HER-2, and cadherin 1 (CDH1). Six hub genes were associated with favorable OS while eight were associated with poor OS. Mechanistically, 2′-5′-oligoadenylate synthetase 1, 3 (OAS1, OAS3) and CDH1 featured high degrees and strong correlations with other hub genes.

Conclusions: This bioinformatics analysis identified key genes and pathways for potential targets and survival predictors for trastuzumab treatment in GC.

Keywords: Differentially expressed genes, Gene ontology, KEGG pathway, Gastric cancer, Trastuzumab, Resistance, Protein-protein interaction

Background

Gastric cancer (GC) remains one of the leading common causes for cancer-related mortality and major global heath challenges [1–4]. Despite the incidence declining in industrialized nations, most new cases are occurred in South America, East Asia, and Eastern Europe [2, 5]. Surgery is the primary treatment for resectable GC [6]. However, the dissection extent of lymph node (D1, D2) remains controversial [3]. Kang et al. reported 46.5% patients who underwent curative surgery experienced recurrence, and half of the recurrence occurred in less than 3 years [7]. In the Dutch Gastric Cancer Group (DGCG) trial, 65% curative resected patients experienced recurrence with 30% overall survival (OS) for D1 and 35% for D2 [8]. Consistently, the Medical Research Council (MRC) trial reported a 34% 5-year OS [9]. Noteworthy, the inclusion of targeted drugs, such as angiogenesis inhibitors (ramucirumab) and epidermal growth factor receptor (EGFR) antibodies (nimotuzumab), have shown encouraging therapeutic benefits in GC patients [10, 11].

* Correspondence: sj11788@rjh.com.cn; zmhtiger@yeah.net
[1]Department of General Surgery, Ruijin Hospital, Shanghai Jiao Tong University, School of Medicine, Shanghai 200025, People's Republic of China
Full list of author information is available at the end of the article

Trastuzumab, a monoclonal antibody targeting epidermal growth factor receptor 2 (HER2) in breast cancer [12], was also among the promising therapeutic management to the GC patients with HER2-positive [13, 14]. It eliminated the activity of HER2 receptor and weakened subsequent multiple signaling pathways [15]. The first randomized prospect trial had shown that a triplet regimen of trastuzumab, cisplatin, and a fluoropyrimidine significantly improved the median OS of GC with HER2 overexpression or amplification [13]. In fact, secondary resistance was acquired within a median of two therapeutic cycles [16]. Until now, the resistance to trastuzumab in GC remains a major obstacle with limited clinical benefits. Efficient biomarkers and underlying mechanism are yet to be fully elucidated.

Hereby, potential biomarkers and pathways associated with trastuzumab resistance were investigated in GC cell lines by the gene expression profile, GSE77346 [17], from the Genetic Expression Omnibus (GEO) database (http://www.ncbi.nlm.nih.gov/geo/). The prognostic values of the biomarkers and potential mechanisms were assessed.

Methods

Gene expression profile from GEO database

The gene expression profile, GSE77346, was retrieved from the Gene Expression Omnibus (GEO) database (http://www.ncbi.nlm.nih.gov/geo/) [18]. The profile was generated by GPL10558, Illumina Human 48 K gene chips (Illumina HumanHT-12 V4.0 Expression BeadChip). The GSE77346 dataset consisted of one trastuzumab-sensitive NCI-N87 cell line and four trastuzumab-resistant cell lines (N87-TR1, N87-TR2, N87-TR3, N87-TR4). Briefly, all the cell lines were maintained in Roswell Park Memorial Institute (RPMI) 1640 medium with 10% heat-inactivated FBS. The green fluorescent protein (GFP) +/luciferase+ NCI-N87 cell lines were harvested and injected into the gastric walls of a nude mice. The tumor-bearing mice were received 20 mg/kg trastuzumab i.p. twice per week when the resulting tumors were detectable (Living Image Software program, Xenogen). The trastuzumab treatments were stopped when the tumors were relapsed. By repeated GFP flow cytometric sorting (FACSAria II sorter, Becton Dickinson), four trastuzumab-resistant cell lines were established [17]. Next, total RNA was retrieved by TRIzol reagent (Ambion, Warrington, UK). The synthesis of biotinylated cRNA (Illumina TotalPrep RNA Amplification Kit, Ambion) and the hybridization (Human HT-12 V4 BeadChip) were performed according to the manufacturer protocols. Probe intensity was obtained and normalized by the Illumina GenomeStudio software (Genome Studio V2011.1) [17]. The gene expression profiles GSE13861, including 84 samples (65 tumors and 19 normal tissues), were used for investigation of mRNAs expression of the hub genes between tumor and normal tissues (Illumina

Human V3) [19]. For external validation on gene expression profiles with other target drugs, we further included GSE19043 and GSE95414. GSE19043 contained 21 samples from DiFi and GTL-16 cell lines, of which biological triplicates of DiFi cells with gefitinib (EGFR inhibition) and DMSO (control) were used in this study for validation. The platform was GPL5104, Sentrix HumanRef-8 v2 Expression BeadChip [20]. GSE95414 contained one parental NCI-N87 cell line and one trastuzumab-DM1 (T-DM1, trastuzumab emtansine)-resistant cell line. T-DM1 is designed to achieve a combinational therapy of trastuzumab and DM1 (a potent microtubule-disrupting drug, a maytansine derivative) [21]. The RNA was processed by Human Transcriptome Array 2.0 arrays (Affymetrix, GPL17586). Given the absence of biological replicates, the fold change between the T-DM1-resistant cell line and parental cell line was used for investigation (original study of GSE95414 is not yet published).

Data processing on DEGs

The differentially expressed genes (DEGs) between the trastuzumab-resistant cell lines and sensitive control were identified by the GEO2R analytical tool [22]. Benjamini and Hochberg method was used for false discovery rate (FDR). The cut-off values of DEGs were defined as adj.p value < 0.05 and log2 fold change (log FC) > 2 or < -2. The DEG expression data were processed for a bidirectional hierarchical clustering plot (FunRich, http://www.funrich.org) [23].

Gene ontology and pathway analysis of DEGs

The Database for Annotation, Visualization, and Integrated Discovery (DAVID, http://david.abcc.ncifcrf.gov/) was employed for the gene ontology (GO) consortium reference, including biological processes (BP), cellular components (CC), and molecular functions (MF) [24, 25]. In addition, DAVID was also employed for pathway enrichment annotations with the data resources from Kyoto Encyclopedia of Genes and Genomes (KEGG, http://www.genome.jp/kegg/) pathway enrichment analysis [24, 26].

Protein-protein interaction (PPI) networks and module analysis

The interaction networks of the DEG-coded proteins were determined by the Search Tool for the Retrieval of Interacting Genes/Proteins (STRING, http://www.string-db.org/) [27]. Node degree ≥ 5 was defined as the cut-off values for further PPI networks visualization by Cytoscape software (version 3.6.0; http://www.cytoscape.org/) [28]. The Molecular Complex Detection (MCODE) program embedded in Cytoscape was used to subcluster the PPI networks with predefined cutoff criterions (max. depth = 100, node score = 0.2 and k-score = 2) [29]. Hub genes were defined by the degree value (paired connections between each node). In addition, the betweenness centrality (defining the fraction of shortest paths involved in a given node) of the hub genes were also added.

Survival analysis of the hub genes

Kaplan-Meier (KM) plotter enables comprehensive analysis of the prognostic values among lists of genes in various cancers based on multiple genomic profiles, including GSE14210, GSE15459, GSE22377, GSE29272, GSE51105, and GSE62254 [30]. The prognostic values of overall survivals (OS) for hub genes were displayed with the hazard ratios (HR) and log-rank p values.

Hub genes correlation in TCGA

The gene expression profiling interactive analysis (GEPIA, http://gepia.cancer-pku.cn) was established for customized genomic analysis based on The Cancer Genome Atlas (TCGA) database [31]. The top 20 hub genes were extracted for interactive networks based on paired gene correlations of the stomach adenocarcinoma (STAD) cohort in TCGA (Pearson correlation coefficients). In addition, the mRNA expressions of the hub genes were also investigated between tumor and normal tissues.

Moreover, the stage-specific expression of each hub gene was also generated by GEPIA. The mRNA expressions of the hub genes of TCGA (STAD) were also retrieved from the Xena system, University of California, Santa Cruz (UCSC) for prognostic analysis [32].

Statistical analysis

Generally, p value < 0.05 was defined as cut-off criterion and considered statistically significant in all cases. SPSS 17.0 (Chicago, IL, USA) and Prism 5.0 (GraphPad Software, San Diego, CA) were used for statistical analysis and illustration.

Results

Identification of DEGs and heat map clustering

A total of 849 DEGs were identified to be associated with trastuzumab resistance, with 374 genes upregulated and 475 downregulated (Fig. 1). A bidirectional hierarchical clustering heat map of the DEGs was illustrated (Fig. 2).

GO enrichment analysis

The GO enrichment analysis was conducted by the DAVID tool. A total of 193 BP terms significantly enriched, including epithelium development/cell surface receptor signaling pathway/locomotion (Table 1). A total of 23 CC terms were significantly enriched, including membrane-bounded vesicle/extracellular region part/extracellular vesicle (Table 1). A total of nine MF terms were significantly enriched, including top-ranked cell adhesion molecular binding/glycoprotein binding/growth factor binding (Table 1). Specifically, in each term, top ranked 10 most

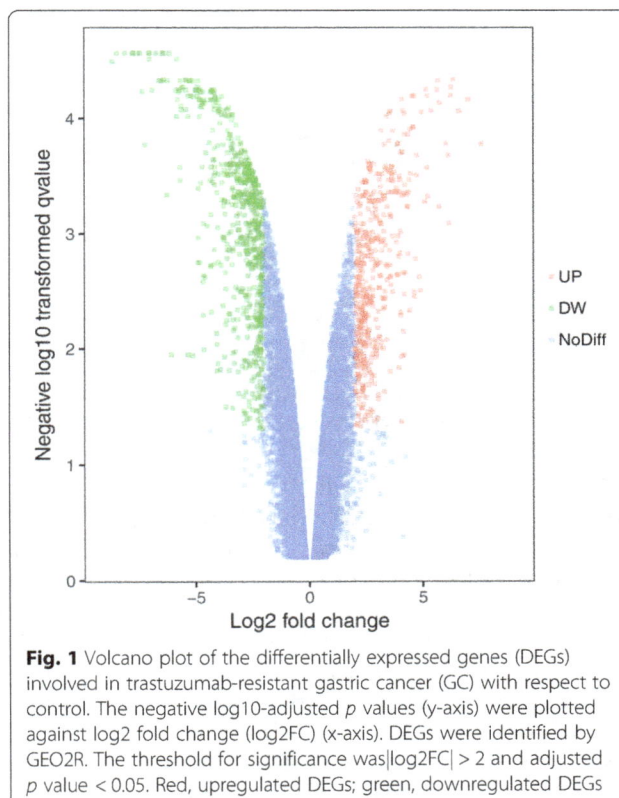

Fig. 1 Volcano plot of the differentially expressed genes (DEGs) involved in trastuzumab-resistant gastric cancer (GC) with respect to control. The negative log10-adjusted p values (y-axis) were plotted against log2 fold change (log2FC) (x-axis). DEGs were identified by GEO2R. The threshold for significance was|log2FC| > 2 and adjusted p value < 0.05. Red, upregulated DEGs; green, downregulated DEGs

significantly enriched gene-ontologies of upregulated and downregulated DEGs were compared (Fig. 3). In BP term, nervous system development and response to type I interferon were significantly enriched in up/downregulated DEGs, respectively (Fig. 3a). In CC term, proteinaceous extracellular matrix and extracellular region part were significantly enriched in up/down regulated DEGs, respectively (Fig. 3b). In MF term, protein dimerization activity and cell adhesion molecule binding were significantly enriched in up/down regulated DEGs, respectively (Fig. 3c).

KEGG pathways analysis

Noteworthy, only two significant signaling pathways were identified in KEGG pathway analysis with cut-off values ($p < 0.05$, FDR < 0.05): pathways in cancer (hsa05200) and ECM-receptor interaction (hsa04512) (Table 2). The top ten enriched signaling pathways in upregulated and downregulated DEGs were illustrated, respectively (Fig. 4). Of note, no significant pathway was identified in upregulated set, and only one, the pathways in cancer (hsa5200), was identified as significant in downregulated set.

PPI network and modules

Next, the PPI networks were initially obtained by the STRING database and visualized by Cytoscape with degrees of each nodes ≥ 5. A total of 291 nodes 1883 edges were included in the PPI networks (Fig. 5). The top 20 hub genes

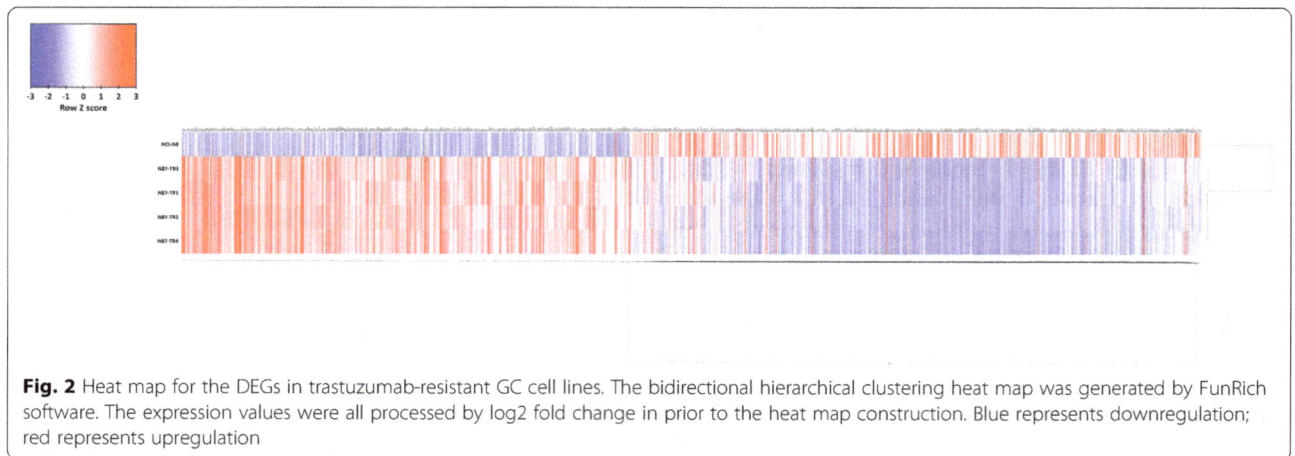

Fig. 2 Heat map for the DEGs in trastuzumab-resistant GC cell lines. The bidirectional hierarchical clustering heat map was generated by FunRich software. The expression values were all processed by log2 fold change in prior to the heat map construction. Blue represents downregulation; red represents upregulation

with highest degrees were determined, including CD44 molecule (CD44), erb-b2 receptor tyrosine kinase 2 (HER2), cadherin 1 (CDH1), 2′-5′-oligoadenylate synthetase 1–3 (OAS1–3), 2′-5′-oligoadenylate synthetase-like (OASL), ISG15 ubiquitin-like modifier (ISG15), bone morphogenetic protein 4 (BMP4), signal transducer and activator of transcription 1 (STAT1), early growth response 1 (EGR1), cyclin D1 (CCND1), vimentin (VIM), Wnt family member 5A (WNT5A), KIT proto-oncogene receptor tyrosine kinase (KIT), bone morphogenetic protein 2 (BMP2), interferon regulatory factor 9 (IRF9), MX dynamin-like GTPase 1 (MX1), FYN proto-oncogene, Src family tyrosine kinase (FYN), and HECT and RLD domain containing E3 ubiquitin protein ligase family member 6 (HERC6) (Fig. 5, Table 3).

In addition, the top scored three modules were determined by MCODE in Cytoscape, with KEGG enrichment results (Fig. 6). Furthermore, the siRNAs of the hub genes were summarized (Additional file 1: Table S1) [33–51].

Prognostic analysis and mRNA expression of hub genes

The prognostic values of the hub genes were assessed by the KM plotter in GC. High HER2, CDH1, OAS1, OAS3, ISG15, BMP4, CCND1, and WNT5A expression levels were associated with poor OS, whereas high CD44, STAT1, EGR1, VIM, KIT, and FYN expression levels were associated with favorable OS. OAS2, OASL, BMP2, IRF9, MX1, and HERC6 were not significantly associated with OS (Fig. 7). The mRNAs expression of CD44, HER2, CDH1,

Table 1 Gene ontology analysis of the DEGs

Category	Term/gene function	Gene count	%	p value	FDR
GOTERM_BP_FAT	GO:0060429~epithelium development	112	13.25444	1.53E−17	3.01E−14
GOTERM_BP_FAT	GO:0007166~cell surface receptor signaling pathway	207	24.49704	2.44E−16	4.33E−13
GOTERM_BP_FAT	GO:0040011~locomotion	134	15.85799	4.27E−14	8.38E−11
GOTERM_BP_FAT	GO:2000026~regulation of multicellular organismal development	145	17.15976	6.52E−14	1.28E−10
GOTERM_BP_FAT	GO:0009887~organ morphogenesis	99	11.71598	9.11E−14	1.79E−10
GOTERM_CC_FAT	GO:0031988~membrane-bounded vesicle	255	30.17751	2.34E−13	3.49E−10
GOTERM_CC_FAT	GO:0044421~extracellular region part	266	31.47929	1.57E−12	2.34E−09
GOTERM_CC_FAT	GO:1903561~extracellular vesicle	206	24.3787	1.08E−11	1.61E−08
GOTERM_CC_FAT	GO:0043230~extracellular organelle	206	24.3787	1.11E−11	1.65E−08
GOTERM_CC_FAT	GO:0070062~extracellular exosome	204	24.14201	2.24E−11	3.34E−08
GOTERM_MF_FAT	GO:0050839~cell adhesion molecule binding	53	6.272189	1.39E−09	2.27E−06
GOTERM_MF_FAT	GO:0001948~glycoprotein binding	20	2.366864	1.71E−07	2.78E−04
GOTERM_MF_FAT	GO:0019838~growth factor binding	21	2.485207	1.31E−06	0.002133
GOTERM_MF_FAT	GO:0098631~protein binding involved in cell adhesion	34	4.023669	4.03E−06	0.006547
GOTERM_MF_FAT	GO:0000982~transcription factor activity, RNA polymerase II core promoter proximal region sequence-specific binding	36	4.260355	7.11E−06	0.011559

As a total of 193 biological processes (BP), 23 cellular components (CC), nine molecular functions (MF) enriched in gene ontology (GO), only the top five in each term according to the false discovery rate (FDR) value were illustrated

DEGs differentially expressed genes

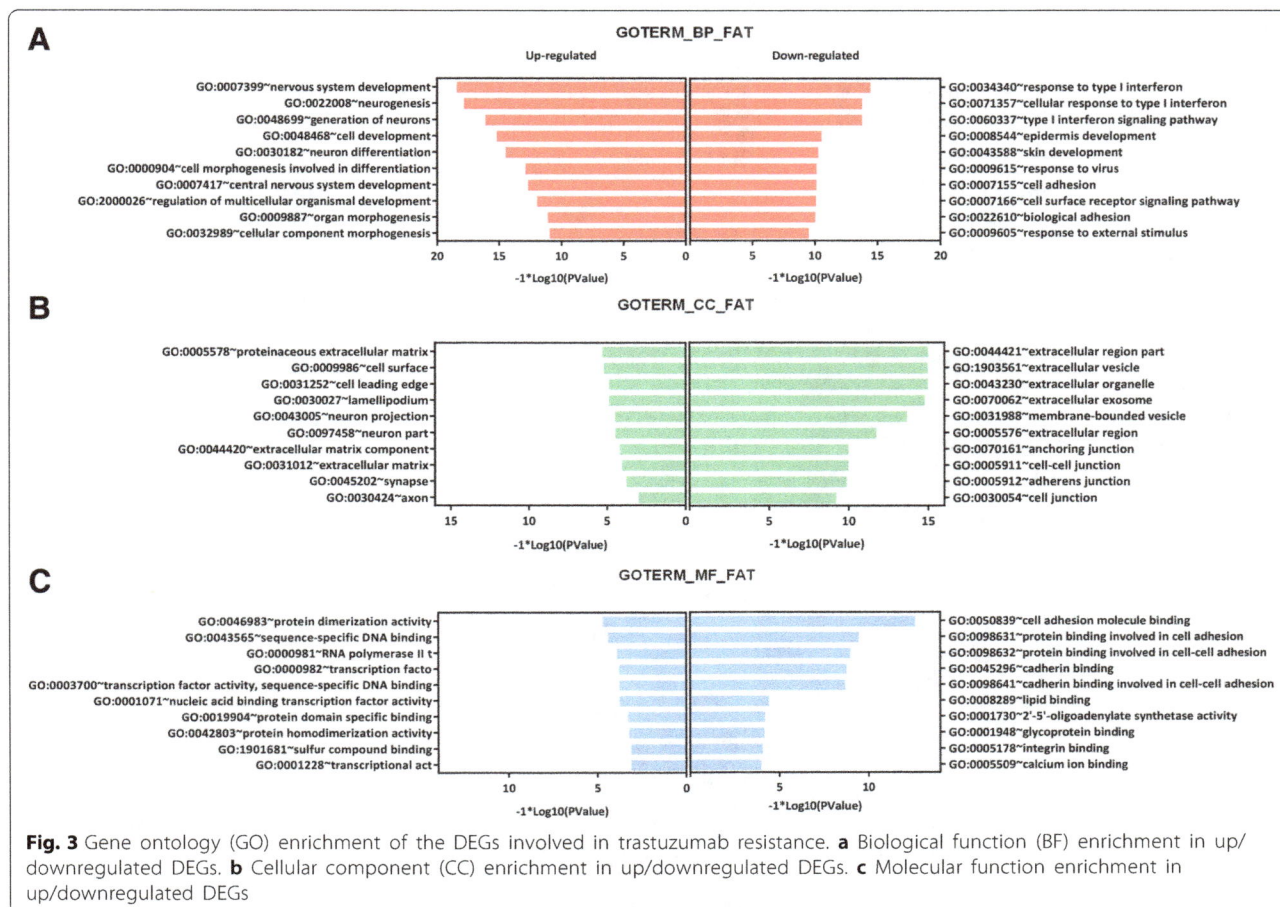

Fig. 3 Gene ontology (GO) enrichment of the DEGs involved in trastuzumab resistance. **a** Biological function (BF) enrichment in up/downregulated DEGs. **b** Cellular component (CC) enrichment in up/downregulated DEGs. **c** Molecular function enrichment in up/downregulated DEGs

OAS1, OAS2, OAS3, OASL, ISG15, STAT1, CCND1, and WNT5A were significantly upregulated in tumor while only KIT was significantly downregulated in tumor (TCGA) compared to normal (TCGA normal + GTEx normal) (Fig. 8a). Next, we further compared the mRNA expression of the hub genes between tumor (TCGA) and normal (TCGA) by the data retrieved from the Xena system. In fact, the results from the Xena (TCGA tumor vs TCGA normal) were different from GEPIA (TCGA tumor vs TCGA normal + GTEx normal). Only five hub genes

Table 2 KEGG pathway enrichment analysis

KEGG pathway	Gene counts	%	p value	FDR	Genes
hsa05200: pathways in cancer	44	5.21	5.95E−08	7.75E−05	GNG4,CCND1,STAT1,LAMB3, JUP,SMAD4,ITGA2,RUNX1, WNT5A,KIT,FGFR3,LAMA4, ITGA3,BCL2L1,FZD8,ADCY7, AXIN2,COL4A1,RAC2, COL4A6,LAMC3,SMO,LPAR5, LAMA1,RXRA,PAS1,FGF20, SLC2A1,ERBB2,ITGA6,WNT11, CDH1,TGFA,BMP2,ADCY1, FZD9,BMP4,GNG7,GNB4,KITLG, LAMC2,FGF9,F2R,LAMA5
hsa04512: ECM-receptor interaction	18	2.13	3.05E−07	3.98E−04	LAMA1,sdc1,LAMB3,ITGA6, ITGA2,ITGB4,ITGA3,LAMA4, THBS1,SV2A,COL4A1,COL6A1, COL4A6,LAMC2,SDC4,CD44, LAMC3,LAMA5

KEGG Kyoto Encyclopedia of Genes and Genome
FDR false discovery rate

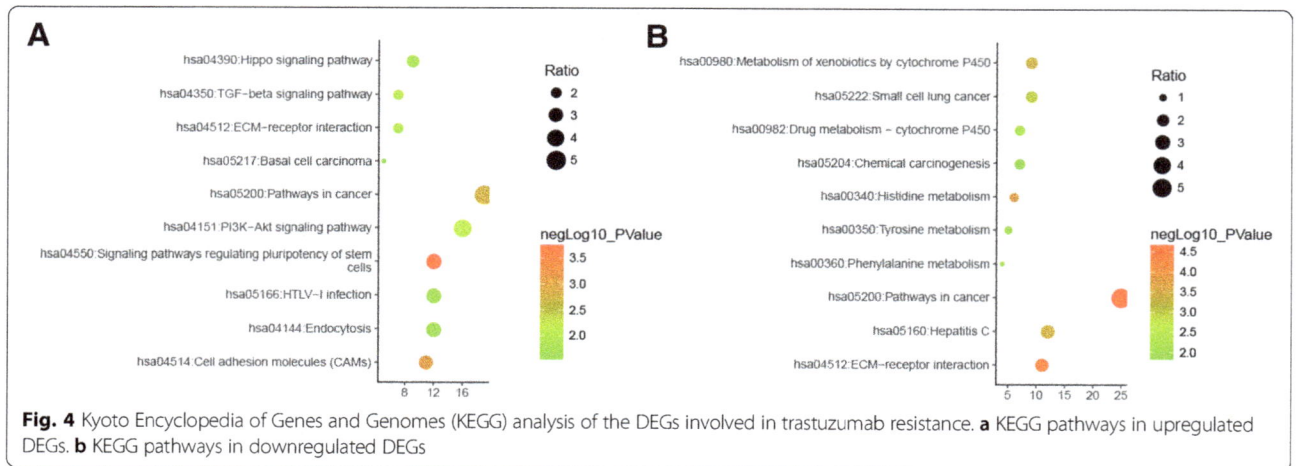

Fig. 4 Kyoto Encyclopedia of Genes and Genomes (KEGG) analysis of the DEGs involved in trastuzumab resistance. **a** KEGG pathways in upregulated DEGs. **b** KEGG pathways in downregulated DEGs

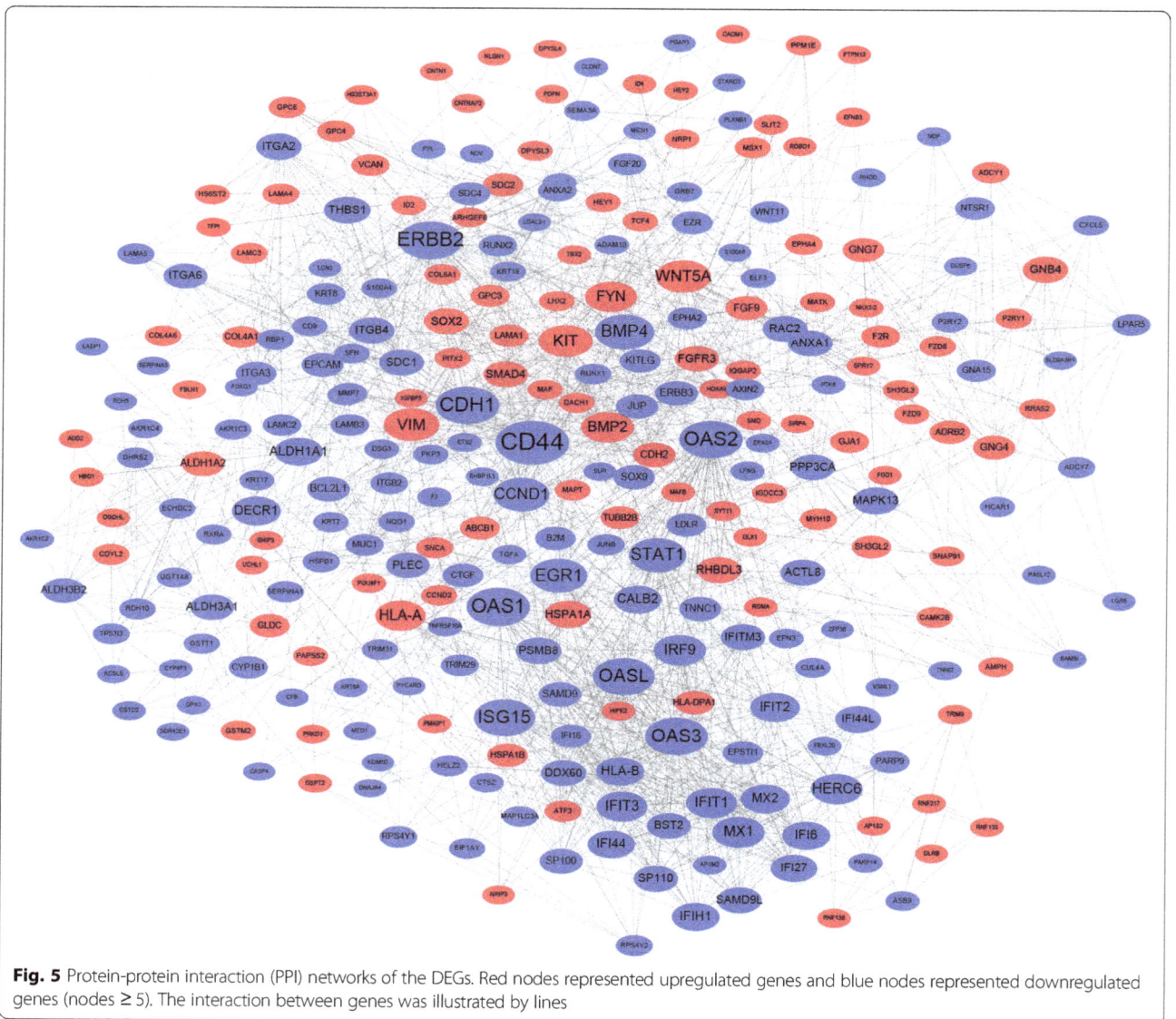

Fig. 5 Protein-protein interaction (PPI) networks of the DEGs. Red nodes represented upregulated genes and blue nodes represented downregulated genes (nodes ≥ 5). The interaction between genes was illustrated by lines

Table 3 Hub genes in the PPI networks

Gene symbols	Gene names	Degrees	Betweenness centrality
CD44	CD44 molecule	68	0.11543115
ERBB2	erb-b2 receptor tyrosine kinase 2	53	0.07513542
CDH1	cadherin 1	52	0.07282977
OAS1	2'-5'-oligoadenylate synthetase 1	52	0.01778379
OAS2	2'-5'-oligoadenylate synthetase 2	52	0.01854906
OAS3	2'-5'-oligoadenylate synthetase 3	51	0.01691589
OASL	2'-5'-oligoadenylate synthetase-like	50	0.01635114
ISG15	ISG15 ubiquitin-like modifier	49	0.02075018
BMP4	Bone morphogenetic protein 4	46	0.04507158
STAT1	Signal transducer and activator of transcription 1	43	0.03737542
EGR1	Early growth response 1	42	0.04589496
CCND1	Cyclin D1	41	0.03727744
VIM	Vimentin	40	0.06221522
WNT5A	Wnt family member 5A	39	0.04301014
KIT	KIT proto-oncogene receptor tyrosine kinase	37	0.03489184
BMP2	Bone morphogenetic protein 2	35	0.02672618
IRF9	Interferon regulatory factor 9	35	0.00398764
MX1	MX dynamin-like GTPase 1	35	0.00512151
FYN	FYN proto-oncogene, Src family tyrosine kinase	34	0.05255568
HERC6	HECT and RLD domain containing E3 ubiquitin-protein ligase family member 6	34	0.02783539

(STAT1, OAS3, OAS2, CDH1, ISG15) significantly exhibited upregulation and two hub genes (KIT and EGR1) exhibited downregulation according to the thresholds (adj.*p* value < 0.05 and |logFC| > 1) (Additional file 2: Table S2). Interestingly, the gene with the most significant logFC value is KIT (logFC = − 2.11514), whereas the gene with the most significant adj.*p* value is STAT1 (adj.*p* value = 8.99E−12).

Furthermore, the mRNA expression of the hub genes (IRF9 was not available) was externally validated in GSE13861 (Additional file 3: Figure S1). Consistently, CD44, OAS3, ISG15, STAT1, and WNT5A were significantly upregulated whereas KIT was significantly downregulated in tumor compared to normal in GSE13861. Moreover, BMP4 was significantly upregulated in tumor in GSE13861. OASL, EGR1, and BMP2 were significantly downregulated in tumor in GSE13861 (Additional file 3: Figure S1). Moreover, the mRNA expression of all the hub genes in specific clinic stages had been analyzed. In fact, only CD44 (*p* = 0.0146), VIM (*p* = 1.07e−05) and KIT (0.00759) exhibited significant stage-specific expression (Additional file 4: Figure S2).

Mechanism of hub genes correlations associated with trastuzumab resistance

To further elucidate the underlying mechanism between the DEGs, the STAD of TCGA data was employed based on GEPIA platform. Of note, 87.8% (65/74) gene-gene correlations were positive. What is more, OAS1, 3, and CDH1 featured high degrees and strong correlations with other hub genes. Additionally, VIM was negatively correlated with CCND1, HER2, and CDH1, respectively. KIT was negatively correlated with HER2, ISG15, and OAS1, respectively (Fig. 8b). Meanwhile, to investigate the potential roles of the hub genes in other target therapies, GSE19043 and GSE95414 were retrieved for external investigation (Additional file 5: Table S3). In GSE19043, none of the hub genes exhibited differential expression between gefitinib group and control, whereas in GSE95414, only six of the hub genes, including VIM, BMP2, CD44, OAS3, KIT, and WNT5A, showed slight fold change values > 1 between T-DM1-resistant cell lines and control (Additional file 6: Figure S3). In summary, the hub genes identified in this study may not be directly involved in gefitinib (EGFR inhibition, GSE95414) and T-DM1 (GSE19043) (Additional file 6: Figure S3).

Discussion

Although the overall mortality and morbidity of GC has been declining over the decades around the globe, it is one of the most common causes for cancer-related deaths. Postoperative recurrence remains high even with curable resection and combinational chemotherapy [7–9]. Trastuzumab, the only approved treatment for GC with HER2 overexpress, had contributed to the encouraging results in GC clinical trials [13, 14]. However, secondary resistance of trastuzumab remained one of the major challenges in treatment courses. Therefore, identification of potential mechanisms and key genes underlying the acquired trastuzumab resistance could distinguish the sensitive subsets and improve overall benefits.

Generally, individual gene rarely dictate either systematic biochemical physiological actions or sophisticated multilevel network interactions. Up to now, genomic data had been stored in large matrix and processed by well-established bioinformatics pipelines for the ultimate conclusive visualization.

This study provided a systematic bioinformatics analysis of the gene expression profile, GSE77346, containing four trastuzumab-resistant cell lines and one sensitive cell line. Pathways in cancer and ECM-receptor interaction were the most significantly enriched for all DEGs. CD44, STAT1, EGR1, VIM, KIT, and FYN were associated with favorable OS while HER2, CDH1, OAS1, OAS3, ISG15, BMP4, CCND1, and WNT5A were associated with poor OS.

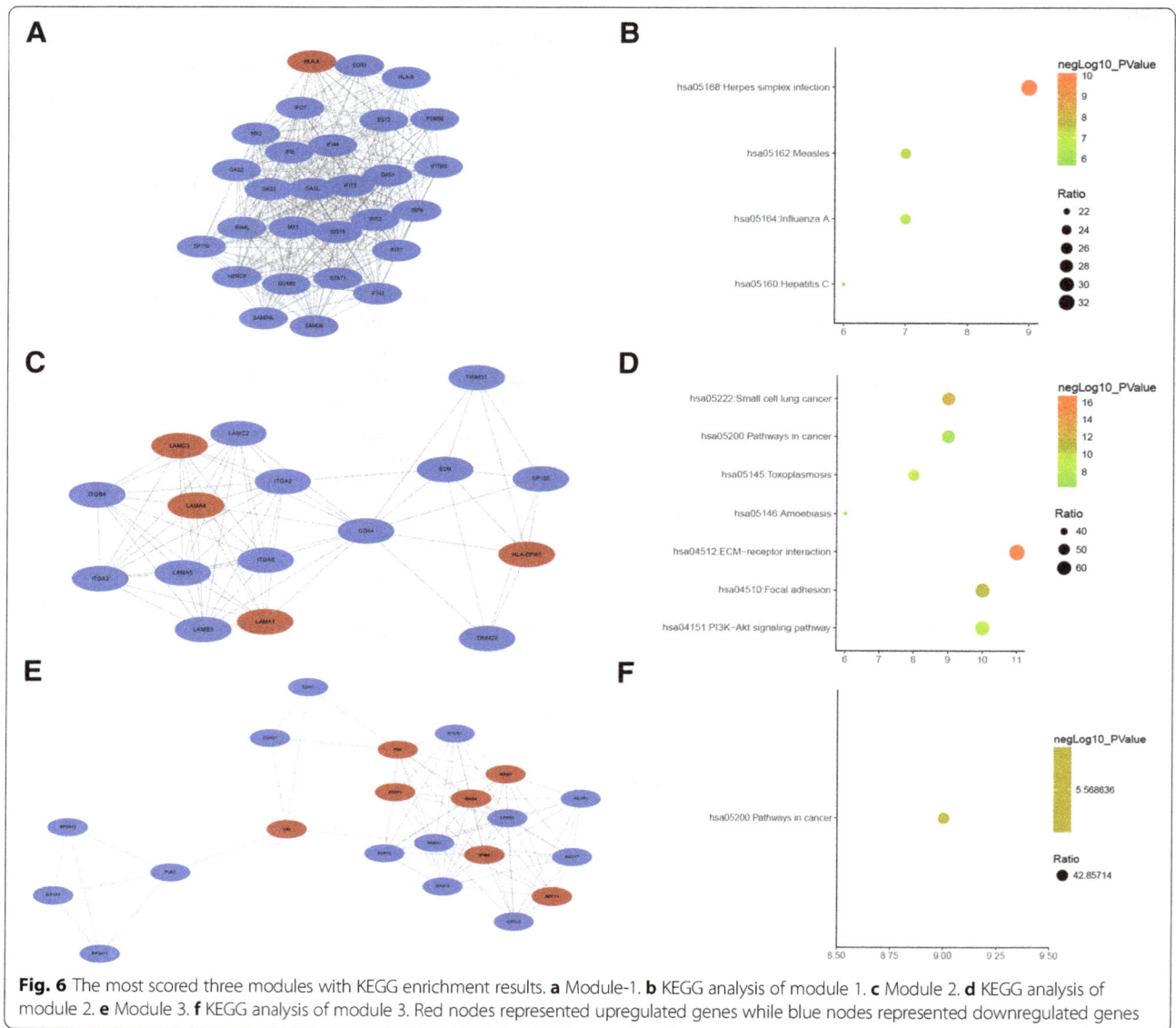

Fig. 6 The most scored three modules with KEGG enrichment results. **a** Module-1. **b** KEGG analysis of module 1. **c** Module 2. **d** KEGG analysis of module 2. **e** Module 3. **f** KEGG analysis of module 3. Red nodes represented upregulated genes while blue nodes represented downregulated genes

Mechanistically, OAS1, OAS3, and CDH1 featured highest degrees among the hub genes, diverse from the nodes (CD44, HER2, and CDH1) with highest degrees in PPI networks.

OAS1 and OAS3, which encode the key enzymes, 2′, 5′-oligoadenylate synthetase (2′5′AS), are involved in viral genome degradation and inhibits protein synthesis [52, 53]. As classic interferon target genes, OAS1 and OAS3 differ in cellular compartment, conformation, and biological functions [54]. Previously, OAS1 and OAS3 had been participated in apoptosis process [55]. Until now, only OAS3 had been associated with the HPV persistence and progression of cervical cancer [56]. No specific study unveiled the association between OAS1 and OAS3 and GC. This is

the first in silico study suggesting the involvement of OAS1and OAS3 in trastuzumab-resistant GC.

CD44, a key cancer stem cell (CSC) marker, was downregulated in trastuzumab-resistant breast cancer and associated with the trastuzumab resistance in GC. [57]. Previously, high expression of CD44 correlated with downregulated HER2 in breast cancer cell lines [58]. SiRNA CD44 led to reduced internalization of trastuzumab, highlighting the involvement of endocytosis and membrane trafficking [58]. Furthermore, Bao et al. revealed that CD44 could directly bind to HER2 and increase invasiveness both in vivo and vitro [59]. Consistently, this study highlighted CD44 as the top hub gene in PPI networks of trastuzumab-resistant GC; however, the correlation between CD44 and HER2 associated with trastuzumab resistance in GC required further validation.

Hub genes	HR(95%CI)		logrank p
CD44	0.73(0.59-0.91)		0.0045
ERBB2	1.22(1-1.48)		0.05
CDH1	1.35(1.08-1.69)		0.0072
OAS1	1.25(1.03-1.51)		0.025
OAS2	0.87(0.64-1.17)		0.3551
OAS3	1.45(1.16-1.82)		0.0009
OASL	0.83(0.67-1.02)		0.0771
ISG15	1.35(1.11-1.64)		0.0025
BMP4	1.38(1.12-1.7)		0.0024
STAT1	0.71(0.57-0.89)		0.0025
EGR1	0.62(0.51-0.77)		4.8E-06
CCND1	1.62(1.31-2)		7.7E-06
VIM	0.7(0.57-0.86)		0.0008
WNT5A	1.76(1.45-2.14)		8.2E-09
KIT	0.73(0.59-0.91)		0.0053
BMP2	1.16(0.93-1.45)		0.1754
IRF9	0.83(0.68-1.01)		0.0615
MX1	0.92(0.74-1.15)		0.4855
FYN	0.73(0.6-0.89)		0.0014
HERC6	1.15(0.95-1.4)		0.1591

0   0.5   1   1.5   2   2.5

Fig. 7 Survival plots of the prognostic values (overall survival) of hub genes involved in trastuzumab-resistant GC. The survival values of the hub genes were generated by the Kaplan-Meier (KM) plotter. The expressions of hub genes were dichotomized by optimal cutoff values. Patients number = 593. p values were calculated by log rank method

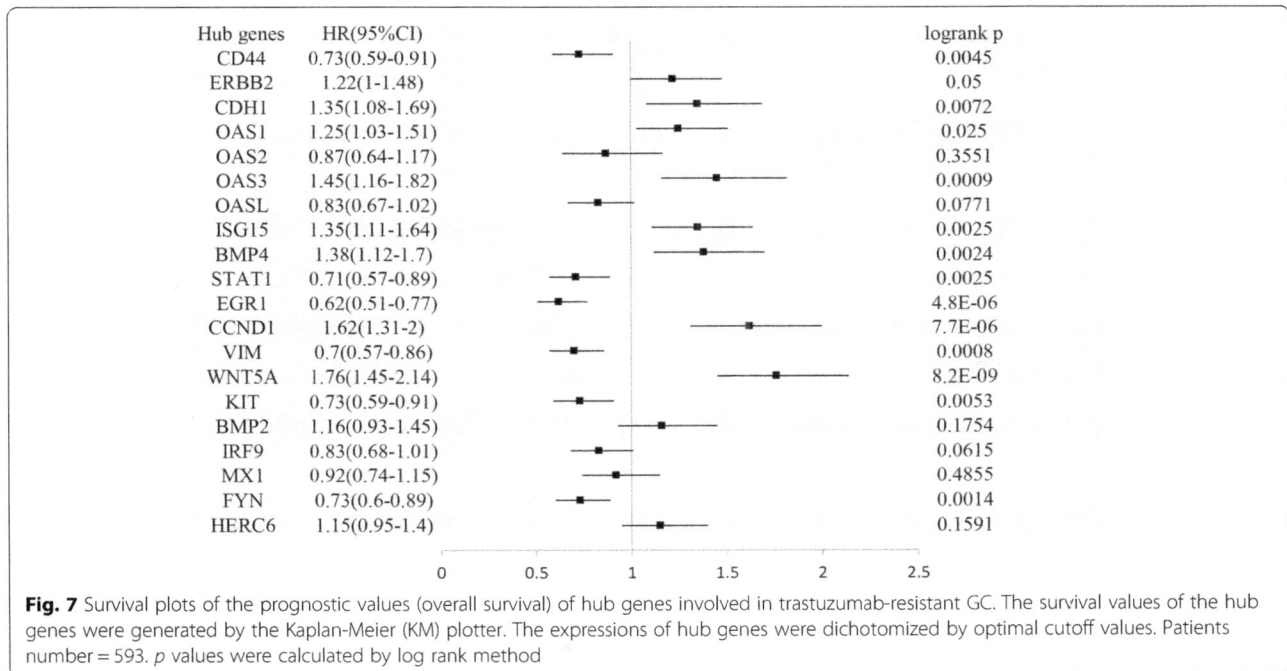

Noteworthy, eight of the 20 hub genes (WNT5A, BMP4, BMP2, CCND1, HER2, CDH1, KIT, STAT1) associated with trastuzumab resistance were commonly enriched in the pathways in cancer (KEGG hsa05200). Thus, the acquired resistance of trastuzumab in GC at least could be partially attributed by the progression of GC itself, if not all. Moreover, the potential impact of the mutations and fusion of the genes in the pathway in cancer on the trastuzumab resistance in GC remains largely unsolved.

In addition, for PPI networks, both degree and betweenness centrality were included for proper evaluation of hub genes. Generally, centrality is not generally equivalent to connectivity. As a local quantity, connectivity does not fully elucidate the importance of certain node in PPI networks. Thus, both connectivity and betweenness centrality were incorporated for a good measurement of hub genes in PPI networks [60].

Remarkably, ion channels, one of the major transmembrane complexes that regulate the communication between the extracellular matrix and intracellular environments, can influence the growth and invasiveness of cancer cells by altered expression or biological activities [61, 62]. In fact, ion channels could be novel molecular targets [62]. Fujimoto et al. indicated that the inhibition of ANO1, a Ca2 + -activated Cl- channel overexpressed in HER2-positive breast cancer, could lead to the transcriptional repression of HER2 in breast cancer cells with resistance to trastuzumab [63]. Another Ca2 + -permeable channel, transient receptor potential canonical 6 (TRPC6), exhibited a vital role in tumor growth, differentiation, and apoptosis with promising pharmaceutic target values [64, 65].

Recently, Huang et al. published a result focusing on the trastuzumab-resistant role of COL4A1 in GC [66]. Validation of COL4A1 in GSE77346 was one of the key steps in their study. However, GSE77346 remained far from fully explored with respect to trastuzumab resistance. In fact, new agents to be discovered against HER2 and other signaling pathways open the way to the improvement of trastuzumab therapy [67].

In breast cancer, trastuzumab remains one of the intensively studied drugs. It has been recommended as combination treatments in breast cancer [67]. In fact, mining the relationships between HER2 signaling pathway and other signaling pathways as well as the potential mechanisms provides greater insights for rational combination therapy. Currently, targets such as mTOR, PI3K, IGF-1R, Akt, HSP90, and VEGF exhibited significant clinical interests in HER2-positive breast cancer [67]. However, insightful evidences to define, refine, and optimize the use of trastuzumab in gastric cancer patients with HER2-positive remain largely lacked. Therefore, this study contributed to the understanding of trastuzumab resistance and the prognostic values of hub genes and opened the way for future research in combination therapy in gastric cancer.

Noteworthy, this was the first in silico study focusing on the bioinformatics analysis of trastuzumab resistance in GC, predicting the key genes and pathways associated with trastuzumab resistance. In addition, this study also investigated the prognostic values of key genes. However, no disease-free survival (DFS) or progression-free survival (PFS) was collected. Further clinical and experimental validation of the study findings was required.

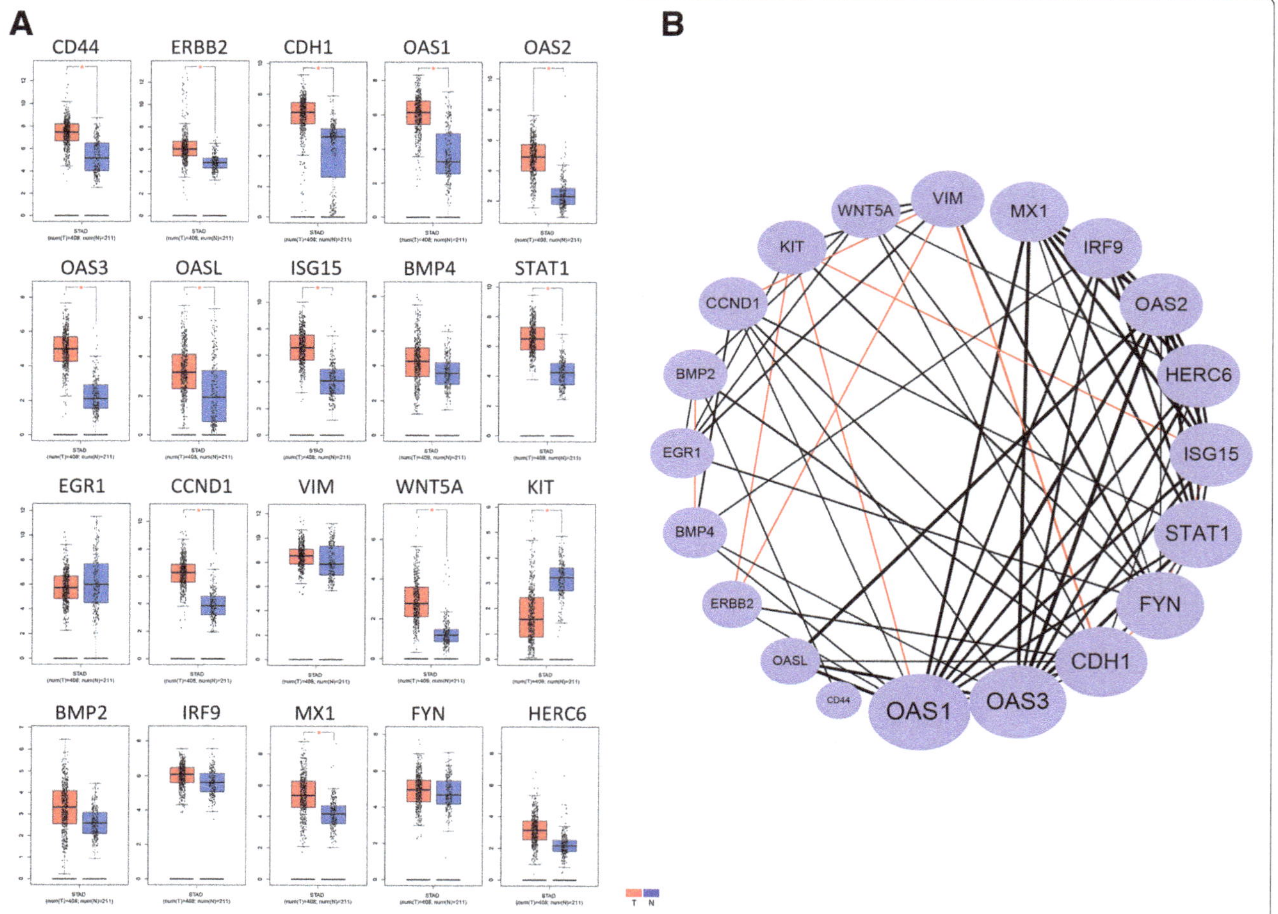

Fig. 8 The mRNA expression and gene-gene correlation of the hub genes associated with trastuzumab-resistant GC. **a** The mRNAs expression of hub genes in tumor and normal tissues in TCGA, red: tumor, blue: normal. **b** the STAD of TCGA was calculated with Pearson's correlation coefficient (− 1 to 1). Red line: negative correlation, black line: positive correlation. Wider line indicated higher correlation value (*p* value < 0.05)

Conclusion

This bioinformatics analysis identified key genes and pathways as potential targets and predictors associated with trastuzumab resistance GC and further opened the way to the improvement of trastuzumab therapy in GC.

Additional files

Additional file 1: Table S1. 20 hub genes with siRNA synthesizers and sequence [34–52].

Additional file 2: Table S2. The adj. *p* value and log fold change (logFC) of the hub genes in TCGA and GSE77346 datasets.

Additional file 3: Figure S1. The mRNA expression of hub genes in GSE13861.

Additional file 4: Figure S2. The mRNA expression of hub genes in clinical stages in TCGA.

Additional file 5: Table S3. Targeted drugs with corresponding GEO datasets for gastric cancer.

Additional file 6: Figure S3. The mRNA expression and the fold change of the hub genes. (A) the mRNA expression of hub genes in GSE19043 (Gefitinib); (B) the fold change of hub genes in GSE95414.

Abbreviations

BP: Biological processes; CC: Cellular components; CI: Confidential intervals; CSC: Cancer stem cell; DAVID: Database for Annotation, Visualization, and Integrated Discovery; DFS: Disease-free survival; EGFR: Epidermal growth factor receptor; FDR: False discovery rate; GC: Gastric cancer; GEO: Gene Expression Omnibus; GFP: Green fluorescent protein; GO: Gene ontology; HER2: Epidermal growth factor receptor 2; HR: Hazard ratio; KEGG: Kyoto Encyclopedia of Genes and Genomes; MCODE: Molecular Complex Detection; MF: Molecular functions; OS: Overall survival; PFS: Progression-free survival; PPI: The protein-protein interaction; RPMI: Roswell Park Memorial Institute; STAD: Stomach Adenocarcinoma; STRING: Search Tool for the Retrieval of Interacting Genes; TCGA: The Cancer Genome Atlas

Acknowledgements

We would like to thank the Shanghai Institute of Digestive Surgery, Ruijin Hospital, Shanghai Jiao Tong University School of Medicine for academic support.

Funding

The study is financially supported by the National Natural Science Foundation of China (NSFC) (81402423, 81572818) and Shanghai Municipal Commission of Health and Family Planning (2017YQ062).

Human participants and animal rights

This article does not contain any studies with human participants or animals performed by any of the authors.

Authors contributions

CY, LZ, PX, and RP carried out data analysis. CY, ZC, ZH, JS, and MZ drafted the manuscript. JS, MZ, and CY participated in the study design and data collection. All authors read and approved the final manuscript.

Competing interests

The authors declare that they have no competing interests.

Author details

[1]Department of General Surgery, Ruijin Hospital, Shanghai Jiao Tong University, School of Medicine, Shanghai 200025, People's Republic of China. [2]Shanghai Minimally Invasive Surgery Center, Ruijin Hospital, Shanghai Jiao Tong University, School of Medicine, Shanghai 200025, People's Republic of China.

References

1. Siegel RL, Miller KD, Jemal A. Cancer statistics, 2016. CA Cancer J Clin. 2016; 66(1):7–30.
2. Chen W, Zheng R, Baade PD, Zhang S, Zeng H, Bray F, Jemal A, Yu XQ, He J. Cancer statistics in China, 2015. CA Cancer J Clin. 2016;66(2):115–32.
3. Ajani JA, Bentrem DJ, Besh S, D'Amico TA, Das P, Denlinger C, Fakih MG, Fuchs CS, Gerdes H, Glasgow RE, Hayman JA. Gastric cancer, version 2.2013. J Natl Compr Cancer Netw. 2013;11(5):531–46.
4. Guggenheim DE, Shah MA. Gastric cancer epidemiology and risk factors. J Surg Oncol. 2013;107(3):230–6.
5. Jemal A, Bray F, Center MM, Ferlay J, Ward E, Forman D. Global cancer statistics. CA Cancer J Clin. 2011;61(2):69–90.
6. Japanese Gastric Cancer Association. Japanese gastric cancer treatment guidelines 2014 (ver. 4). Gastric Cancer. 2017;20(1):1–9.
7. Kang WM, Meng QB, Yu JC, Ma ZQ, Li ZT. Factors associated with early recurrence after curative surgery for gastric cancer. World J Gastroenterol: WJG. 2015;21(19):5934.
8. Hartgrink HH, Van de Velde CJ, Putter H, Bonenkamp JJ, Klein Kranenbarg E, Songun I, Welvaart K, Van Krieken JH, Meijer S, Plukker JT, Van Elk PJ. Extended lymph node dissection for gastric cancer: who may benefit? Final results of the randomized Dutch gastric cancer group trial. J Clin Oncol. 2004;22(11):2069–77.
9. Cuschieri A, Weeden S, Fielding J, Bancewicz J, Craven J, Joypaul V, Sydes M. Patient survival after D 1 and D 2 resections for gastric cancer: long-term results of the MRC randomized surgical trial. Br J Cancer. 1999;79(9–10):1522.
10. Wilke H, Muro K, Van Cutsem E, Oh SC, Bodoky G, Shimada Y, Hironaka S, Sugimoto N, Lipatov O, Kim TY, Cunningham D. Ramucirumab plus paclitaxel versus placebo plus paclitaxel in patients with previously treated advanced gastric or gastro-oesophageal junction adenocarcinoma (RAINBOW): a double-blind, randomised phase 3 trial. Lancet Oncol. 2014;15(11):1224–35.
11. Satoh T, Lee KH, Rha SY, Sasaki Y, Park SH, Komatsu Y, Yasui H, Kim TY, Yamaguchi K, Fuse N, Yamada Y. Randomized phase II trial of nimotuzumab plus irinotecan versus irinotecan alone as second-line therapy for patients with advanced gastric cancer. Gastric Cancer. 2015;18(4):824–32.
12. Seidman A, Hudis C, Pierri MK, Shak S, Paton V, Ashby M, Murphy M, Stewart SJ, Keefe D. Cardiac dysfunction in the trastuzumab clinical trials experience. J Clin Oncol. 2002;20(5):1215–21.
13. Bang YJ, Van Cutsem E, Feyereislova A, Chung HC, Shen L, Sawaki A, Lordick F, Ohtsu A, Omuro Y, Satoh T, Aprile G. Trastuzumab in combination with chemotherapy versus chemotherapy alone for treatment of HER2-positive advanced gastric or gastro-oesophageal junction cancer (ToGA): a phase 3, open-label, randomised controlled trial. Lancet. 2010;376(9742):687–97.
14. Lordick F, Janjigian YY. Clinical impact of tumour biology in the management of gastroesophageal cancer. Nat Rev Clin Oncol. 2016;13(6):348.
15. Xu W, Yang Z, Lu N. Molecular targeted therapy for the treatment of gastric cancer. J Exp Clin Cancer Res. 2016;35(1):1.
16. Okines AF, Cunningham D. Trastuzumab in gastric cancer. Eur J Cancer. 2010;46(11):1949–59.
17. Piro G, Carbone C, Cataldo I, Di Nicolantonio F, Giacopuzzi S, Aprile G, Simionato F, Boschi F, Zanotto M, Mina MM, Santoro R. An FGFR3 autocrine loop sustains acquired resistance to trastuzumab in gastric cancer patients. Clin Cancer Res. 2016;22(24):6164–75.
18. Edgar R, Domrachev M, Lash AE. Gene Expression Omnibus: NCBI gene expression and hybridization array data repository. Nucleic Acids Res. 2002; 30(1):207–10.
19. Cho JY, et al. Gene expression signature–based prognostic risk score in gastric cancer. Clin Cancer Res. 2011;17(7):1850-57.
20. Bertotti A, Burbridge MF, Gastaldi S, Galimi F, Torti D, Medico E, Giordano S, Corso S, Rolland-Valognes G, Lockhart BP, Hickman JA. Only a subset of Met-activated pathways are required to sustain oncogene addiction. Sci Signal. 2009;2(100):ra80.
21. Junttila TT, Li G, Parsons K, Phillips GL, Sliwkowski MX. Trastuzumab-DM1 (T-DM1) retains all the mechanisms of action of trastuzumab and efficiently inhibits growth of lapatinib insensitive breast cancer. Breast Cancer Res Treat. 2011;128(2):347–56.
22. Davis S, Meltzer PS. GEOquery: a bridge between the Gene Expression Omnibus (GEO) and BioConductor. Bioinformatics. 2007;23(14):1846–7.
23. Pathan M, Keerthikumar S, Ang CS, Gangoda L, Quek CY, Williamson NA, Mouradov D, Sieber OM, Simpson RJ, Salim A, Bacic A. FunRich: an open access standalone functional enrichment and interaction network analysis tool. Proteomics. 2015;15(15):2597–601.
24. Huang DW, Sherman BT, Lempicki RA. Systematic and integrative analysis of large gene lists using DAVID bioinformatics resources. Nat Protoc. 2008;4(1):44.
25. Ashburner M, Ball CA, Blake JA, Botstein D, Butler H, Cherry JM, Davis AP, Dolinski K, Dwight SS, Eppig JT, Harris MA. Gene ontology: tool for the unification of biology. Nat Genet. 2000;25(1):25.
26. Kanehisa M, Goto S. KEGG: Kyoto encyclopedia of genes and genomes. Nucleic Acids Res. 2000;28(1):27–30.
27. Szklarczyk D, Franceschini A, Wyder S, Forslund K, Heller D, Huerta-Cepas J, Simonovic M, Roth A, Santos A, Tsafou KP, Kuhn M. STRING v10: protein–protein interaction networks, integrated over the tree of life. Nucleic Acids Res. 2014;43(D1):D447–52.
28. Shannon P, Markiel A, Ozier O, Baliga NS, Wang JT, Ramage D, Amin N, Schwikowski B, Ideker T. Cytoscape: a software environment for integrated models of biomolecular interaction networks. Genome Res. 2003;13(11): 2498–504.
29. Bader GD, Hogue CW. An automated method for finding molecular complexes in large protein interaction networks. BMC Bioinformatics. 2003;4(1):2.
30. Lánczky A, Nagy Á, Bottai G, Munkácsy G, Szabó A, Santarpia L, Győrffy B. miRpower: a web-tool to validate survival-associated miRNAs utilizing expression data from 2178 breast cancer patients. Breast Cancer Res Treat. 2016;160(3):439–46.
31. Tang Z, Li C, Kang B, Gao G, Li C, Zhang Z. GEPIA: a web server for cancer and normal gene expression profiling and interactive analyses. Nucleic Acids Res. 2017;45(W1):W98–102.
32. Goldman M, Craft B, Zhu J, Haussler D. The UCSC Xena system for cancer genomics data visualization and interpretation [abstract]. In: Proceedings of the American Association for Cancer Research Annual Meeting 2017. Washington, DC,: Philadelphia: AACR; 2017. Cancer Res 2017;77(13 Suppl): Abstract nr 2584.
33. Subramaniam V, Vincent IR, Gilakjan M, Jothy S. Suppression of human colon cancer tumors in nude mice by siRNA CD44 gene therapy. Exp Mol Pathol. 2007;83(3):332–40.
34. Tan WB, Jiang S, Zhang Y. Quantum-dot based nanoparticles for targeted silencing of HER2/neu gene via RNA interference. Biomaterials. 2007;28(8): 1565–71.
35. Herrero-Mendez A, Almeida A, Fernández E, Maestre C, Moncada S, Bolaños JP. The bioenergetic and antioxidant status of neurons is controlled by continuous degradation of a key glycolytic enzyme by APC/C–Cdh1. Nat Cell Biol. 2009;11(6):747.

36. Zhao J, Feng N, Li Z, Wang P, Qi Z, Liang W, Zhou X, Xu X, Liu B. 2ng P, oligoadenylate synthetase 1 (OAS1) inhibits PRRSV replication in Marc-145 cells. Antivir Res. 2016;132:268–73.

37. Bin L, Howell MD, Kim BE, Streib JE, Hall CF, Leung DY. Specificity protein 1 is pivotal in the skin's antiviral response. J Allergy Clin Immunol. 2011;127(2):430–8.

38. Lin W, Zhu C, Hong J, Zhao L, Jilg N, Fusco DN, Schaefer EA, Brisac C, Liu X, Peng LF, Xu Q. The spliceosome factor SART1 exerts its anti-HCV action through mRNA splicing. J Hepatol. 2015;62(5):1024–32.

39. Zheng S, Zhu D, Lian X, Liu W, Cao R, Chen P. Porcine 2ction-oligoadenylate synthetases inhibit Japanese encephalitis virus replication in vitro. J Med Virol. 2016;88(5):760–8.

40. Chua PK, McCown MF, Rajyaguru S, Kular S, Varma R, Symons J, Chiu SS, Cammack N, Najera I. Modulation of alpha interferon anti-hepatitis C virus activity by ISG15. J Gen Virol. 2009;90(12):2929–39.

41. Xia Y, Paul BY, Sidis Y, Beppu H, Bloch KD, Schneyer AL, Lin HY. Repulsive guidance molecule RGMa alters utilization of bone morphogenetic protein (BMP) type II receptors by BMP2 and BMP4. J Biol Chem. 2007;282(25):18129–40.

42. Lin W, Choe WH, Hiasa Y, Kamegaya Y, Blackard JT, Schmidt EV, Chung RT. Hepatitis C virus expression suppresses interferon signaling by degrading STAT1. Gastroenterol. 2005;128(4):1034–41.

43. Ogishima T, Shiina H, Breault JE, Terashima M, Honda S, Enokida H, Urakami S, Tokizane T, Kawakami T, Ribeiro-Filho LA, Fujime M. Promoter CpG hypomethylation and transcription factor EGR1 hyperactivate heparanase expression in bladder cancer. Oncogene. 2005;24(45):6765.

44. Oridate N, Kim HJ, Xu X, Lotan R. Growth inhibition of head and neck squamous carcinoma cells by small interfering RNAs targeting eIF4E or cyclin D1 alone or combined with cisplatin. Cancer Biol Ther. 2005;4(3):318–23.

45. Walsh N, O'Donovan N, Kennedy S, Henry M, Meleady P, Clynes M, Dowling P. Identification of pancreatic cancer invasion-related proteins by proteomic analysis. Proteome Sci. 2009;7(1):3.

46. Yang L, et al. siRNA-mediated silencing of Wnt5a regulates inflammatory responses in atherosclerosis through the MAPK/NF-kappaB pathways. Int J Mol Med. 2014;34(4):1147–52.

47. Lefevre G, et al. Roles of stem cell factor/c-Kit and effects of Glivec/STI571 in human uveal melanoma cell tumorigenesis. J Biol Chem. 2004;279(30):31769-79.

48. Morrow AN, Schmeisser H, Tsuno T, Zoon KC. A novel role for IFN-stimulated gene factor 3II in IFN-γ signaling and induction of antiviral activity in human cells. J Immunol. 2010:1001359.

49. Toyokawa K, Leite F, Ott TL. Cellular localization and function of the antiviral protein, ovine Mx1 (oMx1): II. The oMx1 protein is a regulator of secretion in an ovine glandular epithelial cell line. Am J Reprod Immunol. 2007;57(1):23–33.

50. Chen S, Charness ME. Ethanol inhibits neuronal differentiation by disrupting activity-dependent neuroprotective protein signaling. Proc Natl Acad Sci. 2008; https://doi.org/10.1073/pnas.0807758105.

51. Arimoto KI, Hishiki T, Kiyonari H, Abe T, Cheng C, Yan M, Fan JB, Futakuchi M, Tsuda H, Murakami Y, Suzuki H. Murine Herc6 plays a critical role in protein ISGylation in vivo and has an ISGylation-independent function in seminal vesicles. J Interf Cytokine Res. 2015;35(5):351–8.

52. Bonnevie-Nielsen V, et al. Variation in antiviral 2',5'- oligoadenylate synthetase (2'5'AS) enzyme activity is controlled by a single-nucleotide polymorphism at a splice-acceptor site in the OAS1 gene. Am J Hum Genet. 2005;76(4):623–33.

53. Bridge AJ, Pebernard S, Ducraux A, Nicoulaz AL, Iggo R. Induction of an interferon response by RNAi vectors in mammalian cells. Nat Genet. 2003;34(3):263.

54. Barkhash AV, Perelygin AA, Babenko VN, Myasnikova NG, Pilipenko PI, Romaschenko AG, Voevoda AG, Brinton MA. Variability in the 2nko A oligoadenylate synthetase gene cluster is associated with human predisposition to tick-borne encephalitis virus-induced disease. J Infect Dis. 2010;202(12):1813–8.

55. Chawla-Sarkar M, Lindner DJ, Liu YF, Williams BR, Sen GC, Silverman RH, Borden EC. Apoptosis and interferons: role of interferon-stimulated genes as mediators of apoptosis. Apoptosis. 2003;8(3):237–49.

56. Wang SS, Gonzalez P, Yu K, Porras C, Li Q, Safaeian M, Rodriguez AC, Sherman ME, Bratti C, Schiffman M, Wacholder S. Common genetic variants and risk for HPV persistence and progression to cervical cancer. PLoS One. 2010;5(1):e8667.

57. Boulbes DR, Chauhan GB, Jin Q, Bartholomeusz C, Esteva FJ. CD44 expression contributes to trastuzumab resistance in HER2-positive breast cancer cells. Breast Cancer Res Treat. 2015;151(3):501–13.

58. Pályi-Krekk Z, Barok M, Isola J, Tammi M, Szöllo J, Nagy P. Hyaluronan-induced masking of ErbB2 and CD44-enhanced trastuzumab internalisation in trastuzumab resistant breast cancer. Eur J Cancer. 2007;43(16):2423–33.

59. Bao W, Fu HJ, Xie QS, Wang L, Zhang R, Guo ZY, Zhao J, Meng YL, Ren XL, Wang T, Li Q. HER2 interacts with CD44 to up-regulate CXCR4 via epigenetic silencing of microRNA-139 in gastric cancer cells. Gastroenterol. 2011;141(6):2076–87.

60. Barthelemy M. Betweenness centrality in large complex networks. Eur Phys J B. 2004;38(2):163–8.

61. Lastraioli E, Iorio J, Arcangeli A. Ion channel expression as promising cancer biomarker. BBA Biomembranes. 2015;1848(10):2685–702.

62. Xia J, Wang H, Li S, Wu Q, Sun L, Huang H, Zeng M. Ion channels or aquaporins as novel molecular targets in gastric cancer. Mol Cancer. 2017;16(1):54.

63. Fujimoto M, Inoue T, Kito H, Niwa S, Suzuki T, Muraki K, Ohya S. Transcriptional repression of HER2 by ANO1 Cl– channel inhibition in human breast cancer cells with resistance to trastuzumab. Biochem Biophys Res Commun. 2017;482(1):188–94.

64. Cai R, Ding X, Zhou K, Shi Y, Ge R, Ren G, Jin Y, Wang Y. Blockade of TRPC6 channels induced G2/M phase arrest and suppressed growth in human gastric cancer cells. Cancer Lett. 2009;125(10):2281–7.

65. Ding M, et al. Pyrazolo [1,5-a] pyrimidine TRPC6 antagonists for the treatment of gastric cancer. Cancer Lett. 2018;432:47-55.

66. Huang R, Gu W, Sun B, Gao L. Identification of COL4A1 as a potential gene conferring trastuzumab resistance in gastric cancer based on bioinformatics analysis. Mol Med Rep. 2018;17(5):6387–96.

67. Arteaga CL, Sliwkowski MX, Osborne CK, Perez EA, Puglisi F, Gianni L. Treatment of HER2-positive breast cancer: current status and future perspectives. Nat Rev Clin Oncol. 2012;9(1):16.

18

P3H4 is correlated with clinicopathological features and prognosis in bladder cancer

Wangjian Li[1], Lihong Ye[1], Yongliang Chen[1] and Peng Chen[2]* ⓘ

Abstract

Background: Genetic alterations play a significant role in the progression of bladder cancer. Identifying novel biomarkers to personalize the therapeutic regimen and evaluate the prognosis of patients with bladder cancer is vital. Prolyl 3-hydroxylase family member 4 (P3H4) is significantly involved in several types of human cancer. However, the effect of P3H4 in bladder cancer remains unknown.

Methods: The mRNA expression of P3H4 was measured in 44 paired tumors and adjacent normal tissues by using real-time reverse transcription-polymerase chain reaction. RNA-Seq data of 389 patients with bladder cancer were downloaded to investigate the effect of P3H4 on bladder cancer from The Cancer Genome Atlas (TCGA) project.

Results: P3H4 was overexpressed in bladder cancer compared with the adjacent normal tissue both in our tissue samples and TCGA samples. The mRNA expression of P3H4 was significantly related to several clinicopathological factors of bladder cancer, including age, race category, histologic grade, tumor histologic subtype, and AJCC stage. The high P3H4 expression group had a shorter overall survival (OS) than the low P3H4 expression group. Univariate Cox regression analysis showed that age, angiolymphatic invasion, lymph node metastasis, tumor histologic subtype, metastasis, AJCC stage, and P3H4 were significantly related to OS. Moreover, multivariate Cox analysis revealed that P3H4, as well as age and AJCC stage, was an independent predictor of poor OS.

Conclusion: Given its tumorigenic role, P3H4 may serve as a promising tumor-promoting gene in bladder cancer.

Keywords: Bladder cancer, P3H4, Clinicopathological features, Prognosis

Background

Bladder cancer is a common cancer worldwide. An estimated 429,800 new cases of bladder cancer and 165,100 deaths were recorded in 2012 [1]. Bladder cancer is also the leading malignancy of the genitourinary system [2]. The median survival of patients with advanced bladder cancer is only about 14 months even after aggressive treatment, including surgery, radiation, and chemotherapy [3].

Cancer progression is a complex process that involves changes in various genes, including oncogenes, tumor suppressor genes, and non-coding sequence. Genetic profiling studies have indicated that many genetic alterations, such as those in TP53, RB1, TSC1, FGFR3, and PIK3CA, play critical roles in bladder cancer [4–10].

Genetic studies have significantly progressed recently, but many areas remain to be explored.

Prolyl 3-hydroxylase family member 4 (P3H4) is a nucleolar protein initially identified as an autoantigen in cases of interstitial cystitis [11]. P3H4 may also play an important role in membranous nephropathy [12]. Another study indicated that P3H4 is a novel endoplasmic reticulum protein that regulates bone mass homeostasis [13]. P3H4 could affect the activity of lysyl-hydroxylase 1 potentially through interactions with the enzyme and/or cyclophilin B [14]. Fossá et al. reported that P3H4 acts as a tumor-associated autoantigen in patients with prostate cancer [15]. Comtesse et al. found that patients with meningioma possess antibodies against P3H4 and may offer a new diagnostic and therapeutic target for meningioma [16]. Overall, P3H4 is involved in several physiological and pathological processes. Nevertheless, the role of P3H4 in bladder cancer remains unknown.

* Correspondence: chenpeng_hch@163.com
[2]Department of Radiation Oncology, Hangzhou Cancer Hospital, Zhejiang, China
Full list of author information is available at the end of the article

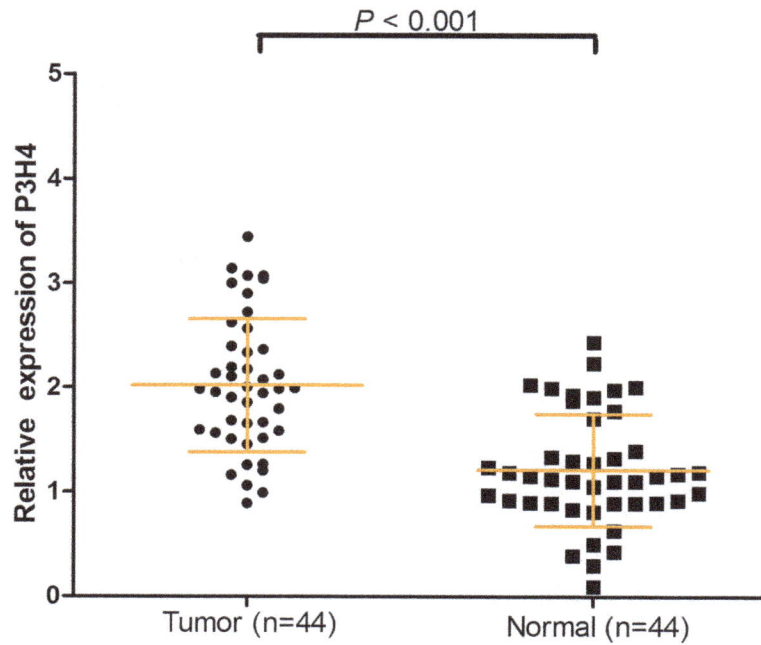

Fig. 1 P3H4 expression in 44 paired bladder cancer samples and adjacent normal tissues was investigated using qRT-PCR. P3H4 expression was significantly upregulated in primary bladder cancer tissues compared with the adjacent normal tissues ($p < 0.001$)

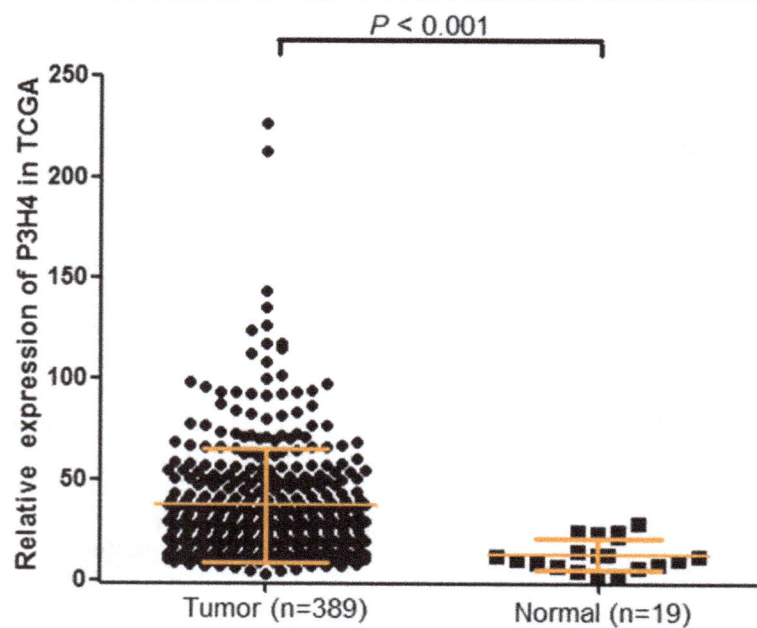

Fig. 2 P3H4 expression in the TCGA cohort, including 389 bladder cancer samples and 19 adjacent normal samples. P3H4 expression was also significantly overexpressed in primary bladder cancer tissue ($p < 0.001$)

The present study analyzed the relationship between P3H4 and bladder cancer. In specific, the relationship between P3H4 and clinicopathological factors of patients with bladder cancer was mainly investigated. The prognostic value of P3H4 was also assessed by Kaplan–Meier and Cox regression analyses.

Methods

Patients

Forty-four bladder cancer and corresponding adjacent normal tissues were obtained from Shaoxing Hospital of China Medical University. Tissue samples were first frozen in liquid nitrogen after resection and stored in a $-80\ °C$ refrigerator until use. The research protocol was approved by the Ethics Committee of Shaoxing Hospital of China Medical University. Moreover, written informed consent for using the tissue samples was obtained from those 44 patients. All samples are muscle invasive bladder cancer (MIBC).

RNA extraction and quantitative real-time polymerase chain reaction

RNA of the tissue samples was extracted using TRIzol reagent in accordance with the manufacturer's instructions (Life Technologies, USA). Quantitative real-time polymerase chain reaction (qRT-PCR) was carried out using Thunderbird SYBR qPCR Mix (Toyobo, Japan) in the Applied Biosystems 7500 Real-Time PCR System (Applied Biosystems, USA). The primers for P3H4 were ACGCGCTGTTCAAGGCTAA (forward) and CCAG CATCCCCTGATAGTAGT (reverse). GAPDH was used as an internal control.

TCGA clinical and P3H4 data

We downloaded TCGA clinical data in "Biotab" format from The Cancer Genome Atlas. Then, the normalized mRNA expression counts of P3H4 were acquired from TCGA and are expressed as RNA-Seq by transcripts per kilobase million values.

Statistical method

Data on normal distribution were expressed as mean ± standard deviation and were then compared with t test. Data on abnormal distribution were compared with Mann–Whitney U test. Chi-square test or Fisher's exact test was used to evaluate the connection between clinicopathological characteristics and P3H4 expression, as appropriate. Kaplan–Meier and Cox regression analyses were performed to assess the prognostic value of P3H4. Statistical significance was considered at $p < 0.05$. All statistical analyses were carried out using SPSS, and GraphPad Prism 5 was used for drafting.

Results

P3H4 was significantly upregulated in bladder cancer

To examine the role of P3H4 in bladder cancer, we investigated the P3H4 expression in 44 primary tumors and their paired adjacent normal tissues using qRT-PCR. P3H4 was upregulated in primary tumor compared with their paired adjacent normal tissues (2.02 ± 0.64 vs 1.21 ± 0.54, $p < 0.001$, Fig. 1). To further confirm the results, we analyzed the expression of P3H4 in 389 bladder

Table 1 The relationship between P3H4 expression and clinicopathological characteristics in the TCGA cohort ($n = 389$)

Characteristics	Expression of P3H4 mRNA, number (%)		
	High ($n = 195$)	Low ($n = 194$)	p value
Age at diagnosis, years	69.25 ± 10.18	66.39 ± 10.87	**0.008**
Gender			0.053
Male	136 (69.74)	152 (78.35)	
Female	59 (30.26)	42 (21.65)	
BMI	26.71 ± 4.78	27.42 ± 6.99	0.277
Race category			**0.001**
White	163 (87.63)	145 (77.54)	
Black or African American	13 (6.99)	9 (4.81)	
Asian	10 (5.38)	33 (17.65)	
Angiolymphatic invasion			0.181
Yes	77 (57.04)	64 (48.85)	
No	58 (42.96)	67 (51.15)	
Extracapsular extension			0.937
Yes	35 (44.30)	31 (43.66)	
NO	44 (55.70)	40 (56.34)	
Karnofsky performance score	84.33 ± 12.46	80.67 ± 15.39	0.146
Histologic grade			**0.001**
High	191 (98.45)	174 (90.63)	
Low	3 (1.55)	18 (9.38)	
Lymph node metastasis			0.454
Yes	59 (38.31)	53 (42.74)	
No	95 (61.69)	71 (57.26)	
Tumor histologic subtype			**0.011**
Non-papillary	141 (73.82)	119 (61.66)	
Papillary	50 (26.18)	74 (38.34)	
Metastasis			0.154
M0	79 (91.86)	110 (97.35)	
M1	7 (8.14)	3 (2.65)	
AJCC stage			**0.006**
I	0 (0)	1 (0.52)	
II	49 (25.13)	79 (41.15)	
III	75 (38.46)	55 (28.65)	
IV	71 (36.41)	57 (29.69)	

Boldface means $p < 0.05$

cancer tissues and 19 adjacent normal tissues from the TCGA database. As shown in Fig. 2, the expression of P3H4 was also significantly upregulated in the TCGA database (37.77 ± 28.27 vs 13.60 ± 7.67, $p < 0.001$). This finding revealed that P3H4 may play a significant role in bladder cancer.

P3H4 expression was associated with clinicopathological features in bladder cancer

To further explore whether P3H4 expression is related to clinicopathological factors of bladder cancer, we divided 389 patients with bladder cancer from the TCGA database into high P3H4 expression ($n = 195$) and low P3H4 expression ($n = 194$) groups according to the median value of P3H4. The results from the TCGA cohort indicated that P3H4 expression was significantly associated with age, race category, histologic grade, tumor histologic subtype, and AJCC stage ($p < 0.05$, Table 1). The average age was greater in the high P3H4 expression group than in the low P3H4 expression group (69.25 ± 10.18 vs 66.39 ± 10.87, $p = 0.008$). Similar results were also found in our local cohort (71.55 ± 7.71 vs 66.32 ± 7.92, $p = 0.032$, Additional file 1: Table S1). Interestingly, the race category was also different between the two groups ($p = 0.001$). The high P3H4 expression group had a higher histologic grade and more non-papillary type percentage than the low P3H4 expression group (98.45% vs 90.63% and 73.82% vs 61.66%, $p = 0.001$ and 0.011, respectively). The most significant finding is that high P3H4 expression corresponded to advanced AJCC stage ($p = 0.005$). Gender, BMI, angiolymphatic invasion, extracapsular extension,

Karnofsky performance score, lymph node metastasis, and metastasis showed no significant correlation with P3H4 expression ($p > 0.05$). Overall, high P3H4 expression may play an important role in bladder cancer.

P3H4 expression was significantly related to prognosis in bladder cancer

To further investigate the prognostic role of P3H4 in bladder cancer, we performed Kaplan–Meier and Cox regression analyses. Kaplan–Meier analysis showed that survival prognosis was different between the high and low P3H4 expression groups. The high P3H4 expression group had a shorter overall survival (OS) than the low P3H4 expression group ($p = 0.009$, Fig. 3). The cumulative 5-year OS in the high P3H4 expression group was 35.1%, which was much lower than that in the low P3H4 expression group (48.3%). Univariate and multivariate Cox regression analyses were then performed. Univariate Cox regression analysis showed that age (hazard ratio (HR) = 1.04, 95% CI = 1.023–1.057, $p < 0.001$), angiolymphatic invasion (HR = 1.619, 95% CI = 1.177–2.226, $p = 0.003$), lymph node metastasis (HR = 2.071, 95% CI = 1.47–2.918, $p < 0.001$), tumor histologic subtype (HR = 0.628, 95% CI = 0.433–0.909, $p = 0.014$), metastasis (HR = 4.507, 95% CI = 2.131–9.532, $p < 0.001$), AJCC stage (HR = 1.708, 95% CI = 1.402–2.08, $p < 0.001$), and P3H4 (HR = 1.504, 95% CI = 1.104–2.048, $p = 0.01$) were associated with OS (Table 2). However, other factors, including gender, BMI, race category, extracapsular extension, Karnofsky performance score, and histologic grade, were not significantly related to OS ($p > 0.05$, Table 2). Moreover, multivariate Cox analysis indicated that

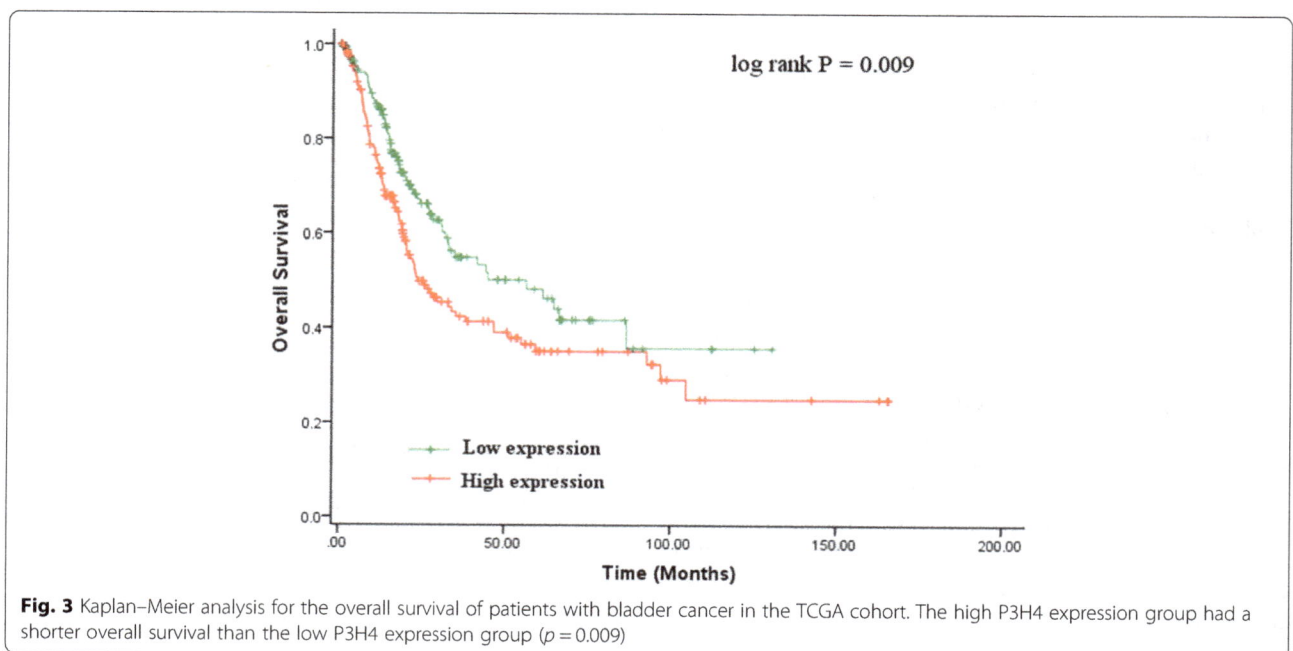

Fig. 3 Kaplan–Meier analysis for the overall survival of patients with bladder cancer in the TCGA cohort. The high P3H4 expression group had a shorter overall survival than the low P3H4 expression group ($p = 0.009$)

Table 2 Univariate Cox regression analysis of P3H4 expression with regard to OS

Clinicopathologic features	HR	95% CI	p value
Age	1.04	1.023–1.057	**< 0.001**
Gender	1.08	0.771–1.513	0.655
BMI	0.994	0.965–1.023	0.683
Race category	1.158	0.862–1.555	0.33
Angiolymphatic invasion	1.619	1.177–2.226	**0.003**
Extracapsular extension	1.359	0.936–1.974	0.107
Karnofsky performance score	0.998	0.976–1.021	0.893
Histologic grade	2.853	0.705–11.542	0.141
Lymph node metastasis	2.071	1.47–2.918	**< 0.001**
Tumor histologic subtype	0.628	0.433–0.909	**0.014**
Metastasis	4.507	2.131–9.532	**< 0.001**
AJCC stage	1.708	1.402–2.08	**< 0.001**
P3H4	1.504	1.104–2.048	**0.01**

Boldface means $p < 0.05$

only age (HR = 1.037, 95% CI = 1.019–1.054, $p < 0.001$), AJCC stage (HR = 1.560, 95% CI = 1.265–1.923, $p < 0.001$), and P3H4 (HR = 1.413, 95% CI = 1.016–1.966, $p = 0.04$) were independent factors of poor OS in bladder cancer (Table 3). Taken together, the results indicate that P3H4 is a poor independent prognostic factor of bladder cancer and worthy of further study.

Discussion

Bladder cancer is the second most common urological cancer worldwide and the most frequent urological cancer in China [17]. Surgical operation is the major treatment for bladder cancer. Despite the recent significant progress in surgical techniques and adjuvant chemotherapy, bladder cancer remains a highly fatal disease [18, 19]. The recurrence rate of this disease after local treatment is high [20]. Owing to the limited prediction abilities of conventional markers, such as clinicopathological characteristics, identifying reliable genetic markers that predict disease progression is vital [21, 22].

In the present study, we studied the association between P3H4 gene expression and bladder cancer. P3H4 is a nucleolar protein initially identified as an autoantigen in interstitial cystitis cases [11]. Previous studies have found that P3H4 may play an important role in several human

Table 3 Multivariate Cox regression analysis of P3H4 expression with regard to OS

Clinicopathologic features	HR	95% CI	p value
Age	1.037	1.019–1.054	**< 0.001**
AJCC stage	1.560	1.265–1.923	**< 0.001**
P3H4	1.413	1.016–1.966	**0.04**

Boldface means $p < 0.05$

diseases, such as membranous nephropathy [12], bone mass homeostasis [13], and Ehlers–Danlos syndrome [23]. Moreover, P3H4 is significantly associated with several types of human cancer. However, the relationship between P3H4 and bladder cancer remains unclear to date.

In the present study, we reported and validated that P3H4 was significantly upregulated in primary tumor compared with their paired adjacent normal tissues in 44 patients with bladder cancer. The differential expression of P3H4 was further confirmed in the TCGA cohort of a large sample size. Furthermore, high P3H4 expression was found to be closely related to several aggressive clinicopathological factors, such as advanced AJCC stage. Moreover, Kaplan–Meier analysis found that the low P3H4 expression group had a better prognosis than the high P3H4 expression group. Univariate and multivariate Cox regression analyses revealed that P3H4 was an independent predictor of poor OS in bladder cancer. Taken together, our findings suggest that P3H4 is involved in the progression of bladder cancer. A systematic literature review revealed that this was the first description of the relationship between P3H4 and bladder cancer.

Despite some encouraging findings, several limitations of our study cannot be ignored. First, although it had been verified by small samples, the relationship between P3H4 expression and bladder cancer should be validated using a large sample data from our local cohort. Second, future studies should conduct in vitro and in vivo experiments to identify the biological roles of P3H4 in bladder cancer. The molecular mechanism of P3H4 in bladder cancer remains to be further studied.

Conclusions

We identified P3H4 as a tumor promotion gene in bladder cancer for the first time. P3H4 was overexpressed in primary tumor tissues compared with their paired adjacent normal tissues. Moreover, high P3H4 expression was associated with aggressive clinicopathological features in bladder cancer. Survival analysis revealed that high P3H4 expression correlated poorly with prognosis in bladder cancer. These results indicate that P3H4 may act as a tumor-promoting gene in bladder cancer.

Abbreviations
HR: Hazard ratio; OS: Overall survival; P3H4: Prolyl 3-hydroxylase family member 4; qRT-PCR: Quantitative real-time polymerase chain reaction; TCGA: The Cancer Genome Atlas

Authors' contributions
PC designed the study. WL collected the data and carried out the experiment. LY and YC performed the statistical analyses. PC and WL wrote the manuscript. All authors read and approved the final manuscript.

Competing interests

The authors declare that they have no competing interests.

Author details

[1]Department of Urology, Shaoxing Hospital of China Medical University, Zhejiang, China. [2]Department of Radiation Oncology, Hangzhou Cancer Hospital, Zhejiang, China.

References

1. Torre LA, Bray F, Siegel RL, Ferlay J, Lortet-Tieulent J, Jemal A. Global cancer statistics, 2012. CA Cancer J Clin. 2015;65:87–108.
2. Burger M, Catto JW, Dalbagni G, Grossman HB, Herr H, Karakiewicz P, Kassouf W, Kiemeney LA, La Vecchia C, Shariat S, Lotan Y. Epidemiology and risk factors of urothelial bladder cancer. Eur Urol. 2013;63:234–41.
3. Antoni S, Ferlay J, Soerjomataram I, Znaor A, Jemal A, Bray F. Bladder cancer incidence and mortality: a global overview and recent trends. Eur Urol. 2017;71:96–108.
4. Choi W, Ochoa A, McConkey DJ, Aine M, Hoglund M, Kim WY, Real FX, Kiltie AE, Milsom I, Dyrskjot L, Lerner SP. Genetic alterations in the molecular subtypes of bladder cancer: illustration in the cancer genome atlas dataset. Eur Urol. 2017;72:354–65.
5. Figueroa JD, Middlebrooks CD, Banday AR, Ye Y, Garcia-Closas M, Chatterjee N, Koutros S, Kiemeney LA, Rafnar T, Bishop T, et al. Identification of a novel susceptibility locus at 13q34 and refinement of the 20p12.2 region as a multi-signal locus associated with bladder cancer risk in individuals of European ancestry. Hum Mol Genet. 2016;25:1203–14.
6. Kim J, Akbani R, Creighton CJ, Lerner SP, Weinstein JN, Getz G, Kwiatkowski DJ. Invasive bladder cancer: genomic insights and therapeutic promise. Clin Cancer Res. 2015;21:4514–24.
7. Maraver A, Fernandez-Marcos PJ, Cash TP, Mendez-Pertuz M, Duenas M, Maietta P, Martinelli P, Munoz-Martin M, Martinez-Fernandez M, Canamero M, et al. NOTCH pathway inactivation promotes bladder cancer progression. J Clin Invest. 2015;125:824–30.
8. Nickerson ML, Dancik GM, Im KM, Edwards MG, Turan S, Brown J, Ruiz-Rodriguez C, Owens C, Costello JC, Guo G, et al. Concurrent alterations in TERT, KDM6A, and the BRCA pathway in bladder cancer. Clin Cancer Res. 2014;20:4935–48.
9. Pietzak EJ, Bagrodia A, Cha EK, Drill EN, Iyer G, Isharwal S, Ostrovnaya I, Baez P, Li Q, Berger MF, et al. Next-generation sequencing of nonmuscle invasive bladder cancer reveals potential biomarkers and rational therapeutic targets. Eur Urol. 2017;72:952–9.
10. Sfakianos JP, Cha EK, Iyer G, Scott SN, Zabor EC, Shah RH, Ren Q, Bagrodia A, Kim PH, Hakimi AA, et al. Genomic characterization of upper tract urothelial carcinoma. Eur Urol. 2015;68:970–7.
11. Ochs RL, Stein TW,J, Chan EK, Ruutu M, Tan EM. cDNA cloning and characterization of a novel nucleolar protein. Mol Biol Cell. 1996;7:1015–24.
12. Cavazzini F, Magistroni R, Furci L, Lupo V, Ligabue G, Granito M, Leonelli M, Albertazzi A, Cappelli G. Identification and characterization of a new autoimmune protein in membranous nephropathy by immunoscreening of a renal cDNA library. PLoS One. 2012;7:e48845.
13. Gruenwald K, Castagnola P, Besio R, Dimori M, Chen Y, Akel NS, Swain FL, Skinner RA, Eyre DR, Gaddy D, et al. Sc65 is a novel endoplasmic reticulum protein that regulates bone mass homeostasis. J Bone Miner Res. 2014;29:666–75.
14. Heard ME, Besio R, Weis M, Rai J, Hudson DM, Dimori M, Zimmerman SM, Kamykowski JA, Hogue WR, Swain FL, et al. Sc65-null mice provide evidence for a novel endoplasmic reticulum complex regulating collagen lysyl hydroxylation. PLoS Genet. 2016;12:e1006002.
15. Fossa A, Siebert R, Aasheim HC, Maelandsmo GM, Berner A, Fossa SD, Paus E, Smeland EB, Gaudernack G. Identification of nucleolar protein No55 as a tumour-associated autoantigen in patients with prostate cancer. Br J Cancer. 2000;83:743–9.
16. Comtesse N, Zippel A, Walle S, Monz D, Backes C, Fischer U, Mayer J, Ludwig N, Hildebrandt A, Keller A, et al. Complex humoral immune response against a benign tumor: frequent antibody response against specific antigens as diagnostic targets. Proc Natl Acad Sci U S A. 2005; 102:9601–6.
17. Witjes JA, Comperat E, Cowan NC, De Santis M, Gakis G, Lebret T, Ribal MJ, Van der Heijden AG, Sherif A, European Association of U. EAU guidelines on muscle-invasive and metastatic bladder cancer: summary of the 2013 guidelines. Eur Urol. 2014;65:778–92.
18. Chaffer CL, Brennan JP, Slavin JL, Blick T, Thompson EW, Williams ED. Mesenchymal-to-epithelial transition facilitates bladder cancer metastasis: role of fibroblast growth factor receptor-2. Cancer Res. 2006;66:11271–8.
19. Kirkali Z, Chan T, Manoharan M, Algaba F, Busch C, Cheng L, Kiemeney L, Kriegmair M, Montironi R, Murphy WM, et al. Bladder cancer: epidemiology, staging and grading, and diagnosis. Urology. 2005;66:4–34.
20. Babjuk M, Burger M, Zigeuner R, Shariat SF, van Rhijn BW, Comperat E, Sylvester RJ, Kaasinen E, Bohle A, Palou Redorta J, et al. EAU guidelines on non-muscle-invasive urothelial carcinoma of the bladder: update 2013. Eur Urol. 2013;64:639–53.
21. Babjuk M, Bohle A, Burger M, Capoun O, Cohen D, Comperat EM, Hernandez V, Kaasinen E, Palou J, Roupret M, et al. EAU guidelines on non-muscle-invasive urothelial carcinoma of the bladder: update 2016. Eur Urol. 2017;71:447–61.
22. van Rhijn BW, Burger M, Lotan Y, Solsona E, Stief CG, Sylvester RJ, Witjes JA, Zlotta AR. Recurrence and progression of disease in non-muscle-invasive bladder cancer: from epidemiology to treatment strategy. Eur Urol. 2009;56:430–42.
23. Hudson DM, Weis M, Rai J, Joeng KS, Dimori M, Lee BH, Morello R, Eyre DR. P3h3-null and Sc65-null mice phenocopy the collagen lysine under-hydroxylation and cross-linking abnormality of Ehlers-Danlos syndrome type VIA. J Biol Chem. 2017;292:3877–87.

19

Progress of preoperative and postoperative radiotherapy in gastric cancer

Nan Zhang[1†], Qian Fei[1,2†], Jiajia Gu[1], Li Yin[1,2] and Xia He[1,2*]

Abstract

Background: Gastric carcinoma, a highly common malignant tumor, is treated mainly by surgery. Meanwhile, radiotherapy is attracting increased attention as a crucial locoregional therapy. However, the application of radiotherapy in gastric carcinoma is still limited and radiation standards remain debatable.

Main body: The use of preoperative radiotherapy for treating gastroesophageal junction cancer has advanced. However, additional phase III clinical trials are needed to further verify the therapeutic value of preoperative radiotherapy for gastric cancer. Patients with D1 or D1 plus lymphadenectomy can benefit from postoperative radiotherapy obviously, and postoperative radiotherapy may be effective for patients with D2 lymphadenectomy with a high N stage. The target volume delineation of preoperative and postoperative radiotherapy should be based on clinical experience and the characteristics of lymphatic drainage.

Conclusions: With the advancement of radiotherapy technology, preoperative and postoperative radiotherapy are becoming increasingly accepted as important auxiliary treatments for gastric cancer.

Keywords: Gastric carcinoma, Radiotherapy, Radiation field, D2 lymph node dissection

Background

The morbidity of gastric cancer has been declining worldwide but remains a highly common malignancy, which is the third leading cause of cancer-related mortality. In 2012, one million new cases occurred around the world, with more than 72,000 deaths [1]. More than 75% newly diagnosed patients were in an advanced stage because of the lack of the typical clinical premonitory symptoms of gastric cancer. Advanced stage means the tumor has invaded the muscle layer or lymph node, and the survival rates of patients in this stage are only 20–50% [2]. Among patients with advanced stage gastric cancer, approximately 50% have lost the chance of surgery. Therefore, comprehensive treatment based on radiotherapy (RT) and chemotherapy has recently received much attention.

In recent years, the application of RT in gastric cancer has become increasingly common with the development of radiation technology. In 2001, John et al. published the results of the INT0116 trial in the New England Journal and caused the RT change from the traditional palliative treatment to important adjuvant therapy in the multidisciplinary treatment for gastric cancer [3].

Preoperative RT

Preoperative RT is mainly used to reduce tumor burden in patients with advanced gastric cancer. This process enables inoperable patients to be eligible for operation. In addition, preoperative RT may play a unique role in controlling micrometastasis, and the pathological response after preoperative RT may provide important prognostic information [4, 5]. The results of several major clinical trials showed that gastroesophageal junction (GEJ) cancer achieves a better therapeutic effect than that of gastric cancer in terms of preoperative RT (Table 1).

In 1998, Chinese researchers found that 370 patients with GEJ cancer treated with preoperative RT significantly improved in tumor resection rate relative to the patients treated with surgery alone (89.5% vs. 74.9%). The local control rates in the two groups were 61% and 45% ($P < 0.05$), and the 10-year survival rates were 20.3%

* Correspondence: hexiabm@163.com
†Nan Zhang and Qian Fei contributed equally to this work.
1Department of Radiation Oncology, Jiangsu Cancer Hospital & Jiangsu Institute of Cancer Research & Affiliated Cancer Hospital of Nanjing Medical University, Nanjing Medical University Affiliated Cancer Hospital, 42 Baiziting, Nanjing 210009, Jiangsu, China
2The Fourth Clinical School of Nanjing Medical University, Nanjing, China

Table 1 Preoperative RT III clinical trials

Study/institute	n	Tumor location	Groups	Local control	Survival
1998 Zhang et al. [6]	370	EGJ	RT+S vs. S	Local control and local recurrence rate 61.4% vs. 51.7%	10-year OS 20.3% vs. 13.3%
2009 Stahl et al. [7]	119	EGJ	CRT+S vs. C+S	Pathological complete response rate 15.6% vs. 2.0%	3-year OS 47.4% vs. 27.7%
2012 Van Hagen et al. [8]	366	EGJ or EC	CRT+S vs. S	Local recurrence rate 14% and 34%	5-year OS 47% vs. 34%
2002 Skoropad et al. [9]	102	GC	RT+S vs. S	No sense	No sense

EGJ esophagogastric junction, *GC* gastric cancer, *EC* esophagus cancer, *RT* radiotherapy, *CRT* concurrent radiotherapy, *S* surgery

and 13.3% ($P = 0.009$), respectively. These results indicate that preoperative RT may be beneficial for improving the local control rate and the overall survival (OS) of patients with GEJ cancer [6]. Stahl revealed that preoperative RT significantly improved the rate of pathological complete response (15.6% vs. 2.0%) of GEJ adenocarcinoma and increased the 3-year OS rate (47.4% vs. 27.7%, $P = 0.07$) [7]. Similarly, Hagen and co-workers investigated 366 cases of gastric cancer or GEJ cancer and found that the patients treated with preoperative radiochemotherapy (carboplatin + paclitaxel, 5 weeks; 41.4 Gy/23 f, 5 days/week) attained a significantly improved rate of tumor resection (92% vs. 69%, $P < 0.001$) and OS (49.4 months vs. 24 months, median survival) relative to those of the patients treated with surgery alone. Besides, preoperative radiochemotherapy was related to a decreased rate of local recurrence (LRRs, 14% and 34%, $P < 0.001$) and distant metastases rates (29% and 35%, $P = 0.025$) relative to surgery [8]. In this study, the regimen above became the recommended treatment program for GEJ adenocarcinoma in the USA.

Compared with the progress of preoperative RT in treating GEJ cancer, the application of preoperative RT still lacks large-scale phase III clinical trials for gastric cancer. In 2002, Skoropad investigated 102 cases of resectable gastric cancer and found that preoperative RT (20 Gy/5 f) did not significantly improve the local control and long-term survival relative to surgery alone (20-year OS rates, 32% and 18%, $P = 0.555$) [9]. In this study, the irradiation technology was regressive despite the follow-up time of 20 years, and the number of cases was minimal. Conversely, some single-arm prospective trials and retrospective analyses confirmed that adopting preoperative chemoradiotherapy (CRT) appeared safe and beneficial for advanced gastric cancer patients [10–16]. Kumagai presented results indicating that patients with gastric or GEJ cancer treated with preoperative RT or CRT attained a higher rate of survival than those patients treated with surgery alone. Simultaneously, he found that adding preoperative RT or CRT did not significantly decrease the rates of postoperative recurrence and mortality [15].

The response of preoperative chemotherapy in gastric cancer has been universally accepted, but whether preoperative concomitant radiochemotherapy can offer survival benefits is unclear relative to preoperative chemotherapy alone [17–19]. The ongoing TOPGEAR clinical trial is designed to address this issue [20]. In addition, a phase II clinical trial (NCT02301481) is being conducted by the Chinese Academy of Medical Sciences to determine whether preoperative radiochemotherapy is superior to preoperative chemotherapy alone for advanced gastric adenocarcinoma patients. A similar clinical study (NCT01815853) is conducted at the Sun Yat-sen University to observe the OS and safety of the preoperative radiochemotherapy. These results of the clinical trials are promising [21].

Postoperative RT

The findings of the INT0116 trial show the important role of postoperative RT in the adjuvant treatment of gastric cancer [3]. However, many deficiencies, such as the lack of the strict control of surgical type (only 10% cases of D2 dissection), the backwardness of radiation technology, and the low treatment compliance, are observed in research. After the Lancet published the 15-year follow-up results of D1 and D2 dissection in 2010, the advantage of reducing the local recurrence caused D2 to gradually become the standard surgical operation of resectable advanced gastric cancer [22]. The following section is mainly based on the current situation of postoperative RT after D2 dissection. The main results of phase III clinical trials in recent years are displayed in Table 2.

In 2012, the 10-year follow-up results of INT0116 showed that postoperative concurrent radiochemotherapy continued its survival benefit and that either the D1 or the D2 subgroup can benefit from this modality [23]. Simultaneously, researchers from South Korea presented results of the ARTIST trial, which showed that the postoperative RT did not significantly improve the rate of disease-free survival (DFS), but for patients with pathologic positive lymph nodes, the postoperative RT demonstrated its survival benefits with no statistical significance ($P = 0.38$)

Table 2 Postoperative RT III clinical trials

Study/institute	n	D2	RT	pN+	III-IV	DFS/RFS	OS	Remarks
2001 INT0116 USA [3]	556	10%	2D	85%	NR	3-year 48% vs. 31% ($p < 0.001$)	3-year 50% vs. 41% ($p = 0.005$)	
2012 INT0116 [23]						10-year similar	10-year similar	D1 and D2 benefit
2012 ARTIST South Korea [24]	458	100%	2D or 3D	86%	41%	3-year 78% vs. 74% ($p = 0.0862$)	NR	N+DFS benefit
2015 ARTIST Final report [25]						5-year 74% vs. 68% ($p = 0.092$)	5-year 75% vs. 73% ($p = 0.527$)	N+ and GC DFS benefit
2012 NCC South Korea [26]	90	100%	2D or 3D	98%	100%	5-year 65% vs. 55% ($p > 0.05$)	5-year 65% vs. 55% ($p > 0.05$)	LRRFS and III stage DFS benefit
2012 IMRT China [27]	351	100%	NR	86%	71%	5-year 45% vs. 36% ($p = 0.029$)	5-year 48% vs. 42% ($p = 0.122$)	

NR not reported, *OS* overall survival, *DFS/RFS* disease-/relapse-free survival, *LRRFS* locoregional failure-free survival, *GC* gastric cancer

[24]. The final results of the ARTIST trial after a 7-year follow-up also yielded similar conclusions [25]. In 2012, two other phase III clinical trials from Korea and China revealed that the postoperative RT after D2 dissection did not improve OS but enhanced the rate of local recurrence-free survival [26, 27]. In 2017, Stumpf et al. analyzed 3656 patients with resected gastric adenocarcinoma from the National Cancer Database in 2004 to 2012 and compared the OS rates between the perioperative chemotherapy group and the postoperative adjuvant radiochemotherapy group. The results of univariate and multivariate analyses suggested that the OS rates in the postoperative adjuvant radiochemotherapy group were superior to those of the perioperative chemotherapy group. In the subgroup analysis, the patients with positive surgical margins benefited more with adjuvant RT [28].

Given the analysis of the above phase III clinical trials, the trend toward negative results for the three trials, which are from the east, may be explained by the wide use of D2 dissection and postoperative chemotherapy. The lymph node dissection is substantial in D2. Hence, for some patients, treatment with D2 dissection plus postoperative chemotherapy is sufficient. On the contrary, the positive results of INT0016 were mainly for the vast majority of patients treated with D1 dissection, in which the lymphatic dissection range is minimal; thus, postoperative RT can play an important role in terms of local control. Hence, patients with gastric cancer require being screened before receiving postoperative RT [1].

In our opinion, whether patients require adding RT after D2 dissection should be determined by the disease stage. Sasako found that for patients with high-stage gastric cancer, postoperative chemotherapy alone cannot improve the RFS [29]. Therefore, adding RT for stage III gastric cancer patients after D2 dissection is necessary. In the ARTIST trial, only 41% of the patients were diagnosed at the III–IV stage, and postoperative RT may be an over-treatment for patients with stages I–II, where postoperative chemotherapy alone was sufficient. Therefore, the patients with pathologically positive lymph nodes in the ARTIST trial did not significantly improve in DFS, whereas for the patients with higher stages, especially stage III, the advantages of postoperative RT for local control were prominent. In an American retrospective review of 23,461 patients with early gastric cancer (IB–II) treated with postoperative RT, Datta concluded that patients in all stages of early gastric cancer can acquire survival benefits [30]. However, the researchers did not clarify whether the surgical patients were treated with D1 or D2 dissection. Well-designed prospective randomized clinical trials are still required to validate whether patients in different stages of gastric cancer with pathologic positive lymph nodes can benefit from postoperative RT.

The latest gastric cancer NCCN guidelines (2018.V1) still recommend postoperative chemotherapy after D2 lymphadenectomy, and postoperative CRT is preferred for surgical patients with a range of resection less than D2. The ARTIST II trial is a phase III randomized trial of adjuvant chemotherapy with compound tegafur–oteracil potassium capsules (S-1) versus S-1/oxaliplatin ± RT for surgical patients with positive nodes [31]. Remarkably, the results of the phase II clinical trial based on S-1 and cisplatin showed that the postoperative concurrent CRT group improved 3 years of DFS relative to the postoperative chemotherapy group, and the toxicities were acceptable [32]. In recent years, several meta-analyses have demonstrated the role of perioperative RT in treating gastric cancer [33–35].

In summary, RT can be used as an important adjuvant therapy during the perioperative period of patients with surgical gastric cancer in an advanced stage, especially for some specific patients after D2 dissection, which effectively improves the PFS and reduces the rate of local recurrence. The value of preoperative RT in gastric cancer still requires further validation, and we anticipate further results of relevant randomized controlled clinical trials. In addition, the screening of tumor-derived radiosensitivity markers has attracted increasing attention in recent years. For example, positive E2F-1 expression and negative HER2 expression may indicate that the patients with gastric cancer treated with postoperative CRT will achieve a good outcome, and in vitro studies have shown that CHK1 overexpression may be associated with radiation resistance [36–38]. Therefore, these markers can be assumed to be used as new risk factors for predicting the survival outcome of gastric cancer patients to select those who may benefit from the perioperative period RT.

Progress of treatment volume range

Preoperative target volume

Previous preoperative target volume includes the whole stomach and large node areas (paraesophageal, extending from the trachea for bifurcation and the lesser curvature of the stomach to the posterior second thoracic vertebra) because of a lack of consolidated phase III clinical trials to define the target volume of gastric cancer. In 2009, EORTC-ROG (European Organization for Research on the Treatment of Cancer) redefined the CTV of GEJ adenocarcinoma and gastric adenocarcinoma, which reduced the error [39]. The therapeutic efficacy of the preoperative RT in gastric cancer has not reached a consensus; therefore, we only analyzed the target volume of GEJ cancer or proximal gastric cancer in this study.

The stomach is a hollow organ, and its position may be influenced by respiratory motion and body movement. The reduction of error of CTV caused by swinging and breathing has become our primary task. Stahl assumed that the CTV includes a 5-cm margin of the proximal primary tumor, a 3-cm margin of the distal primary tumor, and a 1-cm margin of all nodal areas at risk [7]. The PTV margin of 8 mm expanded in all directions from the CTV to reduce the systematic error and target displacements. Hagen et al. defined PTV as the 4-cm margin of the primary tumor [8]. In 2009, the expert opinions of specialists in EORTC-ROG highlighted their definition of PTV as the 1-cm margin of the proximal and transverse CTV, which is the 1.5-cm margin of the distal CTV, to reduce the error; this definition is similar to those of the above two studies, given the lack of sufficient evidence to set the criteria for the target volume [39].

In accordance with Siewert's classification, the opinions of specialists in EORTC-ROG (2009) proposed a lymphatic drainage in different types of GEJ cancer; this proposal provided clinicians with a reference for delineating the target volume. However, the opinions failed to combine with computed tomography (CT) scans or other radiographic studies. Additionally, the patterns of local regional recurrence for gastric cancer were disregarded.

In 2014, on the basis of the study of Hagen, Oppedijk suggested patterns of recurrence for esophageal or GEJ cancer after preoperative radiochemotherapy [40]. After at least 24 months of follow-up, the overall recurrence rates of the surgery group and the CRT plus surgery group were 58% and 35%, respectively. The LRR of the CRT+S group reduced from 34 to 14%. A total of 5% of the patients of the preoperative CRT group experienced local relapse within the irradiated field; 2% experienced a local relapse at the edge of the irradiated field; 6% experienced local relapse outside the irradiated field. In this study, disease relapse mainly occurred in the celiac lymph nodes, para-aortic lymph nodes, and peritoneum, which were associated with the distal esophagus and esophagogastric junction (EGJ) cancer. However, the patients with EGJ cancer only constituted one-fourth, which may have an implication in delineating the high-risk areas of recurrence in EGJ cancer.

Oppedijk found that the incidence of local relapse outside the irradiated field remains high, and expanding the target volume for preoperative RT is necessary. Furthermore, we still lack reliable evidence for delineating the clinical target volume for preoperative RT in GEJ adenocarcinoma, and large-scale clinical trials on regional lymph node recurrence and failure modes are required.

Postoperative target volume

Developing a uniform standard for the delineation of the postoperative RT target volume is difficult because of the different sites, stages, and lymphatic metastases in gastric cancer; the various surgical methods, and the dissimilar conditions of postoperative cutting edge. The earliest guideline for defining the target volume for postoperative RT that was based on the primary tumor sites and the pathway of lymph node metastasis was proposed by Smalley and Tepperin [41, 42]. However, the guideline was recommended for D1 or D1 + lymphadenectomy and during the era of 2D RT techniques with adverse reactions and low local control rates. This article mainly discusses the target volume after D2 lymphadenectomy.

Nam retrospectively analyzed 291 patients after D2 dissection. A total of 83 target volumes of patients included the gastric stump, whereas the remaining 208 did not. The results showed that no significant differences in 5-year OS and DFS existed between these two groups. However, 3–4 grade diarrhea was more common in the patients with target volumes that included the gastric remnant. Therefore, Nam suggested that the target volume should exclude the gastric stump for patients treated with D2 dissection [43]. As found previously, the ARTIST trial also excluded the gastric stump from the irradiated field. Aside for the temporary adverse effects, the long-term survival of patients, especially the occurrence of gastric stump cancer, must also be monitored. Ohira found that the average interval of occurrence of gastric stump cancer was 6.8–18.8 years, but the follow-up period was only 5 years in the study of Nam [44]. The occurrence of postoperative gastric stump carcinoma should be of particular concern, although no report has explored the relationship between postoperative RT and gastric stump cancer. Furthermore, the study of Nam adopted the traditional 2D RT with added adverse reactions, but modern radiation technology has a unique advantage in reducing adverse reactions. In the NCC trial, the patients with irradiated fields that included the gastric stump obtained a high dose in the left renal area. Another study from China, namely, the intensity-modulated radiation therapy (IMRT) trial, demonstrated that with advanced IMRT technology, the toxic side effects caused by radiation exposure to the remnant stomach can be controlled.

Except for the ARTIST trial, almost all the phase III trials defined node nos. 1–16 as node areas at risk (Table 3, Fig. 1). The node areas at risk in the ARTIST trial only included node nos. 7–9 and 12–16, which received a reduced dose exposure to the intestinal tract. Besides, no difference existed between surgery plus RT and chemotherapy alone in adverse reactions. This result implies that the traditional node areas at risk may be exceedingly large for gastric cancer. Selective RT to high-risk lymph nodes should agree with the patterns of lymph nodes (LNs) recurrence after D2 dissection, which further optimizes the target volume. In 2012, Chang retrospectively investigated 357 gastric cancer patients with stage III after D2 or D3 dissection [45]. The results showed that the peritoneum was the most common site of recurrence, and the most common recurrent LNs was outside the field of D2 dissection (node nos. 12–16). Node nos. 16a as well as 16b are the most common recurrent lymph node whatever the site of primary tumor is.

Yoon retrospectively analysed the follow-up records from 91 stage III gastric carcinoma patients with the N3 disease, who were diagnosed with the first regional relapse after D2 dissection [46]. This study suggested that vessel-based delineations of rnGTVs (recurrent nodal gross tumor volume) on CT images depend on the recurrent sites of LNs from the follow-up records after D2 lymphadenectomy. The results showed that no. 16a (58.2%) and 16b (61.5%) were the most commonly affected first recurrent LNs. In addition, node nos. 9, 12, 13, and 14 were involved in 15.4%, 28.6%, 15.4%, and 19.8% of patients, respectively. Conversely, node nos. 11 (7.0%), 8 (3.0%), 2 (2.0%), and 10 (1.0%) were less commonly involved. When tumor involved the proximal third of stomach, the most commonly involved LNs were nos. 9 (30%), 10 (10%), and 13 (10%) lymph nodes. Nos. 12 and 14 were the most commonly involved LNs, when tumor involved the middle third stomach (26% and 13%, respectively). When tumor involved the distal third stomach, nos. 12, 13, 14, 9, and 11 were the commonly involved metastatic LNs (39%, 27.0%, 20.0%, 20.0%, and 10%, respectively). Nos. 14, 12, 11, 9, and 2 were the commonly involved metastatic LNs (41%, 24.0%, 12%, 12%, and 12%, respectively), when tumor involved more than two-thirds of the stomach. It showed that, in this study, the recurrent sites of lymph nodes such as splenic hilum, perigastric area, and below IMA were uncommon. The treatment volume can exclude the liver hilum (no. 12), perigastric area (nos. 1–6), and anterior part of the SMA (no. 14) when tumor involved the proximal third of the stomach; nevertheless, if CTV encompassed the splenic hilum (no. 10), it should also contain the splenic artery region. The treatment volume should include the perigastric region (nos. 1–6), the splenic hilum (no. 10), and the splenic artery region (no. 11) in the middle or distal third stomach. In addition, when patients with extensive tumor involved more than two-thirds of the stomach were only treated with

Table 3 Postoperative RT III clinical trials, toxic reactions, and target volume

Study/institute	RT dose (Gy)	Intervention	Severe toxicity	Target volume	Completed rate
2001 INT0116 USA [3]	45	CRT, 45Gy, 5FU +LV	Grade 3+, 41%, Grade 4+,32%	Tumor bed, regional node (nos. 1–16)	63%
2012 ARTIST South Korea [24]	45	CT-CRT-CT, CRT: Capecitabine; CT: XP	Similar to chemotherapy alone	Tumor bed in T4 LN (nos. 7–9 and 12–16)	82%
2012 NCC South Korea [26]	45	CRT, 5FU+LV	Grade 3+ hematologic toxicities; 20% vs. 25% G3+GI; 17% vs. 11%	Tumor bed, regional node (nos. 1–16)	87%
2012 IMRT China [27]	45	CRT, 45Gy, 5FU +LV	Similar toxicity mostly well tolerated	Tumor bed, regional node (nos. 1–16)	91%

CRT chemoradiotherapy, CT chemotherapy, 5-FU 5-fluorouracil, LV leucovorin, XP capecitabine plus cisplatin, 2D 2-dimentional irradiation, 3D 3-dimensional conformal radiation therapy, IMRT intensity-modulated radiation therapy

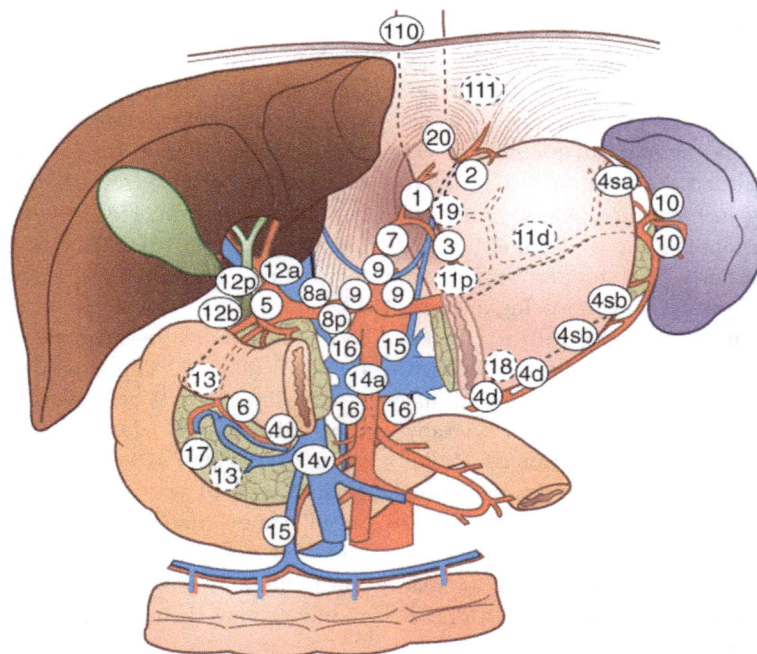

Fig. 1 Schematic diagram of lymph node station. LN, lymph node; 1 right cardiac nodes; 2 left cardiac nodes; 3 nodes along the lesser curvature; 4 nodes along the greater curvature; 5 suprapyloric nodes; 6 infrapyloric nodes; 7 nodes along root left gastric artery; 8 nodes along common hepatic artery; 9 nodes around celiac axis; 10 nodes at splenic hilum; 11 lymph nodes along the proximal SA; 12 nodes at the hepatoduodenal ligament; 13 nodes on the posterior surface of the pancreatic head; 14 lymph nodes along the SMA or superior mesenteric vein; 15 nodes along the middle colic vein; 16a lymph nodes around the abdominal aorta for the upper margin of the celiac trunk to the lower margin of the LRV; 16b lymph nodes around the abdominal aorta from the upper margin of the LRV to the aortic bifurcation; 110 lymph nodes in the lower thoracic paraesophageal; 20 lymph nodes in the esophageal hiatus of the diaphragm [46]

subtotal gastrectomy, no. 2 LNs should be contained in CTV.

Current studies recommended that the target volume for postoperative RT in gastric cancer covered all nodal recurrence sites. Node nos. 1–6, 10, and 11 can be excluded from the treatment volume because of the extremely low recurrence rate after surgery. Jeong reassessed the ARTIST trial depending on the patterns of postoperative recurrence and the definition of the target volume [30]. The study found that the ARTIST trial was similar to the study of Yoon in failure patterns, and the postoperative concomitant radiochemotherapy significantly decreased the recurrence rate of node nos. 16a/b, 13, and 14 compared with chemotherapy alone. This result indicates that RT has advantages in the control of high-risk lymph node.

According to Yoon, if the tumor involved the proximal third stomach, then the lymph nodes for target volume should include 9, 10, 13, and 16a/b. If the gastric cancer involved the middle third stomach, then the extent should include 12, 14, and 16a/b. If the tumor involved the distal third stomach, then the extent should include 9, 11–14, and 16a/b. If the gastric cancer involved more than two-thirds of stomach, then 2,

9, 11, 12, 14, and 16a/b should be included (Table 4). In the present study, a preliminary plan can be recommended. The anastomotic site should be included because of a high rate of recrudesce. Whether the residual stomach should be irradiated remains controversial, and IMRT can reduce the adverse reactions. The tumor bed should be included for the T4 stage. No deal exists either on the extent of lymph nodes for RT.

Additionally, a phase II trial from China provides a new method to contouring the target volumes of lymph node for postoperative RT in gastric cancer [47]. Compared with the traditional surgical-based division system, the stomach is segmented into the upper third-fundus, the middle third-body, and the lower third-pylorus. They

Table 4 Radiation range of lymph nodes after D2 dissection from Yoon

Primary site	Radiation range
Proximal third stomach	9, 10, 13, and 16a/b
Middle third stomach	12, 14, and 16a/b
Distal third stomach	9, 11–14, and 16a/b
More than two-thirds of the stomach	2, 9, 11, 12, 14, and 16a/b

advised that the target volumes should always contain the perigastric LNs (nos. 1–6) and the lymphatics in the gastric wall and the LNs around the celiac artery. The other LNs should be irradiated on the basis of their lymphatic drainage.

A preliminary plan from our hospital advises the following points. The gastric cancer involving the proximal third stomach should include 110, 20, 1–3, 7–11, and 16a/b. The gastric cancer involving the middle third stomach should include 1, 3, 5, 9, 11p, 12, 13, 14 (T4 or pancreas involved), and 16a/b. The gastric cancer involving the distal third stomach should include 3, 5, 9, 11p, 12, 13, 14 (T4 or pancreas involved), and 16a/b (Table 5). The effect of this plan has not been reported, and researchers can enlighten the updating path of delineating lymph node target volumes.

An improved plan for target volumes delineation should be on the basis of clinical experience and the characteristics of lymphatic drainage. Currently, the study of Yoon et al. is the only research on delineating the rnGTV, but they analyzed only the patients with stage III (N3) gastric cancer. The study of Yu provides a new idea for delineating lymph node target volumes; however, the research is single-arm, phase II, and non-randomized. Phase III trials are still necessary to validate the conclusion. The guidelines for the delineation of target volumes for postoperative RT entail further consensus.

Conclusion

Preoperative RT has progressed in treating GEJ cancer; however, the application of preoperative RT still lacks large-scale phase III clinical trials for gastric cancer. In addition, patients with D1 or D1 plus lymphadenectomy can benefit from postoperative RT obviously, and postoperative RT may be beneficial for some patients with D2 lymphadenectomy. Multicenter randomized controlled trials are still required to confirm the value of RT in patients with this disease.

RT is a promising prospect as a local treatment option; future efforts should be directed to defining the target volume, determining the optimal multimodality protocol, and improving the technology of RT. Screening for novel biomarkers of radiosensitivity will also help patients of gastric cancer benefit from personalized therapy.

Table 5 Radiation range of lymph nodes after D2 dissection from the Chinese Academy of Medical Sciences

Primary site	Radiation range
Proximal third stomach	110, 20, 1–3, 7–11, and 16a/b
Middle third stomach	1, 3, 5, 9, 11p, 12, 13, 14*, and 16a/b
Distal third stomach	3, 5, 9, 11p, 12, 13, 14*, and 16a/b

*T4 or pancreas involved

Abbreviations

2D: 2-Dimentional irradiation; 3D: 3-Dimensional conformal radiation therapy; 5-FU: 5-Fluorouracil; CRT: Chemoradiotherapy; CT: Chemotherapy; DFS/RFS: Disease-/relapse-free survival; EC: Esophagus cancer; EGJ: Esophagogastric junction; GC: Gastric cancer; GEJ: Gastroesophageal junction; IMRT: Intensity-modulated radiation therapy; LNs: Lymph nodes; LRRFS: Locoregional failure-free survival; LV: Leucovorin; NR: Not reported; OS: Overall survival; RT: Radiotherapy; S: Surgery; XP: Capecitabine plus cisplatin

Authors' contributions

NZ, QF, and XH contributed to the study conception and design. JJG and LY performed the collection of data and conducted the data interpretation. All authors contributed to the manuscript writing. All authors read and approved the final manuscript.

Competing interests

The authors declare that they have no competing interests.

References

1. Ferlay J, Soerjomataram I, Dikshit R, Eser S, Mathers C, Rebelo M, Parkin D, Forman D, Bray F. Cancer incidence and mortality worldwide: sources, methods and major patterns in GLOBOCAN 2012. Int J Cancer. 2015;136: E359–86.
2. Edge SB, Compton CC. The American Joint Committee on Cancer: the 7th Edition of the AJCC Cancer Staging Manual and the Future of TNM. Ann Surg Oncol. 2010;17:1471.
3. Macdonald JS, Smalley SR, Benedetti J, Hundahl SA, Estes NC, Stemmermann GN, Haller DG, Ajani JA, Gunderson LL, Jessup JM. Chemoradiotherapy after surgery compared with surgery alone for adenocarcinoma of the stomach or gastroesophageal junction. N Engl J Med. 2001;345:725–30.
4. Tormo FV, Andreu Martínez FJ, Cardenal MR, Pomares AA. Evaluation of the toxicity of the combined treatment of chemoradiotherapy, according to the scheme of Macdonald, after radical surgery in patients diagnosed of gastric cancer. Clin Transl Oncol. 2006;8:611.
5. Yao JC, Mansfield PF, Pisters PW, Feig BW, Janjan NA, Crane C, Ajani JA. Combined-modality therapy for gastric cancer. Semin Surg Oncol. 2003;21:223.
6. Zhang ZX, Gu XZ, Yin WB, Huang GJ, Zhang DW, Zhang RG. Randomized clinical trial on the combination of preoperative irradiation and surgery in the treatment of adenocarcinoma of gastric cardia (AGC)--report on 370 patients. Int J Radiat Oncol Biol Phys. 1998;42:929–34.
7. Stahl M, Walz MK, Stuschke M, Lehmann N, Meyer HJ, Rieraknorrenschild J, Langer P, Engenhartcabillic R, Bitzer M, Königsrainer A. Phase III comparison of preoperative chemotherapy compared with chemoradiotherapy in patients with locally advanced adenocarcinoma of the esophagogastric junction. J Clin Oncol Off J Am Soc Clin Oncol. 2009;27:851.
8. Van HP, Hulshof MC, van Lanschot JJ, Steyerberg EW, Mi VBH, Wijnhoven BP, Richel DJ, Nieuwenhuijzen GA, Hospers GA, Bonenkamp JJ. Preoperative chemoradiotherapy for esophageal or junctional cancer. N Engl J Med. 2012;367:737–42.
9. Skoropad V, Berdov B, Zagrebin V. Concentrated preoperative radiotherapy for resectable gastric cancer: 20-years follow-up of a randomized trial. J Surg Oncol. 2002;80:72–8.
10. JA A, PF M, N J JM, PW P, PM L, B F RM, R N DSC, LL G. Multi-institutional trial of preoperative chemoradiotherapy in patients with potentially resectable gastric carcinoma. J Clin Oncol Off J Am Soc Clin Oncol. 2004;22:2774.
11. Ajani JA, Mansfield PF, Crane CH, Wu TT, Lunagomez S, Lynch PM, Janjan N, Feig B, Faust J, Yao JC. Paclitaxel-based chemoradiotherapy in localized gastric carcinoma: degree of pathologic response and not clinical parameters dictated patient outcome. J Clin Oncol Off J Am Soc Clin Oncol. 2005;23:1237.
12. Balandraud P, Moutardier V, Giovannini M, Giovannini MH, Lelong B, Guiramand J, Magnin V, Houvenaeghel G, Delpero JR. Locally advanced adenocarcinomas of the gastric cardia: results of pre-operative chemoradiotherapy. Gastroenterol Clin Biol. 2004;28:651.

13. Klautke G, Foitzik T, Ludwig K, Ketterer P, Klar E, Fietkau R. Neoadjuvant radiochemotherapy in locally advanced gastric carcinoma. Strahlenther Onkol. 2004;180:695–700.

14. Lowy AM, Feig BW, Janjan N, Rich TA, Pisters PW, Ajani JA, Mansfield PF. A pilot study of preoperative chemoradiotherapy for resectable gastric cancer. Ann Surg Oncol. 2001;8:519.

15. Kumagai K, Rouvelas I, Tsai JA, Mariosa D, Lind PA, Lindblad M, Ye W, Lundell L, Schuhmacher C, Mauer M. Survival benefit and additional value of preoperative chemoradiotherapy in resectable gastric and gastro-oesophageal junction cancer: a direct and adjusted indirect comparison meta-analysis. Eur J Surg Oncol J Eur Soc Surg Oncol Br Assoc Surg Oncol. 2015;41:282–94.

16. Fiorica F, Cartei F, Enea M, Licata A, Cabibbo G, Carau B, Liboni A, Ursino S. The impact of radiotherapy on survival in resectable gastric carcinoma: a meta-analysis of literature data. Cancer Treat Rev. 2007;33:729.

17. Cunningham D, Allum WH, Stenning SP, Thompson JN, Cj VDV, Nicolson M, Scarffe JH, Lofts FJ, Falk SJ, Iveson TJ. Perioperative chemotherapy versus surgery alone for resectable gastroesophageal cancer. J Evid Based Med. 2008;355:11.

18. Ychou M, Boige V, Pignon JP, Conroy T, Bouché O, Lebreton G, Ducourtieux M, Bedenne L, Fabre JM, Saintaubert B. Perioperative chemotherapy compared with surgery alone for resectable gastroesophageal adenocarcinoma: an FNCLCC and FFCD multicenter phase III trial. J Clin Oncol Off J Am Soc Clin Oncol. 2011;29:1715–21.

19. Schuhmacher C, Gretschel S, Lordick F, Reichardt P, Hohenberger W, Eisenberger CF, Haag C, Mauer ME, Hasan B, Welch J. Neoadjuvant chemotherapy compared with surgery alone for locally advanced cancer of the stomach and cardia: European Organisation for Research and Treatment of Cancer Randomized Trial 40954. J Clin Oncol Off J Am Soc Clin Oncol. 2010;28:5210–8.

20. Australasian Gastro-Intestinal Trials Group. Trial of preoperative therapy for gastric and esophagogastric junction adenocarcinoma (TOPGEAR) [http://clinicaltrials.gov/show/NCT01924819]. Accessed 1 Aug 2017.

21. Zhou Z. Pre-operative chemoradiotherapy or chemotherapy following surgery and adjuvant chemotherapy in patients with gastric cancer [http://clinicaltrials.gov/ct2/show/NCT01815853]. Accessed 1 Aug 2017.

22. Songun I, Putter H, Kranenbarg EM, Sasako M, Cj VDV. Surgical treatment of gastric cancer: 15-year follow-up results of the randomised nationwide Dutch D1D2 trial. Lancet Oncol. 2010;11:404–5.

23. Smalley SR, Benedetti JK, Haller DG, Hundahl SA, Estes NC, Ajani JA, Gunderson LL, Goldman B, Martenson JA, Jessup JM. Updated analysis of SWOG-directed intergroup study 0116: a phase III trial of adjuvant radiochemotherapy versus observation after curative gastric cancer resection. J Clin Oncol Off J Am Soc Clin Oncol. 2012;30:2327–33.

24. Lee J, Lim DH, Kim S, Park SH, Park JO, Park YS, Lim HY, Min GC, Sohn TS, Noh JH. Phase III trial comparing capecitabine plus cisplatin versus capecitabine plus cisplatin with concurrent capecitabine radiotherapy in completely resected gastric cancer with D2 lymph node dissection: the ARTIST Trial. J Clin Oncol Off J Am Soc Clin Oncol. 2012;30:268–73.

25. Park SH, Sohn TS, Lee J, Lim DH, Hong ME, Kim K, Sohn I, Jung SH, Choi MG, Lee JH. Phase III trial to compare adjuvant chemotherapy with capecitabine and cisplatin versus concurrent chemoradiotherapy in gastric cancer: final report of the adjuvant chemoradiotherapy in stomach tumors trial, including survival and subset analyses. J Clin Oncol Off J Am Soc Clin Oncol. 2015;33:3130–6.

26. Kim TH, Park SR, Ryu KW, Kim YW, Bae JM, Lee JH, Choi IJ, Kim YJ, Kim DY. Phase 3 trial of postoperative chemotherapy alone versus chemoradiation therapy in stage III–IV gastric cancer treated with R0 gastrectomy and D2 lymph node dissection. Int J Radiat Oncol Biol Phys. 2012;84:585–92.

27. Zhu WG, Xua DF, Pu J, Zong CD, Li T, Tao GZ, Ji FZ, Zhou XL, Han JH, Wang CS. A randomized, controlled, multicenter study comparing intensity-modulated radiotherapy plus concurrent chemotherapy with chemotherapy alone in gastric cancer patients with D2 resection. Radiother Oncol J Eur Soc Ther Radiol Oncol. 2012;104:361–6.

28. Amini A, Jones BL, Stumpf P, Leong S, Lieu CH, Weekes C, Davis SL, Messersmith WA, Purcell WT, Ghosh D, et al. Patterns of care for locally advanced pancreatic adenocarcinoma using the National Cancer Database. Pancreas. 2017;46:904–12.

29. Sasako M, Sakuramoto S, Katai H, Kinoshita T, Furukawa H, Yamaguchi T, Nashimoto A, Fujii M, Nakajima T, Ohashi Y. Five-year outcomes of a randomized phase III trial comparing adjuvant chemotherapy with S-1

versus surgery alone in stage II or III gastric cancer. J Clin Oncol Off J Am Soc Clin Oncol. 2011;29:4387.

30. Datta J, Mcmillan MT, Ruffolo L, Lowenfeld L, Mamtani R, Plastaras JP, Dempsey DT, Karakousis GC, Drebin JA, Fraker DL. Multimodality therapy improves survival in resected early stage gastric cancer in the United States. Ann Surg Oncol. 2016;23:1–10.

31. Phase III randomized trial of adjuvant chemotherapy with S-1 vs. S-1/oxaliplatin ± radiotherapy for completely resected gastric adenocarcinoma: the ARTIST II trial (ARTIST-II) [http://clinicaltrials.gov/ct2/show/NCT01761461]. Accessed 1 Aug 2017.

32. Shim HJ, Kim KR, Hwang JE, Bae WK, Ryu SY, Park YK, Nam TK, Chung IJ, Cho SH. A phase II study of adjuvant S-1/cisplatin chemotherapy followed by S-1-based chemoradiotherapy for D2-resected gastric cancer. Cancer Chemother Pharmacol. 2016;77:605–12.

33. Ohri N, Garg MK, Aparo S, Kaubisch A, Tome W, Kennedy TJ, Kalnicki S, Guha C. Who benefits from adjuvant radiation therapy for gastric cancer? A meta-analysis. Int J Radiat Oncol Biol Phys. 2013;86:330–5.

34. Pang X, Wei W, Leng W, Chen Q, Xia H, Chen L, Li R. Radiotherapy for gastric cancer: a systematic review and meta-analysis. Tumour Biol J Int Soc Oncodev Biol Med. 2014;35:387–96.

35. Soon YY, Leong CN, Tey JC, Tham IW, Lu JJ. Postoperative chemo-radiotherapy versus chemotherapy for resected gastric cancer: a systematic review and meta-analysis. J Med Imaging Radiat Oncol. 2014;58:483.

36. Lee J, Park CK, Park JO, Lim T, Park YS, Lim HY, Lee I, Sohn TS, Noh JH, Heo JS. Impact of E2F-1 expression on clinical outcome of gastric adenocarcinoma patients with adjuvant chemoradiation therapy. Clin Cancer Res. 2008;14:82.

37. Gordon MA, Gundacker HM, Benedetti J, Macdonald JS, Baranda JC, Levin WJ, Blanke CD, Elatre W, Weng P, Zhou JY. Assessment of HER2 gene amplification in adenocarcinomas of the stomach or gastroesophageal junction in the INT-0116/SWOG9008 clinical trial. Ann Oncol. 2013;24:1754.

38. Bargielaiparraguirre J, Pradomarchal L, Fernandezfuente M, Gutierrezgonzález A, Morenorubio J, Muñozfernandez M, Sereno M, Sanchezprieto R, Perona R, Sanchezperez I. CHK1 expression in gastric cancer is modulated by p53 and RB1/E2F1: implications in chemo/radiotherapy response. Sci Rep. 2016;6:21519.

39. Matzinger O, Gerber E, Bernstein Z, Maingon P, Haustermans K, Bosset JF, Gulyban A, Poortmans P, Collette L, Kuten A. EORTC-ROG expert opinion: radiotherapy volume and treatment guidelines for neoadjuvant radiation of adenocarcinomas of the gastroesophageal junction and the stomach. Radiother Oncol J Eur Soc Therap Radiol Oncol. 2009;92:164–75.

40. Oppedijk V, van der Gaast A, van Lanschot JJ, van Hagen P, van Os R, van Rij CM, van der Sangen MJ, Beukema JC, Rütten H, Spruit PH. Patterns of recurrence after surgery alone versus preoperative chemoradiotherapy and surgery in the CROSS trials. J Clin Oncol Off J Am Soc Clin Oncol. 2014;32:385.

41. Smalley SR, Gunderson L, Tepper J, Jr MJ, Minsky B, Willett C, Rich T. Gastric surgical adjuvant radiotherapy consensus report: rationale and treatment implementation. Int J Radiat Oncol Biol Phys. 2002;52:283–93.

42. Tepper JE, Gunderson LL. Radiation treatment parameters in the adjuvant postoperative therapy of gastric cancer. Semin Radiat Oncol. 2002;12:187.

43. Nam H, Lim-Do H, Kim S, Kang W, Sohn T, Noh J, Kim Y, Park C, Park C, Ahn Y, Huh S. A new suggestion for the radiation target volume after a subtotal gastrectomy in patients with stomach cancer. Int J Radiat Oncol Biol Phys. 2008;71:448–55.

44. Ohira M, Toyokawa T, Sakurai K, Kubo N, Tanaka H, Muguruma K, Yashiro M, Onoda N, Hirakawa K. Current status in remnant gastric cancer after distal gastrectomy. World J Gastroenterol. 2016;22:2424.

45. Chang JS, Lim JS, Noh SH, Hyung WJ, An JY, Lee YC, Rha SY, Lee CG, Koom WS. Patterns of regional recurrence after curative D2 resection for stage III (N3) gastric cancer: implications for postoperative radiotherapy. Radiother Oncol J Eur Soc Therap Radiol Oncol. 2012;104:367–73.

46. Yoon HI, Chang JS, Lim JS, Noh SH, Hyung WJ, An JY, Lee YC, Rha SY, Kim KH, Koom WS. Defining the target volume for post-operative radiotherapy after D2 dissection in gastric cancer by CT-based vessel-guided delineation. Radiother Oncol J Eur Soc Therap Radiol Oncol. 2013;108:72–7.

47. Haijun Y, Qiuji W, Zhenming F, Yong H, Zhengkai L, Conghua X, Yunfeng Z, Yahua Z. A new approach to delineating lymph node target volumes for post-operative radiotherapy in gastric cancer: a phase II trial. Radiother Oncol J Eur Soc Therap Radiol Oncol. 2015;116:245.

20

Molecular pathological expression in malignant gliomas resected by fluorescein sodium-guiding under the YELLOW 560 nm surgical microscope filter

Ningning Zhang[1,2*†], Zhende Shang[2†], Zhigang Wang[1], Xianbing Meng[2], Zheng Li[2], Hailong Tian[1], Dezhang Huang[1], Xin Yin[1], Bin Zheng[2] and Xinhua Zhang[2*]

Abstract

Background: This study aimed to analyze the relationship between molecular pathologic expression of GFAP and Ki-67 and fluorescence levels, and to provide molecular pathological basis for the removal of malignant gliomas (MG) by Fluorescein Sodium (FLS) navigation under the YELLOW 560 nm surgical microscope filter.

Methods: A retrospective analysis of clinical data of 18 MG cases confirmed by the postoperative pathology was performed. All cases were resected by FLS guiding under the YELLOW 560 nm filter. Hematoxylin-eosin (HE) staining, molecular pathology markers GFAP, and Ki-67 immunohistochemical staining of the specimens were performed. The relationship between fluorescence staining levels and GFAP positive rate, Ki-67 proliferation index, and WHO grades was studied.

Results: There were 69 pathological specimens with fluorescence levels of "bright" fluorescence ($n = 32$), "low" fluorescence ($n = 18$), and "no" fluorescence ($n = 19$). Immunohistochemical staining showed GFAP-positive expression in both tumor cells and normal glial cells. The staining levels of the specimens in the fluorescence regions were higher than that in the non-fluorescence regions. GFAP expression was positive in 61 specimens and negative in 8 specimens. Comparison of Ki-67 proliferation index using chi-square test showed different fluorescence levels had different Ki-67 proliferation indexes ($x^2 = 14.678$, $p = 0.005$). With high proliferation index of specimens, fluorescence level was brighter. WHO grade had no correlation with fluorescence levels ($x^2 = 3.531$, $p = 0.171$).

Conclusion: FLS-guided resection of MG is safe and effective. In the boundary area of MG, fluorescence levels and Ki-67 proliferation index showed correlation. FLS-guided resection achieved the function of "reducing tumor cell," thus reducing the proliferation index in the lesion area.

Keywords: Fluorescein sodium, YELLOW 560 nm, Malignant glioma, GFAP, Ki-67

Background

Malignant gliomas (MG) are graded as WHO grade III or IV gliomas. Glioblastoma is the most common malignant primary tumor of the skull. Adult glioblastoma accounted for 15.4% of all primary brain tumors and 45.6% of primary malignant tumors [1]. The treatment

* Correspondence: 276278529@qq.com; zhangxinhuazs@163.com
†Ningning Zhang and Zhende Shang contributed equally to this work.
[1]Department of Neurosurgery, Shandong University Qilu Hospital, Qingdao, Shandong, China
[2]Department of Neurosurgery, Affiliated Hospital of Taishan Medical University, Tai An, Shandong, China

of glioblastoma remained difficult, demonstrating poor prognosis, high recurrence rate, high mortality rate, and low cure rate. Recently, several treatment strategies have been developed, including microsurgical treatment, chemotherapy, radiotherapy, and other modern therapeutic models, but the prognosis improvement still remained difficult. The increased total resection rate can improve the progression-free survival (PFS) and the overall survival (OS) rate of the patients with MG [2, 3]. The key treatment for this type of tumor is to maximize safe resection of the tumor. The pathological occurrence of glioma involves multiple-sources and is highly malignant and invasive. The boundary between the tumor and normal brain tissue is indistinctive and remains difficult for the complete removal of tumor cells. Several experimental studies both in vivo and in vitro have confirmed [4–6] that even 2 cm residual area outside glioblastoma can cause tumor recurrence and poor prognosis. Many surgical techniques have been developed, including neuronavigation, intraoperative ultrasound, electrophysiological monitoring during operation, magnetic resonance during surgery, fluorescence guided surgery, and so on, to improve the total resection rate and improve the patients' disease progressive-free and overall survival rate. The technique of Fluorescein Sodium (FLS) navigation for the resection of MG is used to mark the tumor during operation and assist the doctors for removing tumor. Although 5-acetyl propionic acid(5-ALA) was also useful in guided resection of glioblastoma, but it had much difficulty in clinical popularization because of many disadvantages, such as not approved by the Committee on Food and Drug Administration, photo-induced toxicity, expensive equipment, and complicated application process. In 2013, K.M. Schebesch et al. [7] reported the use of FLS under YELLOW 560 nm to resect intracranial tumors in 35 cases. This study supported the use of FLS navigation resection as a safe and effective method for MG. However, there is a lack of quantitative study on the fluorescence intensity of FLS navigation of MG as these are different from other malignant tumors, and MG rarely metastasize to other different organs. These in turn often lead to death by invading the underlying brain tissues and resistance to modern treatment strategies.

Histological grading of glioma is based on modern histological features, including necrosis, cell nuclear polymorphism, nuclear fission ability, angiogenesis, and so on. The molecular pathology and immunohistochemistry were applied clinically to investigate individually and monitor the patients from the gene and protein levels. Immunohistochemical study of molecular markers has been more accurate and added practical value in the pathological diagnosis and prognostic judgment. Many molecular markers are used for guiding diagnosis, differential diagnosis, tumor malignancy, treatment guidance, and prognosis evaluation.

In this study, glial fibrillary acidic protein (GFAP) and proliferation-related protein Ki67 were selected as the classic markers of glioma, and the different fluorescence level specimens were analyzed by immunohistochemical pathology and operation. Our study aimed to further investigate the differential expression of molecular pathology of MG under different fluorescence levels to provide a basis for the use of FLS in the navigation of the MG cells and more effective identification of the

boundary between the tumor and the brain. We hope to better guide the application of FLS navigation, protect the normal brain tissue, improving the surgical resection rate and prognosis.

Methods
Data collection
Retrospective analysis of the 18 cases of pathologically confirmed MG resected by FLS guiding under the YELLOW 560 nm filter from the neurosurgery department of Shandong University Qilu Hospital (Qingdao) between January 2014 and December 2016 (Table 1).

Selected criteria [8]
Patients 1, age ranged between 18 and 75 years; 2, who were newly diagnosed, untreated or have relapsed MG, with certain pathological results after postoperative confirmation; 3, according to the surgery after 24–72 h of intracranial MRI examination; 4, according to the enhancement area of postoperative MRI, the surgeon and the imaging department evaluates the total resection of the tumor.

Exclusion standard
(1) Patients under 18 years old and more than 75 years old were excluded; (2) tumors originating from the brain stem; (3) excluding patients who are suffering low-level gliomas or non-tumors whose MRI showed enhancement areas; (4) renal insufficiency of patients; (5) patients with hepatic insufficiency; (6) other parts of the body with active malignant tumor patients; (7) preoperative tumor MRI enhancement and postoperative pathology proved to be metastatic tumor patients; (8) according to the operation, a single specimen retention of the case should be excluded.

Definition description
Total resection criteria for surgery and post-operation
Total resection of the glioblastoma during surgery was based on the surgeon and the navigational judgment of the operation. Total resection was according to complete disappearance of the FLS staining of tumor tissues, and complete disappearance of the enhanced tumor tissues under neuronavigated operation. While postoperative total resection according to the postoperative brain enhanced MRI after 24–72 h, less than $0.175 \ cm^3$ volume of the residual postoperative enhancement was considered as total resection [8, 9]. Some cases of total resection were performed larger than the postoperative-enhanced MRI region; these cases could be called as extended resection or ultra-total resection.

Table 1 Clinical characteristics in summary

No	Age/sex	Symptoms/signs	Localization	Tumor size (cm^3)	Pathology	% of resection	No. of biopsies
1	42/M	Seizure	RF	15.732	AA (WHO III)	100	4
2	71/F	Headache, somnolence	RT/P	126.759	GBM	100	2
3	49/M	Recurrent	RF	26.4	DA (partial AA, WHO III)	100	7
4	62/F	Aphasia, right prosopolegia	LF	68.04	GBM	100	3
5	48/F	Headache, left hemiparesis	LF/T/I	84.48	GBM	100	5
6	66/M	Headache, somnolence	LP/O	122.4	GBM	88.6	6
7	36/F	Headache, IICP	RF/T	28.7	GA (partial AA, WHO III)	100	2
8	50/F	Headache, left hemiparesis, IICP	RF	37.44	GBM	100	2
9	71/F	Left hemiparesis	LF/P	36	GBM	100	5
10	49/M	Seizure	RF	70.119	OD (WHO III)	100	5
11	35/M	Seizure	LF	49.02	OD (WHO III)	100	2
12	49/F	Recurrent	RF/T/I	94.875	rGBM	99.6	4
13	41/F	Headache, aphasia	LF/T/P	81.567	AA (WHO III)	100	3
14	61/F	Seizure	RF/T/I	21.06	DA (partial AA, WHO III)	100	2
15	26/F	Seizure	LF	44	OD (WHO III)	100	4
16	34/F	Recurrent	LF	13.888	rGBM	100	8
17	45/M	Seizure, left hemiparesis	RP	36	AA (WHO III)	100	2
18	32/M	Seizure, right tendon hyperreflexia	LF	13.32	GBM	100	3

F female, *M* male, *L* left, *R* right, *T* temporal lobe, *P* parietal lobe, *O* occipital lobe, *I* insular lobe, *GBM* glioblastoma multiforme, *rGBM* reccurent glioblastoma multiforme, *AA* anaplastic astrocytoma, *DA* diffuse astrocytomas, *OD* oligodendrogliomas

Standard for postoperative tumor imaging recurrence

The MRI findings showed that the area of tumor resection was larger than 0.175 cm^3, which was considered to be recurrent [8, 9].

The method of developing FLS in operation

Twenty percent fluorescent sodium was obtained from Guangzhou Baiyun Mountain Ming Xing Pharmaceutical Co., Ltd. (National Drug Code: H44023400). Before the use of 20% FLS, diluted to 3%, skin test was performed with 5 ml deep vein injection to observe the patient's vital signs and rashes and other abnormalities, and then diluted to 1%. The dosage was in accordance with the patient's weight, i.e., 2–3 mg/kg. Drug delivery time: injected the drug just before skin cut after anesthesia induction was begun. Drug delivery: single dose intravenous injection.

Procedure control

The use of neuronavigation in surgery

This procedure uses the frame-free brainlab neural navigation. Routine brain MRI scans were performed in the 1 week before operation. Neuronavigation was recorded using gadolinium-enhanced T1WI sequence, and a surgical plan was established to enhanced boundaries with T1WI. The boundary of neuronavigation was not used as a major criterion for complete resection of tumors. For central sulcus MG, the scanning of diffused tensor imaging (DTI) was used to assess the adjacent relationship between tumor and subcortical fibrous bundles.

Combined use of electrophysiological monitoring in operation [10]

MG in the central sulcus area maximize safe resection of tumors while ensuring the integrity of the patient's movement and sensory function. During the operation, the neural electrophysiological monitoring was performed to complete the resection of the tumor while protecting the vital nerve function as intact as possible.

Tumor resection during surgery

After exposing the tumor tissue, the Pentero 900 microscope was used to adjust the filter to the YELLOW 560 nm mode. Most of the time, the surgeon can remove the tumor tissue in YELLOW 560 nm mode, and it is convenient in the YELLOW 560 nm mode to be converted to white light mode by switching the button when it required to stop bleeding or to obtain a pathological specimen. During the operation, the surgeon uses the suction device to absorb the blood from the field of vision as far as possible in order to avoid the situation that leads to blurred vision. Sometimes, in order to avoid damage to the normal brain tissue, ultrasound absorbers from the internal and external absorption of tumor tissues were used until the fluorescence staining of the tumor tissue is completely removed.

Retention of pathological specimens

During the operation, under the real-time YELLOW 560 mode, regardless of tumor location, according to the yellow staining degree of the tissue specimen is labeled as "no yellow dye," "low yellow dye," and "bright yellow dye" levels. All tissue specimens were removed and immediately applied with 10% formalin fixation and embedded for pathological analysis. In the tumor boundary area, pathological specimens obtained randomly from each patient were marked as "no,", "low," and "bright" yellow according to the yellow fluorescence staining levels.

Experiment main reagents

GFAP and Ki-67 were purchased from Fuzhou Mai Xin Company.

Sheep anti-rat/rabbit IgG (KIT-5030) were purchased from Fuzhou Mai Xin Company.

Experimental main equipment

Leica RM2235 type electric paraffin slicer (German Leica Company).

Leica BONDTM Automatic IHC dyeing system (German Leica Company).

Specimen treatment

All specimens were fixed with 10% formalin, conventional paraffin embedding, slicing machine adjusted to thickness of 4 μm, and sliced continuously. After slicing, HE was stained conventionally and GFAP and Ki67 were stained by immunohistochemistry.

Immunohistochemical staining (en vision method)

The 4 μm paraffin sections were fixed and washed, and extreme care must be taken to avoid peeling off the sections. The slides were specially repaired by citric acid working fluid (for Ki67) by incubating at 120 °C temperature for 2 min. And GFAP was no need to be repaired.

Results interpretation and evaluation

GFAP staining of tissue cell cytoplasm of yellow or brown-yellow granules were considered positive, and no color or faint yellowish granules were considered negative.

Compute the Ki-67 labeling index (Ki-67 LI). Ki-67 LI is defined as the percentage of the total number of cells that are Ki-67 positive. For the region of necrosis and vascular endothelial cells, cells can be differentiated when the nucleus that is less than 2 mm is not counted. In view of less than 1 cell per low magnification, LI is considered to be less than 0.1% , is not visible under the microscope, and is calculated as 0 [4].

Postoperative follow-up

The follow-up of outpatients, inpatients was done through cell phone, SMS, interview, WeChat, Tencent

QQ, and email. Imaging evaluations were performed at 1 month, 3 months after surgery, and every 6 months. All patients underwent MRI scanning and contrast-enhancement (CE) of the brain in 24–72 h after operation, 1 month after operation, 3 months, and every 6 months. The associated complications were observed from elevated blood pressure, seizures, tracheal spasms, or allergic reactions following the injection of FLS.

Statistical analysis

Continuous variables are described in average, median, and standard deviation. SPSS19.0 statistical software was used and χ^2 test with multiple composition ratios were used. $p < 0.05$ was considered statistically different.

Results

General information results

The patients included in this study were 18 cases, including 7 male cases and 11 female cases. The average age was 48.2 years (26–71 years old). Main symptoms and postoperative pathological classification had been listed in Table 1.

Fluorescence imaging results

One percent FLS was intravenously injected before skin incision after induction of general anesthesia. The first 17 cases were administered with 3 mg/kg weight of FLS, followed by 2 mg/kg weight, and both obtained the same effect (see Fig. 1 and Fig. 2). After opening the dura, i.e., intravenous FLS injection for 20–40 min, it gathers tumor tissue without spilling into normal brain tissue. After craniotomy, all tumors were stained by FLS in YELLOW 560 nm mode. The tumor tissue showed a bright fluorescent color (see Fig. 1b (a)), especially in the MRI-enhanced area. But in the necrotic region of the tumor or in the area where the MRI was not enhanced, it showed a "low" or "none" fluorescent staining (see Fig. 1d (b)). The liquid region of cystic tumors can still be shown as bright fluorescence in color and obviously lighter than that in the cerebrospinal fluid. Even at very low concentrations of FLS (2 mg/kg), the YELLOW 560 nm model of the Pentero 900 microscope can easily differentiate between fluorescent and non-fluorescent tissues.

Surgical results

The average tumor volume was 53.88 cm^3 (13.32–126.759 cm^3). The total resection was performed in 16 cases (see Fig. 3 and Fig. 2). The 69 pathological specimens were randomly obtained from 18 cases (32 bright-, 18 low-, 19 non-fluorescence). The postoperative KPS score was slightly higher than before, though no statistically significant difference (average preoperative 82 vs. postoperative 83, $p = 0.566$). Five patients reported a short KPS score reduction (cases 4, 6, 8, 13, and 17) after surgery. In addition, eighth case had permanent mild

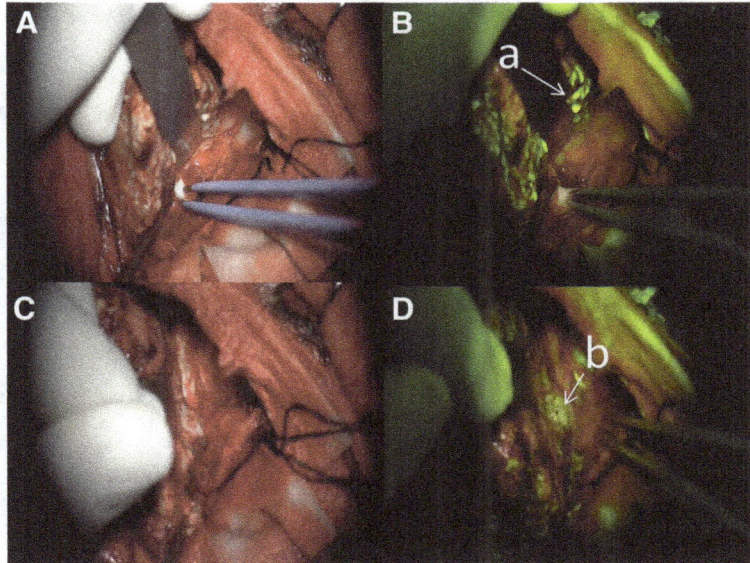

Fig. 1 Case 16. Comparison between white light and YELLOW 560 nm mode under Pentero 900 microscope was developed. **a**, **c** For white light, the boundary display was not clear, especially the direction of the bipolar, and difficult to distinguish. **b**, **d** Two figures showed the YELLOW 560 nm mode of development, where the dyed bright fluorescent color of the tumor tissue and the surrounding non-fluorescent tissue boundaries were clear, facilitating the removal of tumors. In **b**, "a" is the "light" fluorescent color, and the bipolar refers to the "none" fluorescent color. In **d**, "b" refers to a "low" fluorescent color and can be easily differentiated from the "none" fluorescent color tissue (indicated by bipolar in **b**)

hemiplegia, with short-term recovery to the preoperative state. No venous thrombosis and pulmonary embolism occurred after operation. The color of the skin, mucus membranes, and urine of the patient after being injected with FLS was yellow and disappeared after about 24 h after the operation. No related serious adverse events were found.

Two patients (case 1 and 18) had epileptic seizures in the early postoperative period (1 month), considering the preoperative state of the patients.

Follow-up results

Sixteen cases were completely followed up (cases 4 and 11 were lost), with a follow-up rate of 88.9% (16/18). Complete radiotherapy and chemotherapy (Stupp regimen) were completed in 10 cases (10/18).3 patients died of tumor progression (cases 5, 6, and 8) and 1 patient died of severe pneumonia.

Pathological examination results

Relationship between the expression of GFAP and fluorescence levels of MG (Table 2, Fig. 4, Fig. 5)

In 69 specimens, 61 were GFAP positive. SPSS 19.0 Statistical software was used to compare the relationship between the positive rate of GFAP expression and the levels of fluorescence of MG, and χ^2 test with multiple composition ratios was used, revealing no statistically significant difference ($\chi^2 = 0.627$, $p = 0.731$).

The relationship between WHO grading and fluorescence levels (Table 2)

Comparing the relationship between the WHO grading and fluorescence levels of MG revealed no statistically significant difference ($\chi^2 = 3.531$, $p = 0.171$).

Ki-67 LI relation to fluorescence levels (Table 3, Fig. 4, Fig. 5)

Comparing the relationship between Ki-67 LI and fluorescence levels of MG revealed statistically significant difference ($\chi2 = 14.678$, $p = 0.0050.014$).

Discussion

Effect of FLS navigation on the removal rate of MG

Nowadays, there were three main fluorescent agents used for guided resection of glioblastoma including indocyanine Green (ICG), FLS, and 5-ALA. The removal of MG by the ICG-guided resection involves a short time, which could be helpfully used to obtain specimens but little useful for continuous navigation monitoring. ICG navigation combined with other navigations (such as 5-ALA) was mainly used for examination of residual tumors involving a short time after resection of MG [11]. 5-ALA had not yet been approved by the Committee on Food and Drug Administration which is an endogenous luminescent agent, with optical instability, partly low sensitivity, and specificity. Because of its "light bleaching," the tumor edge was not clearly displayed [12]. 5-ALA also had the disadvantages of

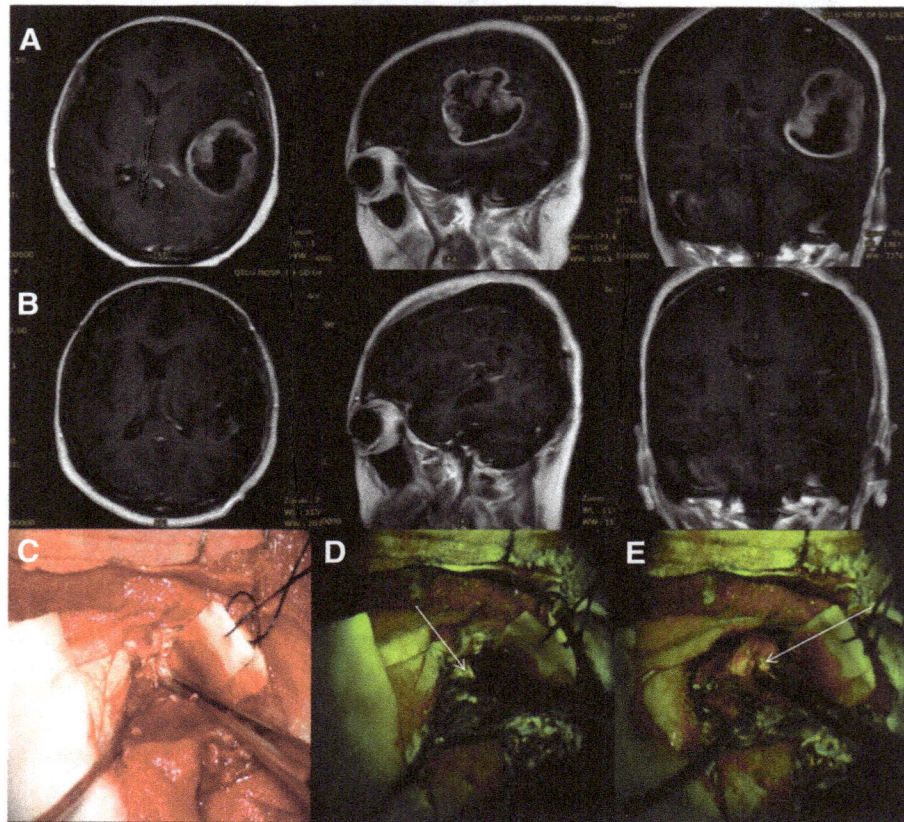

Fig. 2 Case 5. **a** T1WI enhancement MRI of the left frontal temporal insular lobe. **b** Postoperative MRI in 24 h. **c** Under Pentero 900, white light showed the tumor boundary, the boundary was unclear, and cannot be distinguished. **d**, **e** Tumor boundaries under YELLOW 560 nm. Fluorescence and non-fluorescent tissues are easily differentiated under the YELLOW 560 mode. **d** Specimens obtained in the boundary of "low" fluorescence color (white arrow). **e** "None" fluorescence to obtain specimen (white arrow)

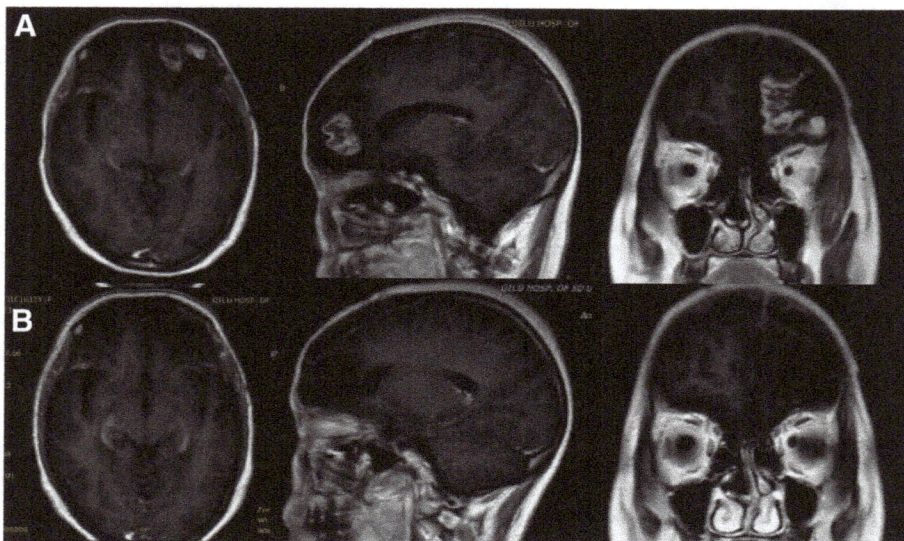

Fig. 3 Case 16. Performed on the axial, sagittal, coronal, and enhanced MRI. **a** Imaging the postoperative recurrence of the left frontal GBM after first operation for 2 years, and the volume was 13.9 cm³. **b** In 72 h, the axial, sagittal, coronal postoperative-enhanced MRI imaging showed no enhanced area residue

Table 2 Relationship between the expression of GFAP, WHO grades, and fluorescence levels of MG

Items	Fluorescence levels			Degree of freedom	x^2	p
	None	Low	Bright			
GFAP (+)	17	15	29	2	0.627	0.731
GFAP (−)	2	3	3			
WHO III	12	7	12	2	3.531	0.171
WHO IV	7	11	20			

photo-induced toxicity, expensive equipment, and complicated application process. Hence, 5-ALA had much difficulty in clinical popularization. FLS in ophthalmic fundus angiography had been safely and effectively used for many years, and was used to identify tumors in neurosurgery [13, 14]. Shinoda et al. [15] reported resection of 32 glioblastomas, and the total resection rate reached 84.4%. Chen B et al. [16] reported 10 cases of MG with complete resection of 80%, while only 33.3% of MG in control group (12 cases). KOC [17] resected 47 cases of glioblastomas demonstrating a total resection of 83% while control group (33 cases) showed 55%. Though there was no significant difference of influencing the lifetime (43.9 weeks and 41.8 weeks). 20 mg/kg FLS obtained clear imaging, and 10 cases of glioblastoma were expected to be resected. Kuroiwa et al. [18] after using special filter, 10 cases of glioblastoma were resected by intravenous injection of 8 mg/kg FLS. F. Acerbi et al. [8] using Pentero microscope intravenously injected 5 mg/kg FLS, then 12 cases of GBM obtained a total resection

of 75%, and the remaining patients with tumor resection volume of 90.5% (82.6–99.9%). In 2013, K.M. Schebesch et al. [7] reported that under the YELLOW 560 nm filter, with intravenous injection of 200mg FLS (3-4mg/kg), 35 cases of intracranial tumors, including 22 cases of MG, were resected. In our preliminary study, the total resection rate of MG under the guidance of FLS was 92.1%. The 6 month-PFS (92.3%) and median survival period (11 months) after the resection of glioblastoma were similar to those of FLUGLIO [8, 19]. Of the 18 cases, the total resection was achieved in 16 cases with multiple regional retentions of specimens according to the postoperative-enhanced MRI. Under the white light mode, the tumor tissue was blurring in the boundary between the tumor and the surrounding tissues. While under YELLOW 560 nm mode, the normal tissue and the tumoral tissue could be clearly identified (Figs. 1 and 2). Postoperative KPS score decreased before operation, and a slight increase after the operation, though the difference was not statistically significant (average preoperative 82 vs. postoperative 83, $p = 0.566$). No postoperative complication was associated with FLS, and thus it was considered safe and effective for the removal of MG by FLS navigation.

The relationship between GFAP expression and the levels of FLS in MG

GFAP, an acidic protein belonging to the family of intermediate silk proteins, is the cytoskeleton protein of specific astrocytes [20], which was first separated from the white matter plaque of multiple sclerosis patients [21].

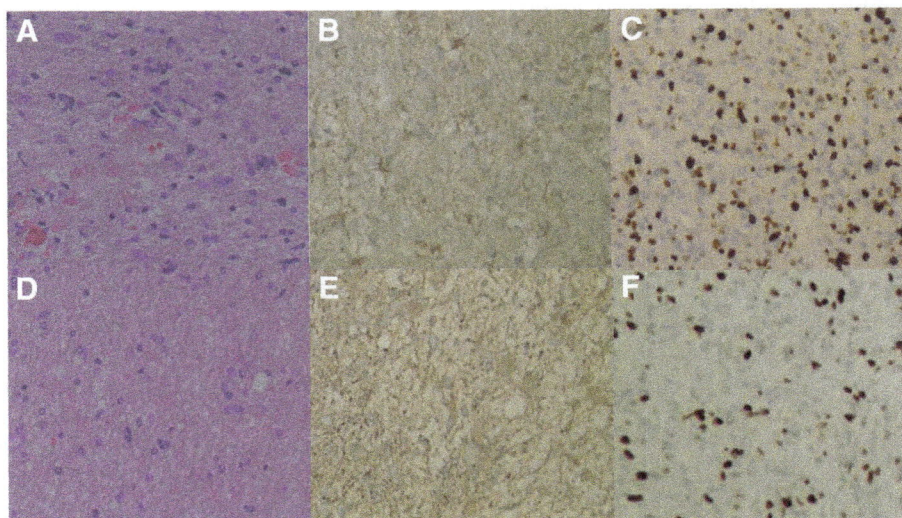

Fig. 4 Case16. **a–c** The biopsies obtained from Fig. 1b (a), stained by HE X200, GFAP X200, and Ki-67 X200, respectively. **d–f** Biopsies obtained from Fig. 1d (b), stained by HE X200, GFAP X200, and Ki-67 X200, respectively. **a** GBM cell nuclear split pleomorphism and was accompanied by a large number of vascular distributions. **b** Lighter color with GFAP staining, which was caused by lesser cytoplasm. **c** Ki-67 LI was 45%. **d** Brain tissue infiltration by tumor cells, nuclear atypia was uncommon as shown in **a**. **e** Deeper color with GFAP staining, which was caused by full cytoplasm. **f** Ki-67 LI was 25%

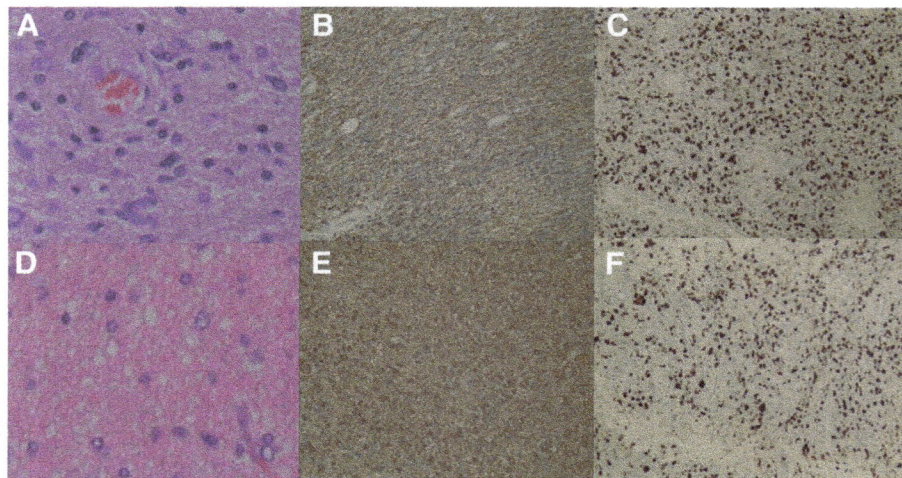

Fig. 5 Case 5. **a–c** Observed HE staining under × 400, GFAP staining under × 200, and Ki-67 staining under × 100 at the specimens obtained from Fig. 2d (white arrow). **d–f** Observed under × 400 of HE staining, under × 200 of GFAP staining, and under × 100 of Ki-67 staining at the specimens obtained from Fig. 2e (white arrow). From **a**, the nuclear split pleomorphism of GBM tumor are seen obviously and accompanied by vascular distribution. The GFAP staining in **b** showed lighter color than **e** caused by less cytoplasm in **b**. **c** Ki-67 LI 50%. **d** Figure contains tumor cells infiltration; abnormity was uncommon. **e** Glial cells were plump, and GFAP staining was darker. **f** Ki-67 LI was 30%

The function of nutritional support neurons plays an important role in shaping and maintaining normal morphology of glial cells [20, 22]. GFAP is normally expressed in astrocytes, ventricular membrane cells, and so on, and is considered as the iconic protein of astrocytes [23]. GFAP-positive expression could be found in astrocytoma, ventricular duct tumor, mixed glioma of the astrocytes line, giant cell astrocytoma, pleomorphic yellow astrocytoma, astrocytoma, glioma sarcoma, and so on [24]. As a reliable protein marker, it was widely used in the clinical immunohistochemical identification of glioma and non-gliomas [25]. In this group, 61 specimens of GFAP were positive. There was no correlation between the expression rate of GFAP and fluorescence levels (Fig. 4b, e and Fig. 5b, e). The result might be due to that (1) the normal glial cells also express GFAP, and our study observed that the same patient had different fluorescence level regions and obtained the different specimens when the color of fluorescence was darker (Fig. 1b (a) vs. Fig. 1d (b), and Fig. 2d white arrow vs. Fig. 2e white arrow) while the color of staining was lighter (Fig. 4b vs. Fig. 4e, and Fig. 5b vs. Fig. 5e). According to the literature, with the increase of the

malignant degree of astrocytoma, the production of GFAP decreased [26]. Immunohistochemistry showed that the GFAP-positive staining rate and staining color of MG were lighter than those of normal brain tissue. We had confirmed this discipline through only using semi-quantitative analysis. (2) Semi-quantitative analysis has a certain degree of bias. It may be more instructive to study the quantitative expression of GFAP in the future. (3) Due to multiple-sources of MG, the positive rate of molecular pathology expression also changed a lot.

Relationship between WHO grading and fluorescence level in MG

The higher the malignant degree of glioma, the worst will be the prognosis, and the higher will be the WHO grading. We supposed that glioma with different malignant degrees might have influence on the developing intensities of FLS. But in this group, there was no significant correlation between the WHO grading and fluorescence levels ($\chi2 = 3.531$, $p = 0.171$). The reason may be due to (1) after injection, FLS transmitted through the destruction of the blood-brain barrier and agglomerated in the extracellular matrix. Diaz and others reported that [27] FLS showed obvious development in gadolinium-enhanced preoperative MRI area. It indicated that the development of FLS was similar to the enhancement mechanism of gadolinium injection, which was related to the damage of blood-brain barrier. However, some studies, including our early observation combined with neuronavigation, found that there was still FLS [28] outside the gadolinium-sprayed amine-enhanced range. So, there are still many unsolved reasons in the

Table 3 Relationship between the expression of GFAP, WHO grades and fluorescence levels of MG

Ki-67 LI %	Fluorescence degree			Degree of freedom	χ^2	p
	None	Low	Bright			
< 20	7	3	2	4	14.678	0.005
20–40	9	8	9			
≧ 40	3	7	21			

distribution mechanism of FLS. (2) This small sample size was not enough to show the relationship between WHO grading and fluorescence levels. (3) WHO grading gradually developed to molecular pathology; many molecular pathology mechanisms are unclear, and different types of MG characteristics according to the molecular pathological diagnosis may be different.

Relationship between Ki-67 and fluorescence levels in MG

Ki-67, a nuclear antigen of proliferating cells, can be detected in the nuclear plasma and mitotic phase of the cell transferring to the chromosome surface. In MG, Ki-67 acts as a cell proliferation marker that was more specific than PCNA [22]. The percentage of Ki-67-positive expression can reflect the degree of malignancy [29]. Ki-67 was expressed in all levels of astrocytoma and showed high expression levels in the higher grades of tumors [30]. Kiss et al. [31] observed that low- and very low-density Ki-67 LI had longer survival rates. Torp et al. [32] also reported that Ki-67 LI was associated with malignancy of astrocytoma, with high levels of Ki-67 LI than with low levels of LI, exhibiting a worse prognosis. Bouvier et al. believed that greater than 5% of Ki-67 LI was considered as a risk factor for tumor progression and poor prognosis [32]. In this group, all the patients showed Ki-67 expression and was graded by Ki-67 proliferation index LI. Ki-67 LI was correlated with fluorescence levels, and the difference was statistically significant ($\chi2 = 14.678$, $p = 0.005$). This suggested that the removal of MG through FLS navigation can reduce the MG cells and reduce Ki-67 LI, improving the prognosis of patients (Fig. 4 and Fig. 5). Bouvier and other studies have also found that Ki-67 Li may not be an independent risk factor, but low levels of Ki-67 and total resection were achieved, and continuous postoperative chemotherapy patients had a better prognosis.

Although the expression of Ki-67 was still observed (Fig. 4f and Fig. 5f) in the near-positive boundary biopsy of FLS staining (Fig. 1d (b) and Fig. 2e white arrow), it had been significantly reduced after surgical resection ($\chi2 = 14.678$, $p = 0.005$). Furthermore, it has been found in our earlier study that there was still fluorescein dye outside the area of MRI enhancement according to preoperative MRI registered by neuronavigation [19]. Thus, the fluorescein-stained regions could be included and larger than the contrast-enhanced regions. More aggressive or super-total resection of MGs could be deemed to the reasonable treatment strategy for MGs [5]. For the development of FLS and to help in glioma resection, more clinical data should be studied and discussed.

Conclusion

FLS navigation was helpful in resecting the MG. In the boundary area, fluorescence levels and GFAP-positive rate, WHO classification level were not correlated. The development of FLS may be related to the destruction of blood-brain barrier, but the mechanism of distribution of FLS still needs further study and discussion. Fluorescence levels and Ki-67 proliferation index has correlation. It is suggested that fluorescein-sodium-guided resection of MG can achieve the function of "reducing tumor cell," which reduces the proliferation index in the lesion area. This subsequently provides better basis for postoperative radiotherapy and chemotherapy, and hope to reduce recurrence and improve prognosis.

Funding

This study was supported by the Research Foundation Project entitled "Correlation Studies between 4IgB7H3 Induce T Cell Incompetence and Glioma Cell Invasion and Migration" of Shandong University Qilu Hospital, Qingdao. The study was supported by the Science and Technology Program of People's Livelihood of the City of Qingdao (no. 17-3-3-36-nsh).

Authors' contributions

NZ and ZS conceived and coordinated the study; designed, performed, and analyzed the experiments; and wrote the manuscript. ZW, HT, DH, NZ, and XM performed the operations. XZ, ZL, XY, and BZ carried out the data collection, data analysis, and revised the manuscript. All authors reviewed the results and approved the final version of the manuscript.

Competing interests

The authors declare that they have no competing interests.

References

1. Ostrom QT, Gittleman H, Liao P, Rouse C, Chen Y, Dowling J, et al. CBTRUS statistical report: primary brain and central nervous system tumors diagnosed in the United States in 2007-2011. Neuro-Oncology. 2014; 16(Suppl 4):iv1-63.
2. Orringer D, Lau D, Khatri S, Zamora-Berridi GJ, Zhang K, Wu C, et al. Extent of resection in patients with glioblastoma: limiting factors, perception of resectability, and effect on survival. J Neurosurg. 2012;117:851-9.
3. Salvati M, Pichierri A, Piccirilli M, Floriana Brunetto GM, D'Elia A, Artizzu S, et al. Extent of tumor removal and molecular markers in cerebral glioblastoma: a combined prognostic factors study in a surgical series of 105 patients. J Neurosurg. 2012;117:204-11.
4. Stummer W, Pichlmeier U, Meinel T, Wiestler OD, Zanella F, Reulen HJ, et al. Fluorescence-guided surgery with 5-aminolevulinic acid for resection of malignant glioma: a randomised controlled multicentre phase III trial. Lancet Oncol. 2006;7:392-401.
5. Li YM, Suki D, Hess K, Sawaya R. The influence of maximum safe resection of glioblastoma on survival in 1229 patients: can we do better than gross-total resection? J Neurosurg. 2016;124:977-88.
6. Stendel R. Extent of resection and survival in glioblastoma multiforme: identification of and adjustment for bias. Neurosurgery. 2009;64:E1206 author reply E.
7. Schebesch KM, Proescholdt M, Hohne J, Hohenberger C, Hansen E, Riemenschneider MJ, et al. Sodium fluorescein-guided resection under the YELLOW 560 nm surgical microscope filter in malignant brain tumor surgery–a feasibility study. Acta Neurochir. 2013;155:693-9.
8. Acerbi F, Broggi M, Eoli M, Anghileri E, Cavallo C, Boffano C, et al. Is fluorescein-guided technique able to help in resection of high-grade gliomas? Neurosurg Focus. 2014;36:E5.
9. Wen PY, Macdonald DR, Reardon DA, Cloughesy TF, Sorensen AG, Galanis E, et al. Updated response assessment criteria for high-grade gliomas: response assessment in neuro-oncology working group. J Clin Oncol. 2010;28:1963-72.
10. Cordella R, Acerbi F, Broggi M, Vailati D, Nazzi V, Schiariti M, et al. Intraoperative neurophysiological monitoring of the cortico-spinal tract in image-guided mini-invasive neurosurgery. Clin Neurophysiol. 2013;124:1244-54.
11. Ferroli P, Acerbi F, Albanese E, Tringali G, Broggi M, Franzini A, et al. Application of intraoperative indocyanine green angiography for CNS tumors: results on the first 100 cases. Acta Neurochir Suppl. 2011;109:251-7.

12. Stummer W, Stocker S, Wagner S, Stepp H, Fritsch C, Goetz C, et al. Intraoperative detection of malignant gliomas by 5-aminolevulinic acid-induced porphyrin fluorescence. Neurosurgery. 1998;42:518–25 discussion 25–6.

13. Moore GE. Fluorescein as an agent in the differentiation of normal and malignant tissues. Science. 1947;106:130–1.

14. Moore GE, Peyton WT, et al. The clinical use of fluorescein in neurosurgery; the localization of brain tumors. J Neurosurg. 1948;5:392–8.

15. Shinoda J, Yano H, Yoshimura S, Okumura A, Kaku Y, Iwama T, et al. Fluorescence-guided resection of glioblastoma multiforme by using high-dose fluorescein sodium. Technical note J Neurosurg. 2003;99:597–603.

16. Chen B, Wang H, Ge P, Zhao J, Li W, Gu H, et al. Gross total resection of glioma with the intraoperative fluorescence-guidance of fluorescein sodium. Int J Med Sci. 2012;9:708–14.

17. Koc K, Anik I, Cabuk B, Ceylan S. Fluorescein sodium-guided surgery in glioblastoma multiforme: a prospective evaluation. Br J Neurosurg. 2008;22:99–103.

18. Kuroiwa T, Kajimoto Y, Ohta T. Development of a fluorescein operative microscope for use during malignant glioma surgery: a technical note and preliminary report. Surg Neurol. 1998;50:41–8 discussion 8-9.

19. Zhang N, Tian H, Huang D, Meng X, Guo W, Wang C, et al. Sodium fluorescein-guided resection under the YELLOW 560 nm surgical microscope filter in malignant gliomas: our first 38 cases experience. Biomed Res Int. 2017;2017:7865747.

20. de Armond SJ, Eng LF, Rubinstein LJ. The application of glial fibrillary acidic (GFA) protein immunohistochemistry in neurooncology. A progress report Pathol Res Pract. 1980;168:374–94.

21. Eng LF, Vanderhaeghen JJ, Bignami A, Gerstl B. An acidic protein isolated from fibrous astrocytes. Brain Res. 1971;28:351–4.

22. Raghavan R, Steart PV, Weller RO. Cell proliferation patterns in the diagnosis of astrocytomas, anaplastic astrocytomas and glioblastoma multiforme: a Ki-67 study. Neuropathol Appl Neurobiol. 1990;16:123–33.

23. Merzak A, Koocheckpour S, Pilkington GJ. CD44 mediates human glioma cell adhesion and invasion in vitro. Cancer Res. 1994;54:3988–92.

24. Baskan O, Silav G, Sari R, Canoz O, Elmaci I. Relationship of intraoperative ultrasound characteristics with pathological grades and Ki-67 proliferation index in intracranial gliomas. J Med Ultrason (2001). 2015;42:231–7.

25. Torp SH. Diagnostic and prognostic role of Ki67 immunostaining in human astrocytomas using four different antibodies. Clin Neuropathol. 2002;21:252–7.

26. Eng LF, Rubinstein LJ. Contribution of immunohistochemistry to diagnostic problems of human cerebral tumors. J Histochem Cytochem. 1978;26:513–22.

27. Kiss R, Dewitte O, Decaestecker C, Camby I, Gordower L, Delbecque K, et al. The combined determination of proliferative activity and cell density in the prognosis of adult patients with supratentorial high-grade astrocytic tumors. Am J Clin Pathol. 1997;107:321–31.

28. Bouvier-Labit C, Chinot O, Ochi C, Gambarelli D, Dufour H, Figarella-Branger D. Prognostic significance of Ki67, p53 and epidermal growth factor receptor immunostaining in human glioblastomas. Neuropathol Appl Neurobiol. 1998;24:381–8.

29. Diaz RJ, Dios RR, Hattab EM, Burrell K, Rakopoulos P, Sabha N, et al. Study of the biodistribution of fluorescein in glioma-infiltrated mouse brain and histopathological correlation of intraoperative findings in high-grade gliomas resected under fluorescein fluorescence guidance. J Neurosurg. 2015;122:1360–9.

30. Neira JA, Ung TH, Sims JS, Malone HR, Chow DS, Samanamud JL, et al. Aggressive resection at the infiltrative margins of glioblastoma facilitated by intraoperative fluorescein guidance. J Neurosurg. 2017;127:111–22.

31. Rodriguez-Pereira C, Suarez-Penaranda JM, Vazquez-Salvado M, Sobrido MJ, Abraldes M, Barros F, et al. Value of MIB-1 labelling index (LI) in gliomas and its correlation with other prognostic factors. A clinicopathologic study. J Neurosurg Sci. 2000;44:203–9 discussion 9-10.

32. Kayaselcuk F, Zorludemir S, Gumurduhu D, Zeren H, Erman T. PCNA and Ki-67 in central nervous system tumors: correlation with the histological type and grade. J Neuro-Oncol. 2002;57:115–21.

21

Ability of the ALBI grade to predict posthepatectomy liver failure and long-term survival after liver resection for different BCLC stages of HCC

Ze-Qun Zhang, Li Xiong, Jiang-Jiao Zhou, Xiong-Ying Miao, Qing-Long Li, Yu Wen* and Heng Zou*[iD]

Abstract

Background: Underlying liver function is a major concern when applying surgical resection for hepatocellular carcinoma (HCC). We aimed to explore the capability of the albumin-bilirubin (ALBI) grade to predict post-hepatectomy liver failure (PHLF) and long-term survival after hepatectomy for HCC patients with different Barcelona Clinic Liver Cancer (BCLC) stages.

Methods: Between January 2010 and December 2014, 338 HCC patients who were treated with liver resection were enrolled. The predictive accuracy of ALBI grade system for PHLF and long-term survival across different BCLC stages was examined.

Results: A total of 26 (7.7%) patients developed PHLF. Patients were divided into BCLC 0/A and BCLC B/C categories. ALBI score was found to be a strong independent predictor of PHLF across different BCLC stages by multivariate analysis. In terms of overall survival (OS), it exhibited high discriminative power in the total cohort and in BCLC 0/A subgroup. However, differences in OS between ALBI grade 1 and 2 patients in BCLC B/C subgroup were not significant ($P = 0.222$).

Conclusion: The ALBI grade showed good predictive ability for PHLF in HCC patients across different BCLC stages. However, the ALBI grade was only a significant predictor of OS in BCLC stage 0/A patients and failed to predict OS in BCLC stage B/C patients.

Keywords: Child-Pugh grade, Post-hepatectomy liver failure, Albumin-bilirubin score, Hepatocellular carcinoma, BCLC classification, Overall survival

Background

As one of the most common and aggressive malignancies, hepatocellular carcinoma (HCC) ranks the second most fatal cancer globally [1]. Although surgical resection is the mainstay therapy for extremely early and early stage HCC, it is not recommended for intermediate and advanced stage HCC as determined by Barcelona Clinic Liver Cancer (BCLC) classification because of the increased risks and limited advantages of the procedure [2]. Recently, due to advances in techniques and perioperative management, surgical resection for HCC has become more aggressive. HCC patients at BCLC B and C stages have been reported to have good prognosis after surgical resection [3–6].

Patients with BCLC B and C HCC often possess a high tumor burden, including an increased tumor size, multiple tumors, and vascular invasion. To achieve microscopically radical resection margins, patients tend to undergo extended liver resection, which increases the chances of post-hepatectomy liver failure (PHLF). This is especially obvious when patients have underlying long-term hepatic disorders, such as hepatic fibrosis and cirrhosis [7–9], which often result in impaired liver

---

* Correspondence: wenyu2861@csu.edu.cn; zhcsuxy@csu.edu.cn
Ze-Qun Zhang and Li Xiong are co-first authors.
Ze-Qun Zhang and Li Xiong contributed equally to this work.
Department of General Surgery, The Second Xiangya Hospital, Central South University, Changsha 410011, Hunan, China

function. As a life-threatening complication with an intrinsic risk of mortality, PHLF is still a major concern for hepatic surgeons in clinical practice. To minimize PHLF and postoperative mortality, development of a simple, objective, and accurate assessment tool for liver function prior to surgery is of vital importance. Recently, the application of albumin-bilirubin (ALBI) grade to evaluate liver function in patients with HCC was proposed [10–12]. The ALBI grade not only offers similar prognostic information as the Child-Pugh (CP) class but also eliminates the necessity of assessing empirical variables such as hepatic encephalopathy and ascites. Several studies have shown that the ALBI grade had a superior predictive value for PHLF and overall survival (OS) in HCC patients following liver resection [13, 14].

The survival of HCC patients undergoing liver resection depends mainly on tumor burden and hepatic function [15]. The ALBI grade was proven to be a reliable hepatic function assessment tool and could accurately predict survival in patients with extremely early or early stage HCC who underwent liver resection [12, 16–19]. However, few studies have examined the role of the ALBI grade in predicting the survival of patients with intermediate and advanced stage HCC after hepatectomy.

Here, we evaluated the effectiveness of the ALBI grade in predicting PHLF and OS across different BCLC stages among HCC patients undergoing liver resection.

Methods
Patients
In this retrospective study, HCC patients who underwent liver resection were enrolled from January 2010 to December 2014 at the Second Xiangya Hospital. The hospital medical database was searched to retrieve baseline parameters. Inclusion criteria included the following: liver function with CP A or B; no other simultaneous malignancies; no therapy for HCC before surgery; and no insufficiency concerning the heart, lung, kidney, and brain before operation. Written informed consent for this retrospective research was waived. This investigation was approved by the ethics committee of the hospital.

Diagnosis and definitions
HCC was diagnosed using histopathological examination of the surgical samples. The HCC stage accorded with the BCLC guidelines [20]. Based on the recommendations of the International Study Group of Liver Surgery (ISGLS), PHLF was defined as a total serum bilirubin value > 50 μmol l^{-1} on day 5 after surgery or hereafter and a prothrombin time index $< 50\%$ (an international normalized ratio (INR) > 1.7) in the meanwhile [21, 22]. Adjustment in clinical administration was not required for grade A PHLF; non-invasive interventions such as fresh-frozen plasma, albumin management, diuretics, and ventilation were applied for grade B PHLF; and invasive interventions such as circulatory and extracorporeal liver support, hemodialysis, intubation, and mechanical ventilation were used barely for grade C PHLF [21]. A relative low platelet count ($< 100 \times 10^9$/l) with splenomegaly and diagnosis of gastric/esophageal varices were used as indicators of clinically significant portal hypertension (CSPH) [23, 24]. Hepatectomy was defined as minor if fewer than three Couinaud segments were resected and major if three liver segments or more were resected. Deaths recorded within 60 days after surgery were considered to represent mortality.

Determination of the CP class was performed according to methods published previously [25]. The model of end-stage liver disease (MELD) score was computed applying the formula: $9.57 \times \ln(\text{creatinine [mg/dl]}) + 11.2 \times \ln(\text{INR}) + 3.78 \times \ln(\text{bilirubin [mg/dl]}) + 6.43$ [26]. The calculation of the ALBI score used this equation: ALBI score $= -0.085 \times (\text{albumin [g l}^{-1}]) + 0.66 \times \log_{10}(\text{total bilirubin [}\mu\text{mol l}^{-1}])$, and was further categorized into three different grades: grade 3 (> -1.39), grade 2 (> -2.60 to ≤ -1.39), and grade 1 (≤ -2.60) [10].

Surgical technique
Before surgery, contrast-enhanced computed tomography (CT) and abdominal ultrasound were routinely conducted to assess tumor condition. Preoperative indocyanine green tests were routinely performed for patients with hepatitis B or C infection. For laparotomy, right subcostal margin incision was chosen. Laparoscopic approach was implemented widely for tumor diameter < 5 cm located in segments 2–6. During operation, the fluid infusion was minimal to maintain a relatively low central venous pressure to reduce bleeding. To precisely determine the relationship between tumors and other tissues as well as assess the orientation of tumors, intraoperative ultrasound was conducted if needed. If resectability had been determined, anatomical resection was performed aiming to excise the tumor's portal territory when future remnant liver functional reserve was sufficient.

Follow-up evaluation
The trace of each patient was done at 1 month following discharge from hospital and at intervals of 3 months during the first year, and at 6-month intervals in following years. Follow-up included liver function tests, determination of α-fetoprotein (AFP) concentration, and abdominal-enhanced CT. The primary endpoints for this study were PHLF and death. OS was from date of resection to last living visit or loss to follow-up. The last visit was done on December 31, 2017.

Statistical analysis

Continuous data were analyzed by t test or Mann-Whitney U test. χ^2 test was used to compare categorical data. Identification of independent predictors of PHLF was achieved by multivariate logistic regression analysis. Receiver operating characteristic (ROC) curve analysis was carried out to determine the cut-off points for the occurrence of PHLF. The area under the ROC curve (AUC) was applied to assess discriminative power. Comparisons between ROC curves were conducted with Delong test. OS was assessed visually through Kaplan-Meier plots, and differences between curves were analyzed by log-rank test. Independent risk factors for OS were identified using multivariate Cox proportional hazard regression models. Statistical significance was considered for a two-tailed value of $P < 0.05$. SPSS 17.0 (Inc., Chicago, IL, USA) was applied for data analysis.

Results

Patient information

A sample of 338 HCC patients was included. Most patients had a CP class of A (308/338, 91.1%), and the remaining 30 were class B (30/308, 8.9%). For ALBI grade 1, there were 39.6% (134/338) patients while grade 2 had 58.6% patients (198/338) and grade 3 had 1.8% (6/338) patients. Table 1 shows the features of the patients.

Postoperative morbidity, PHLF, and mortality

Of the 338 patients, 142 (42.0%) developed complications after surgery. Pneumonia which had the highest frequency occurred in 39 patients (11.5%), followed by plural effusion and ascites in 37 (10.9%). PHLF occurred in 26 patients (7.7%), among them, 8 patients (2.4%) had grade A PHLF, 13 patients (3.8%) had grade B, and 5 patients (1.5%) had grade C. During 60 days after operation, 15 patients died, resulting in a postoperative mortality rate of 4.4%.

Correlation between PHLF and CP class or ALBI grade

PHLF occurred in 16 of the 308 (5.2%) CP class A patients and in 10 of the 30 (33.3%) CP class B patients ($P < 0.001$). Among the total cohort, 3 of 134 (2.2%) ALBI grade 1 patients had PHLF, while 19 of 198 (9.6%) ALBI grade 2 patients fell into PHLF ($P = 0.008$). Four of 6 (66.7%) ALBI grade 3 patients developed PHLF. Higher ALBI grade led to higher risk of grade C PHLF (Fig. 1a). The incidence of grade C PHLF was higher in patients with ALBI grade 3 compared to those with ALBI grade 2 ($P = 0.003$) or ALBI grade 1 ($P = 0.001$). Moreover, patients with BCLC B/C HCC were more likely to suffer from grade C PHLF than those with BCLC 0/A HCC ($P = 0.027$, Fig. 1b).

Multivariate analyses of PHLF across the BCLC stages of HCC

The entire cohort was categorized into two subgroups in the multivariate logistic regression analysis. For the total cohort, ALBI score, CP score, and major hepatectomy were identified significant. In the BCLC 0/A subgroup, ALBI score, CP score, and major hepatectomy were identified significant. In the BCLC B/C subgroup, platelet count, ALBI score, and CP score were identified significant (Table 2).

Discriminative power of ALBI score to predict PHLF across the BCLC stages of HCC

Figure 2a shows the predictive power of -ALBI scores for PHLF as determined by the ROC curve analyses which were the total cohort (AUC, 0.782; 95% CI, 0.701–0.862, $P < 0.001$), BCLC 0/A subgroup (AUC, 0.780; 95% CI, 0.670–0.889; $P < 0.001$), and BCLC B/C subgroup (AUC, 0.790; 95% CI, 0.680–0.900; $P = 0.002$). For the total cohort, the -ALBI score had a greater AUC than CP score (AUC, 0.656; 95% CI, 0.527–0.784; $P = 0.008$) ($P = 0.005$, Delong test) and MELD score (AUC, 0.669; 95% CI, 0.566–0.771; $P = 0.004$) ($P = 0.013$, Delong test) (Fig. 2b). The -ALBI score had an optimal cut-off value of 2.44 (that was to say, the cut-off point of ALBI score lay in – 2.44, the same below), presenting a specificity and a sensitivity of 56.1% and 88.5% respectively.

We divided the entire cohort into two subgroups, BCLC 0/A and BCLC B/C, to minimize the potential confounding bias caused by tumor characteristics. The cut-off value of the former group was 2.41, with a specificity and a sensitivity of 60.3% and 81.3% respectively, while the cut-off value of the latter group was 2.36, with a sensitivity of 90.0% and a specificity of 60.2%. In the BCLC 0/A group, the AUC of -ALBI score was greater than MELD and CP scores (Fig. 2c). Same result could be obtained in BCLC B/C subgroup (Fig. 2d).

Discriminative power of the ALBI grade for OS at different BCLC stages of HCC

A total of 183 HCC deaths (54.1%) occurred throughout the follow-up (with a median of 31.5 months). The OS rate in the total cohort at 1, 2, and 3 years were 78.1%, 55.3%, and 49.4%, in that order. The OS rate in patients with ALBI grade 1 at 1, 2, and 3 years were 83.6%, 68.7%, and 61.2%, respectively, which were higher compared to patients with ALBI grade 2 (74.7%, 47.0%, and 41.9%, respectively) ($P = 0.003$) (Fig. 3a). We did not analyze the OS of the ALBI grade 3 cohort because there were few patients (6 patients) in this group. Four of these patients died within 2 years after the operation. In the BCLC 0/A subgroup, the OS rate of ALBI grade 2 patients was lower compared to that of ALBI grade 1 patients ($P = 0.008$)

Table 1 Baseline characteristics of 338 HCC patients

Variables	Total cohort (n = 338)	BCLC 0/A HCC (n = 205)	BCLC B/C HCC (n = 133)
Age, years[†]	52 (44–66)	52 (44–60)	52 (43–60)
Male gender[‡]	299 (88.5)	180 (87.5)	119 (89.5)
Positive HBsAg[‡]	278 (82.2)	170 (82.9)	108 (81.2)
Total bilirubin, μmol/l[†]	14.0 (13.4–19.4)	13.9 (10.0–19.6)	14.4 (10.6–18.7)
Albumin, g/l[†]	37.9 (35.1–40.8)	38.0 (35.4–41.0)	37.6 (34.0–40.7)
ALT, U/l[†]	36.1 (25.8–52.0)	34.3 (24.7–53.0)	37.9 (26.4–51.0)
Prothrombin time, s[†]	13.2 (12.0–14.1)	13.2 (12.0–14.1)	13.2 (12.1–14.1)
INR[†]	1.04 (0.95–1.14)	1.04 (0.94–1.14)	1.05 (0.95–1.14)
Platelet count, × 10^9/l[†]	155 (110–205)	155 (110–211)	154 (113.5–201.5)
Maximum tumor size, cm[†]	6.0 (4.2–10.0)	6.0 (3.5–9.2)	8 (5.0–11.0)
Serum AFP, ng/ml[‡]			
≥ 400	141 (41.7)	73 (35.6)	68 (51.1)
< 400	197 (58.3)	132 (64.4)	65 (48.9)
CSPH[‡]	56 (16.6)	34 (16.6)	22 (16.5)
ALBI score[†]	− 2.460 (− 2.704− − 2.192)	− 2.518 (− 2.719− − 2.236)	− 2.399 (− 2.702− − 2.136)
ALBI grade[‡]			
1	134 (39.6)	89 (43.4)	45 (33.8)
2	198 (58.6)	114 (55.6)	84 (63.2)
3	6 (1.8)	2 (1.0)	4 (3.0)
MELD score (range)	7 (6–18)	7 (6–18)	7 (6–17)
MELD score[‡]			
≥ 9	88 (26.0)	47 (22.9)	41 (30.8)
< 9	250 (74.0)	158 (77.1)	92 (69.2)
Child-Pugh grade[‡]			
A	308 (91.1)	190 (92.7)	118 (88.7)
B	30 (8.9)	15 (7.3)	15 (11.3)
C	0 (0)	0 (0)	0 (0)
BCLC stage[‡]			
0	12 (3.6)	–	–
A	193 (57.1)	–	–
B	82 (24.3)	–	–
C	51 (15.1)	–	–

HCC hepatocellular carcinoma, *HBsAg* hepatitis B surface antigen, *ALT* alanine aminotransferase, *INR* international normalized ratio, *AFP* α-fetoprotein, *CSPH* clinically significant portal pressure, *ALBI* albumin-bilirubin, *BCLC* Barcelona Clinic Liver Cancer
†Values are median (interquartile range)
‡Values are number (%)

(Fig. 3c). However, in BCLC B/C subgroup, OS did not differ between ALBI grade 2 patients and ALBI grade 1 patients ($P = 0.222$) (Fig. 3e). The OS exhibited little difference between patients with CP class A and those with CP class B in the total cohort ($P = 0.052$) (Fig. 3b), BCLC 0/A subgroup ($P = 0.052$) (Fig. 3d) and BCLC B/C subgroup ($P = 0.911$) (Fig. 3f). Moreover, comparison of OS between MELD scores < 9 and ≥ 9 also showed no statistical difference ($P = 0.784$) (Additional file 1: Figure S1).

Multivariate cox regression analyses of OS across BCLC stages

Multivariate analyses revealed that the ALBI score, platelet count, tumor size, microvascular invasion (MVI), and differentiation grade were significant risk factors for OS in the total cohort. We further performed multivariate analysis in the two subgroups (Table 3). In the BCLC 0/A subgroup, we observed similar results as in the total cohort (Table 3). Interestingly, the ALBI score was not a

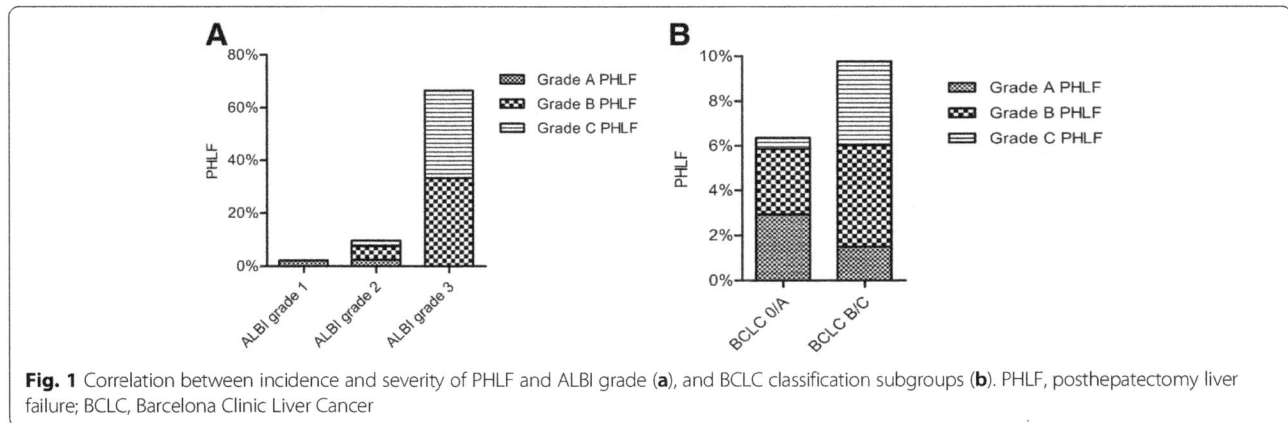

Fig. 1 Correlation between incidence and severity of PHLF and ALBI grade (**a**), and BCLC classification subgroups (**b**). PHLF, posthepatectomy liver failure; BCLC, Barcelona Clinic Liver Cancer

significant predictor, only MVI and differentiation grade remained independent predictors of OS in the BCLC B/C subgroup (Table 3).

Discussion

Surgical resection is extensively performed for HCC patients with a favorable liver functional reserve. However, PHLF remains a serious complication of hepatic resection and a main cause of postoperative mortality [7, 27]. To improve the survival of patients with PHLF, early diagnosis and therapy are imperative. Many previous reports have provided evidence that the ALBI grade is an effective predictor of PHLF after liver resection in patients with HCC [13, 14]. However, few studies have focused on the role of the ALBI score in predicting PHLF for patients with intermediate and advanced HCC. We found that the ALBI score could predict PHLF not only in the total cohort but also in the BCLC 0/A and BCLC B/C subgroups. BCLC B/C patients have a relatively higher tumor burden and often possess a larger tumor size, satellite nodes, or portal/hepatic vein tumor thrombosis. To achieve a radical cure, patients are inclined to

undergo extensive or major hepatectomy in clinical practice, which increases the probability of occurrence of PHLF, especially for patients suffering from chronic hepatic disorders. For these reasons, accurate assessment of hepatic function prior to surgery is of great clinical significance for these patients.

To determine whether ALBI score can predict PHLF accurately, we used a stage-stratified approach. Patients with BCLC B/C HCC owned a greater possibility of occurring severer PHLF than those with BCLC 0/A HCC. Several facts may contribute to this result. On the one hand, generally, BCLC B/C HCC own a heavier tumor burden, it is easy to make extensive hepatectomy to achieve radical resection. On the other hand, BCLC B/C HCC have a longer time of tumor progression, so the liver function of these patients might be worse than that of BCLC 0/A patients. ROC curve analyses demonstrated that the AUC values of MELD and CP scores were lower compared to that of the -ALBI score in predicting PHLF in the total cohort and the BCLC stage subgroups, implying that the ALBI score might have better prognostic value for PHLF among

Table 2 Multivariate logistic regression analyses for posthepatectomy liver failure across BCLC stages

Variable	Multivariate logistic regression					
	Total cohort		BCLC 0/A		BCLC B/C	
	OR (95% CI)	P	OR (95% CI)	P	OR (95% CI)	P
Prothrombin time > 14 s	1.19 (0.39–3.63)	0.765	1.39 (0.35–5.47)	0.635	0.48 (0.04–6.60)	0.584
Platelet count < 100 × 10⁹/l	2.82 (0.97–8.19)	0.056	0.45 (0.07–2.94)	0.405	132.70 (6.04–916.91)	0.002
Tumor size > 5 cm	0.65 (0.21–2.01)	0.456	0.50 (0.11–2.23)	0.361	0.49 (0.04–6.52)	0.587
ALBI score > −2.44	3.43 (1.11–10.57)	0.032	2.33 (1.09–9.19)	0.046	30.48 (1.36–682.73)	0.031
Child-Pugh score > 6	6.47 (2.10–19.94)	0.001	5.50 (1.23–24.50)	0.025	43.21 (2.43–767.29)	0.010
Blood loss > 400 ml	2.13 (0.83–5.44)	0.115	1.75 (0.55–5.57)	0.346	5.86 (0.53–64.72)	0.149
Major hepatectomy	5.51 (1.86–16.29)	0.002	7.23 (1.73–30.57)	0.007	12.02 (0.97–149.04)	0.053
MELD score > 8	0.67 (0.21–2.11)	0.496	0.90 (0.21–3.78)	0.885	0.35 (0.03–3.62)	0.378

OR odds ratio, *CI* confidence interval, *BCLC* Barcelona Clinic Liver Cancer, *ALBI* albumin-bilirubin, *MELD* model for end-stage liver disease

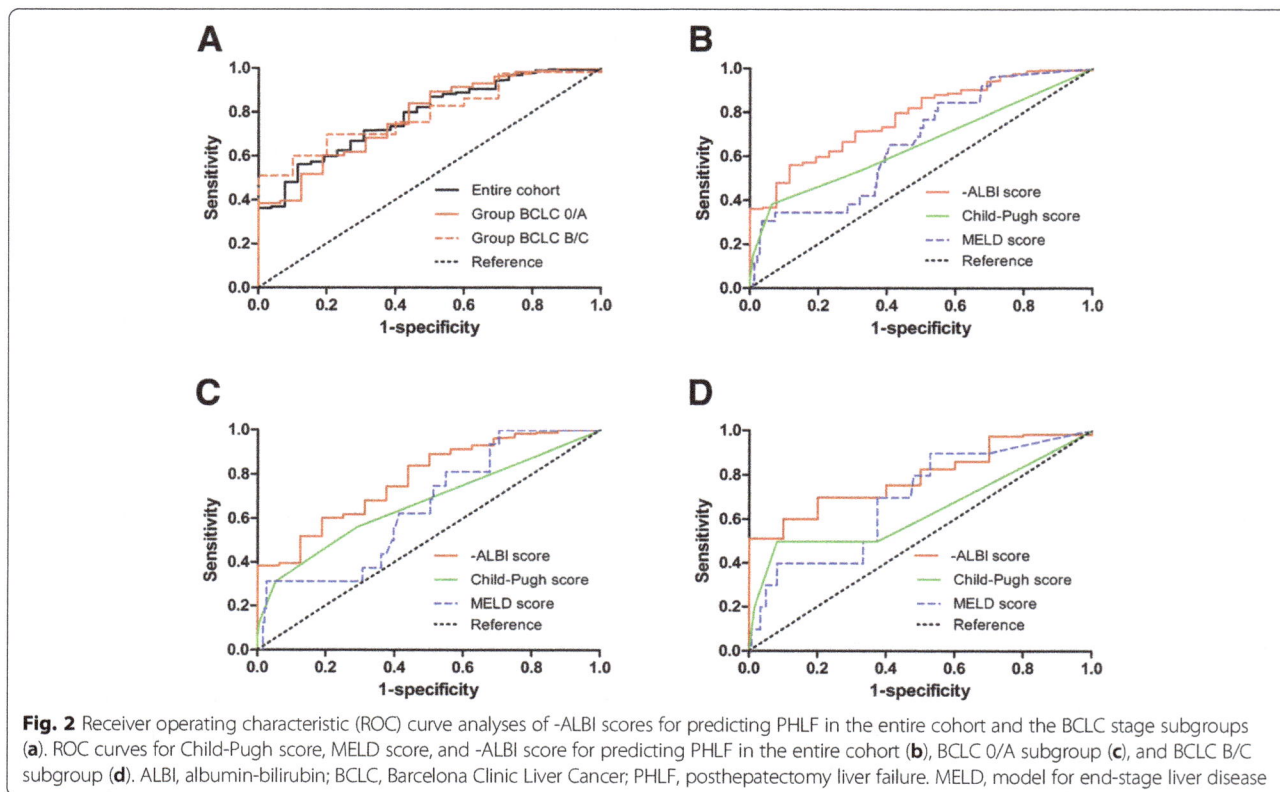

Fig. 2 Receiver operating characteristic (ROC) curve analyses of -ALBI scores for predicting PHLF in the entire cohort and the BCLC stage subgroups (**a**). ROC curves for Child-Pugh score, MELD score, and -ALBI score for predicting PHLF in the entire cohort (**b**), BCLC 0/A subgroup (**c**), and BCLC B/C subgroup (**d**). ALBI, albumin-bilirubin; BCLC, Barcelona Clinic Liver Cancer; PHLF, posthepatectomy liver failure. MELD, model for end-stage liver disease

patients undergoing liver resection. This was consistent with previous reports [13, 14].

In addition, our results revealed that the -ALBI grade had an AUC of 0.790 for predicting PHLF in BCLC B/C patients, which indicates a relatively good prognostic value. The ROC curve showed that optimal cut-off value of -ALBI calculated by the ROC curve was 2.36 in BCLC B/C HCC subgroup. This suggested that for patients with an ALBI score > − 2.36 in BCLC B/C stage, increased attention should be given by hepatic surgeons to avoid PHLF. Additionally, the ALBI score showed a favorable prognostic value for PHLF in the total cohort and in the BCLC 0/A subgroup, which is consistent with the earlier studies [16, 17]. This study indicated that the ALBI score might be helpful in choosing eligible candidates who may benefit from surgery, especially among BCLC B/C patients with a small-sized liver after resection. Moreover, we found MELD score showed no significance in the multivariate analysis for PHLF in this research. On the one hand, this might be on account of the small sample size from a single center. On the other hand, MELD score maybe suffers some limitations itself. For example, several other studies reported that MELD score showed no predictive power for perioperative outcomes in HCC patients without cirrhosis [28–30]. And interestingly, we found that the platelet count was an

effective predictor of PHLF only in BCLC B/C patients, but not in BCLC 0/A patients. The platelet count is commonly thought to be correlated with the severity of portal hypertension [31]. Therefore, portal hypertension might play a more important role in predicting PHLF for BCLC B/C patients than in those with early stage HCC, but further study is required to verify this conclusion.

The survival of HCC patients was partly impacted by the underlying liver function. Consistent with the previous studies [16–18], we found that the ALBI score was a significant risk factor for OS in both the total cohort and the BCLC 0/A subgroup. Moreover, the OS rate was higher in ALBI grade 1 patients compared to that in ALBI grade 2 patients both in the total cohort and in the BCLC 0/A subgroup. However, OS showed little difference among CP classes in the total cohort and the two subgroups. These results suggested that the ALBI grade might have a greater discriminative ability than the CP class for predicting the OS of HCC patients after liver resection in a curative setting.

Furthermore, the prognostic value of ALBI scores was evaluated for BCLC B/C patients. According to the BCLC staging system in most Western countries, hepatectomy is not recommended for this unique group of patients [20]. However, recent studies have demonstrated that intermediate and advanced HCCs were not

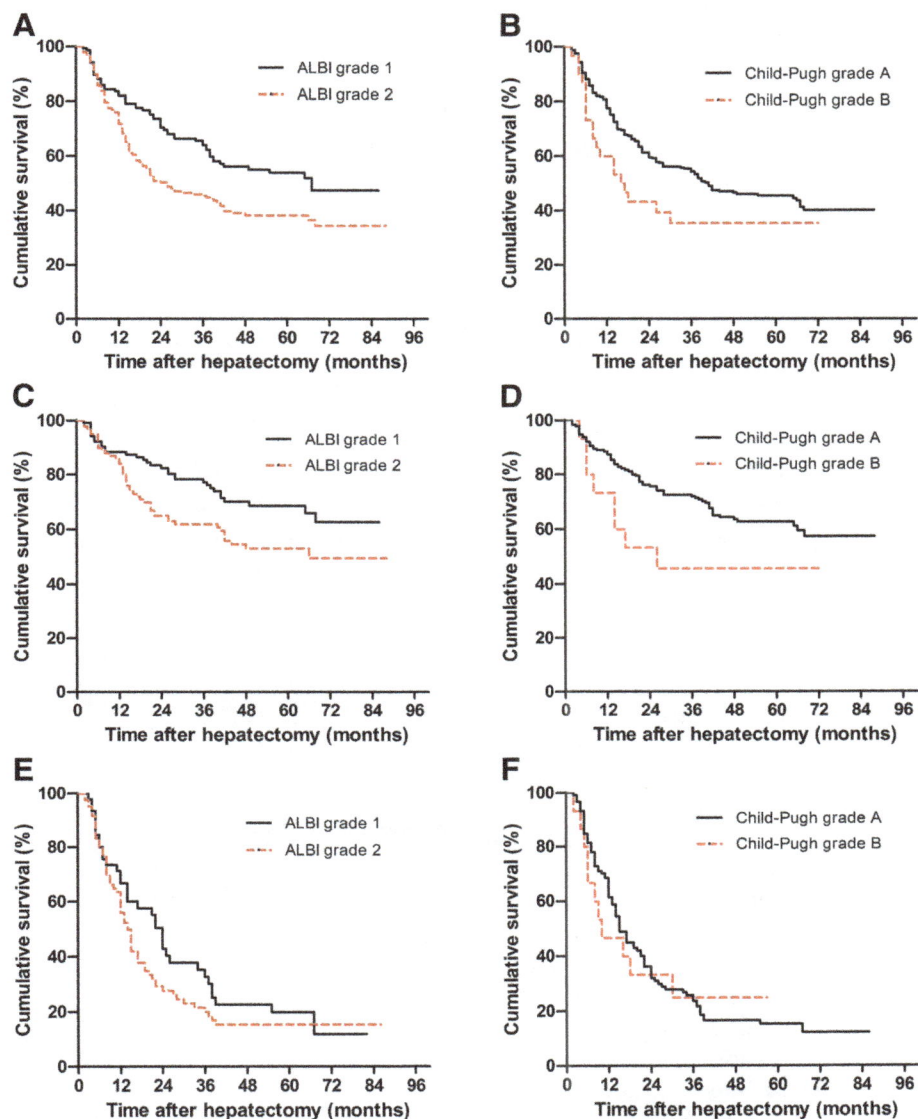

Fig. 3 Kaplan-Meier curves demonstrating overall survival according to the **a** ALBI grade in the total cohort, **b** Child-Pugh class in the total cohort, **c** ALBI grade in the BCLC 0/A subgroup, **d** Child-Pugh class in the BCLC 0/A subgroup, **e** ALBI grade in the BCLC B/C subgroup, and **f** Child-Pugh class in the BCLC B/C subgroup. ALBI, albumin-bilirubin; BCLC, Barcelona Clinic Liver Cancer

absolute contradictions for surgical resection, which could provide significant survival benefits for carefully selected patients [6]. Importantly, we found that OS showed little difference between ALBI grade 2 and ALBI grade 1 patients in this cohort ($P = 0.222$). Moreover, multivariate Cox regression model revealed that the ALBI score showed no predictive ability in the BCLC B/C subgroup ($P = 0.122$).

Prognoses of HCC patients are largely dependent on the tumor characteristics at the time when they undergo surgery. We found differentiation grade and MVI were significant predictors in the Cox regression model.

Compared to patients with early stage HCC, patients with BCLC B/C HCC generally have heavier tumor burdens, as indicated by large tumor sizes, poor differentiation, and vascular invasion [32]. Vascular invasion is an independent risk factor of recurrence and OS, directly correlated with the size of the main nodule and histological differentiation [33, 34]. Differentiation grade indicates a greater likelihood of malignant behavior, resulting in a higher risk of recurrence and metastasis, significantly affect OS. Interestingly, AFP level showed no significance in predicting OS in our study, despite this marker has been reported to predict reaction to locoregional treatments and

Table 3 Multivariate analyses of factors affecting overall survival across BCLC stage

| Variable | Multivariable Cox regression | | | | | |
| | Total cohort | | BCLC 0/A | | BCLC B/C | |
	HR (95% CI)	P	HR (95% CI)	P	HR (95% CI)	P
Age, years	1.03 (0.72–1.48)	0.868	1.08 (0.61–1.93)	0.791	0.79 (0.49–1.29)	0.343
Male gender	0.86 (0.53–1.40)	0.541	1.10 (0.51–2.37)	0.803	0.85 (0.44–1.65)	0.626
Platelet count, ×10⁹/l	1.62 (1.10–2.38)	0.014	1.90 (1.02–3.53)	0.043	1.26 (0.75–2.11)	0.383
Prothrombin time, sec	1.00 (0.89–1.12)	0.938	0.92 (0.76–1.11)	0.362	1.07 (0.92–1.25)	0.379
Serum AFP, ng/ml	1.09 (0.80–1.49)	0.594	1.22 (0.72–2.05)	0.457	0.92 (0.61–1.39)	0.677
Tumor size, cm	1.71 (1.21–2.44)	0.003	1.95 (1.15–3.32)	0.014	1.58 (0.95–2.64)	0.079
ALBI score	1.62 (1.18–2.22)	0.003	2.29 (1.39–3.78)	0.001	1.42 (0.91–2.20)	0.122
Major hepatectomy	1.33 (0.93–1.88)	0.115	1.02 (0.53–1.95)	0.965	1.33 (0.86–2.08)	0.201
MVI	2.10 (1.49–2.97)	< 0.001	1.91 (1.13–3.01)	0.028	1.53 (0.89–2.83)	0.046
Differentiation grade	1.69 (1.24–2.30)	0.001	1.77 (1.08–2.89)	0.024	2.03 (1.28–3.23)	0.003
MELD score	0.98 (0.90–1.08)	0.727	0.98 (0.84–1.15)	0.803	1.00 (0.88–1.14)	0.989

HR hazard ratio, *CI* confidence interval, *BCLC* Barcelona Clinic Liver Cancer, *AFP* α-fetoprotein, *ALBI* albumin-bilirubin, *MVI* microvascular invasion, *MELD* model for end-stage liver disease

outcome of untreated advanced HCC [35, 36]. To summarize, tumor burden is likely to play a more significant role in determining survival time than the underlying liver function in this group of patients. Thus, the ALBI grade alone may not be sufficient to predict OS in BCLC B/C stage HCC patients who undergo liver resection. A possible solution may be integrating the ALBI grade and tumor characteristics to generate a more accurate model to predict OS for this population, which should be performed in the future.

Several limitations exist in the present research. First, most of the patients had an infection of hepatitis B virus as the cause of HCC in the current research. Our results may not be applicable to Western countries, where hepatitis C virus infection and alcoholic steatohepatitis are the predominant etiologies of HCC. Second, the reliability of the present research was weakened by its retrospective specialty, single-center data, and comparably small sample capacity. Third, limited by the relatively small sample size, we did not include some variables which might have an effect on PHLF in order to increase the stability of statistical models and the credibility of results. A prospective study design with a large sample and effective controls is needed to expand our findings.

Conclusions

In summary, our study has verified that the ALBI grade is a significant prognostic factor for PHLF in HCC patients across different BCLC stages. However, for the first time, we found the ALBI grade was only a significant predictor of OS in BCLC stage 0/A patients and was not a good predictor in BCLC stage B/C patients.

Abbreviations
AFP: α-fetoprotein; ALBI: Albumin-bilirubin; BCLC: Barcelona Clinical Liver Cancer; CP: Child-Pugh; CSPH: Clinically significant portal pressure; HCC: Hepatocellular carcinoma; INR: International normalized ratio; MELD: Model of end-stage liver disease; OS: Overall survival; PHLF: Post-hepatectomy liver failure

Authors' contributions
The manuscript was drafted by ZZQ and revised by XL, ZH, and ZZQ. ZH and WY designed the clinical study. ZZQ and ZH conducted the data analysis and produced the figures and tables. ZJJ, LQL, and MXY conceived the conception and assisted its design. All authors read and approved the final manuscript.

Competing interests
The authors declare that they have no competing interests.

References
1. Torre LA, Bray F, Siegel RL, Ferlay J, Lortet-Tieulent J, Jemal A. Global cancer statistics, 2012. CA Cancer J Clin. 2015;65:87–108.
2. de Lope CR, Tremosini S, Forner A, Reig M, Bruix J. Management of HCC. J Hepatol. 2012;56(Suppl 1):S75–87.
3. Yin L, Li H, Li AJ, et al. Partial hepatectomy vs. transcatheter arterial chemoembolization for resectable multiple hepatocellular carcinoma beyond Milan criteria: a RCT. J Hepatol. 2014;61:82–8.
4. Kokudo T, Hasegawa K, Matsuyama Y, et al. Survival benefit of liver resection for hepatocellular carcinoma associated with portal vein invasion. J Hepatol. 2016;65:938–43.
5. Kokudo T, Hasegawa K, Matsuyama Y, et al. Liver resection for hepatocellular carcinoma associated with hepatic vein invasion: a Japanese nationwide survey. Hepatology. 2017;66:510–7.
6. Ho MC, Hasegawa K, Chen XP, et al. Surgery for intermediate and advanced hepatocellular carcinoma: a consensus report from the 5th Asia-Pacific primary liver cancer expert meeting (APPLE 2014). Liver Cancer. 2016;5:245–56.
7. Farges O, Malassagne B, Flejou JF, Balzan S, Sauvanet A, Belghiti J. Risk of major liver resection in patients with underlying chronic liver disease: a reappraisal. Ann Surg. 1999;229:210–5.

8. Belghiti J, Hiramatsu K, Benoist S, Massault P, Sauvanet A, Farges O. Seven hundred forty-seven hepatectomies in the 1990s: an update to evaluate the actual risk of liver resection. J Am Coll Surg. 2000;191:38–46.

9. Yamanaka N, Okamoto E, Kuwata K, Tanaka N. A multiple regression equation for prediction of posthepatectomy liver failure. Ann Surg. 1984; 200:658–63.

10. Johnson PJ, Berhane S, Kagebayashi C, et al. Assessment of liver function in patients with hepatocellular carcinoma: a new evidence-based approach-the ALBI grade. J Clin Oncol. 2015;33:550–8.

11. Hiraoka A, Michitaka K, Kumada T, et al. Validation and potential of albumin-bilirubin grade and prognostication in a nationwide survey of 46,681 hepatocellular carcinoma patients in Japan: the need for a more detailed evaluation of hepatic function. Liver Cancer. 2017;6:325–36.

12. Li MX, Zhao H, Bi XY, et al. Prognostic value of the albumin-bilirubin grade in patients with hepatocellular carcinoma: validation in a Chinese cohort. Hepatol Res. 2017;47:731–41.

13. Wang YY, Zhong JH, Su ZY, et al. Albumin-bilirubin versus child-Pugh score as a predictor of outcome after liver resection for hepatocellular carcinoma. Br J Surg. 2016;103:725–34.

14. Zou H, Wen Y, Yuan K, Miao XY, Xiong L, Liu KJ. Combining albumin-bilirubin score with future liver remnant predicts post-hepatectomy liver failure in HBV-associated HCC patients. Liver Int. 2018;38:494–502.

15. Liu PH, Hsu CY, Hsia CY, et al. Prognosis of hepatocellular carcinoma: assessment of eleven staging systems. J Hepatol. 2016;64:601–8.

16. Pinato DJ, Sharma R, Allara E, et al. The ALBI grade provides objective hepatic reserve estimation across each BCLC stage of hepatocellular carcinoma. J Hepatol. 2017;66:338–46.

17. Toyoda H, Lai PB, O'Beirne J, et al. Long-term impact of liver function on curative therapy for hepatocellular carcinoma: application of the ALBI grade. Br J Cancer. 2016;114:744–50.

18. Chong CC, Chan AW, Wong J, et al. Albumin-bilirubin grade predicts the outcomes of liver resection versus radiofrequency ablation for very early/early stage of hepatocellular carcinoma. Surgeon. 2018;16:163–70.

19. Dong ZR. Zou J, Sun D, et al. Preoperative albumin-bilirubin score for postoperative solitary hepatocellular carcinoma within the Milan criteria and child-Pugh a cirrhosis. J Cancer. 2017;8:3862–7.

20. Bruix J, Sherman M. Management of hepatocellular carcinoma: an update. Hepatology. 2011;53:1020–2.

21. Rahbari NN, Garden OJ, Padbury R, et al. Posthepatectomy liver failure: a definition and grading by the International Study Group of Liver Surgery (ISGLS). Surgery. 2011;149:713–24.

22. Balzan S, Belghiti J, Farges O, et al. The "50-50 criteria" on postoperative day 5: an accurate predictor of liver failure and death after hepatectomy. Ann Surg. 2005;242:824–8 discussion 28–9.

23. Forner A, Llovet JM, Bruix J. Hepatocellular carcinoma. Lancet. 2012;379: 1245–55.

24. Chen X, Zhai J, Cai X, et al. Severity of portal hypertension and prediction of postoperative liver failure after liver resection in patients with Child-Pugh grade a cirrhosis. Br J Surg. 2012;99:1701–10.

25. Pugh RN, Murray-Lyon IM, Dawson JL, Pietroni MC, Williams R. Transection of the oesophagus for bleeding oesophageal varices. Br J Surg. 1973;60: 646–9.

26. Butt AA, Ren Y, Lo Re V 3rd, Taddei TH, Kaplan DE. Comparing child-Pugh, MELD, and FIB-4 to predict clinical outcomes in hepatitis C virus-infected persons: results from ERCHIVES. Clin Infect Dis. 2017;65:64–72.

27. Schroeder RA, Marroquin CE, Bute BP, Khuri S, Henderson WG, Kuo PC. Predictive indices of morbidity and mortality after liver resection. Ann Surg. 2006;243:373–9.

28. Teh SH, Sheppard BC, Schwartz J, Orloff SL. Model for end-stage liver disease score fails to predict perioperative outcome after hepatic resection for hepatocellular carcinoma in patients without cirrhosis. Am J Surg. 2008; 195:697–701.

29. Stockmann M, Lock JF, Riecke B, et al. Prediction of postoperative outcome after hepatectomy with a new bedside test for maximal liver function capacity. Ann Surg. 2009;250:119–25.

30. Lin XJ, Yang J, Chen XB, Zhang M, Xu MQ. The critical value of remnant liver volume-to-body weight ratio to estimate posthepatectomy liver failure in cirrhotic patients. J Surg Res. 2014;188:489–95.

31. Augustin S, Millan L, Gonzalez A, et al. Detection of early portal hypertension with routine data and liver stiffness in patients with asymptomatic liver disease: a prospective study. J Hepatol. 2014;60:561–9.

32. Sasaki K, Morioka D, Conci S, et al. The tumor burden score: a new "metro-ticket" prognostic tool for colorectal liver metastases based on tumor size and number of tumors. Ann Surg. 2018;267:132–41.

33. Roayaie S, Blume IN, Thung SN, et al. A system of classifying microvascular invasion to predict outcome after resection in patients with hepatocellular carcinoma. Gastroenterology. 2009;137:850–5.

34. Sumie S, Kuromatsu R, Okuda K, et al. Microvascular invasion in patients with hepatocellular carcinoma and its predictable clinicopathological factors. Ann Surg Oncol. 2008;15:1375–82.

35. Llovet JMPC, Shan M, Lathia C, Bruix J. Biomarkers predicting outcome of patients with advanced hepatocellular carcinoma (HCC) randomized in the phase III SHARP trial. Presidential plenary session, AASLD 59th annual meeting, San Francisco. Hepatology. 2008;48:372A.

36. Llovet JM, Bruix J. Systematic review of randomized trials for unresectable hepatocellular carcinoma: chemoembolization improves survival. Hepatology. 2003;37:429–42.

22

Association between the sonographer's experience and diagnostic performance of IOTA simple rules

Chun-ping Ning[1], Xiaoli Ji[2], Hong-qiao Wang[1], Xiao-ying Du[1], Hai-tao Niu[3*] and Shi-bao Fang[3*]

Abstract

Background: To validate the clinical value of simple rules in distinguishing malignant adnexal masses from benign ones and to explore the effect of simple rules for experienced and less-experienced sonographers.

Methods: Patients with persistent adnexal masses were enrolled between November 2013 and December 2015. All masses were proven through histological examinations. Five sets of diagnoses were made and compared with one another. Diagnosis 1 was made, according to the simple rules, by a trainee with little clinical diagnostic experience. Diagnoses 2 and 3 were made by experienced and less-experienced sonographers, respectively, according to their clinical experiences. With diagnosis 1 as a reference, the two sonographers were asked to provide a second diagnosis, which were diagnoses 4 and 5. The efficiency of the five sets of diagnoses was compared using ROC curves.

Results: In total, 75 malignant (37.7%) and 124 benign lesions (62.3%) were enrolled in this study. The mean diameter of the benign masses was obviously smaller than that of the malignant ones (6.8 ± 3.4 cm vs. 9.3 ± 4.9 cm, $p < 0.01$). The malignant ratio in postmenopausal women was much higher (66.1%) than that in the premenopausal population (25.7%) ($p < 0.0001$). Totally, 156 of the 199 cases (79.4%) resulted in conclusive diagnoses. Sensitivity and specificity were 98.4% and 73.9%, respectively, among the conclusive cases. The area under the ROC curve (Az) for the simple rule diagnosis was significantly lower than that for the experienced sonographer diagnosis (0.85 vs. 0.96, $p < 0.0001$); compared with the less-experienced sonographer, this difference was not significant (0.85 vs. 0.86, $p = 0.9776$). No significant difference was found in the comparison between the diagnoses made by the experienced sonographer before and after referencing the simple rule diagnosis (Az, 0.96 vs. 0.97, $p = 0.2055$). Using diagnosis 1 as a reference, the diagnostic performance of the less-experienced sonographer increased (from 0.86 to 0.92, $p = 0.012$); however, it was still lower than that of the experienced sonographer (Az, 96% vs. 92%, $p = 0.0241$).

Conclusions: The simple rules was an appealing method for discriminating malignant masses from benign ones, particularly for a less-experienced sonographer.

Keywords: Ultrasound, Adnexal, Mass, Diagnosis

Background

Numerous diseases both benign and malignant can present as adnexal masses, such as ovarian cancers, hydrosalpinx, chocolate cysts, ectopic pregnancy, and adnexal abscess. Plenty of treatment options were proposed thanks to the surgical advances. A wise selection relies on the correct evaluation of the mass before the operation. However, the noninvasive preoperative assessment remains a major challenge for gynecologists.

Ultrasound, particularly transvaginal ultrasound, has been considered as the first-line examination in gynecology. An experienced sonographer was able to distinguish benign from malignant masses according to the subjective evaluation of ultrasound findings [1, 2]. However, a great diversity of the examiner's experience was noticed which could influence the diagnostic performance significantly [3]. Most of the time, the expertise of differential diagnoses was a kind of instinct,

* Correspondence: ningchunping1222@163.com; fsb-62@163.com
[3]Urology Department, Affiliated Hospital of Qingdao University, No. 16 of Jiangsu Road, Qingdao, Shandong, China
Full list of author information is available at the end of the article

and it was quite difficult to be transferred directly to an examiner with less experience from an experienced sonographer. Plenty of efforts were made during the last decades to improve the diagnostic ability of transvaginal sonography, such as proposing a scoring system establishing a logistic regression model, using the support vector machines, and so on [4–7]. However, none of the methods was convenient enough to be used universally.

"Simple rules" was a new method proposed by a group of researchers in the International Tumor Analysis Association (IOTA). The main aim of the proposal was to increase the diagnostic performance of ultrasound [8]. The rules contained ten ultrasound examination features, five of which were benign and five of which were malignant. Thus far, several papers have validated the clinical value of the rules [9–12]. However, the IOTA simple rules have not been tested in the Chinese population. In China, sonographers are responsible for both scanning and diagnosing, and the expertise of sonographers varies a lot. Therefore, the question is whether there are any differences when the simple rules were used by different sonographers and how the simple rules affect diagnoses made by sonographers with different experience levels.

This study had two aims: first, to validate the clinical value of simple rules in differentiating malignant adnexal masses from benign ones, and second, to explore the effect of simple rules on experienced and less-experienced sonographers.

Methods

The study was conducted between November 2013 and December 2015. The protocol for using the patients' ultrasonic images and pathological results to assess the efficacy of IOTA simple rules in distinguishing benign adnexal masses from malignant ones was approved by the Ethics Committee. All participants provided written consent to participate in the research.

Patients

Patients who were admitted to the gynecological department of the Affiliated Hospital of Qingdao University and who were scheduled for surgeries because of adnexal masses (detected by gynecologic examination with/without ultrasonography, previously) were included in this study. When a patient had more than one adnexal mass, the larger or more complex mass was included. When the masses were similar both in volume and texture, we selected the one that was more easily accessible through transvaginal ultrasound.

The following exclusion criteria were followed: (1) pregnant women; (2) patients who refused both transvaginal and transrectal ultrasound examinations; (3) patients whose surgery date exceeded 30 days from the date of the ultrasound scan; (4) patients who accepted adjuvant therapy, such as chemotherapy or radiotherapy, before the surgery; and (5) patients whose masses were surgically removed at other medical centers.

Image storing

The study was conducted using advanced ultrasound equipment (Voluson E8 ultrasound machine, GE Medical Systems). According to the protocol, all participants underwent transvaginal or transrectal (for virgins or patients who refused transvaginal ultrasound examination) ultrasound examinations with a transvaginal probe (frequency, 6~13 MHz). When the mass was too large to be viewed entirely by transvaginal ultrasound, transabdominal ultrasound was employed (frequency, 3~5 MHz). All examinations were performed by an experienced sonographer, who has been working in the gynecologic ultrasound department for 5 years. The sonographer was asked to fully scan the adnexal mass following the guidance proposed by IOTA [13]. Digital images and video clips of the masses were stored in a hard drive for further evaluations. At least eight images and three clips were stored for each patient. The size of the mass was measured in real-time.

Diagnoses

A total of five sets of diagnoses were made and analyzed in this study. One set was made using the simple rules, and the other four sets were based on subjective assessments of the sonographers.

Diagnosis based on simple rules

The simple rule diagnosis (diagnosis 1) was made by an ultrasound trainee who had studied in the ultrasonic department for approximately 1 year and accepted a 3-month real-time ultrasound training period under the supervision of an expert examiner. Before the evaluation, the trainee had undergone a theoretical course, including the terms, definitions, and measurements of the sonographic features [13], according to the simple rules proposed by IOTA [8].

The simple rules included two groups of features (M features and B features) and three rules. Rule 1—a "malignant" diagnosis was made when a mass was found conformed to one or more "M" features without any "B" features. Rule 2—a mass was considered benign if it has one or more B features and no M feature. Rule 3—if both M features and B features were present, or if none of the features was present, the simple rules yield an "inconclusive" result. Here, the features were listed in Table 1.

Diagnoses based on subjective assessments

Two sonographers, one with 11 years of experience and the other with 3 years of experience, were invited to

Table 1 Malignant and benign features of the "simple rules"

M features	B features
1 Irregular solid tumor	Unilocular cyst
2 Ascites	Acoustic shadows
3 At least four papillary structures	Smooth multilocular tumor
4 Irregular multilocular solid tumor with the largest diameter of at least 100 mm	The presence of solid components for which the largest solid component is < 7 mm in the largest diameter
5 Very high color content on color Doppler examination	No detectable blood flow on Doppler examination

review the images and perform a diagnosis (diagnoses 2 and 3), respectively. They were asked to classify the masses into five groups, according to the ultrasonic features: benign, possibly benign, undetermined, possibly malignant, and malignant. The two reviewers were blinded to the clinical and pathological information when they were assessing the cases. The diagnoses were locked as soon as they were made and could not be changed afterwards. Two months later, the two sonographers were asked to review the stored images (order disturbed) again and perform a second diagnosis (diagnoses 4 and 5), respectively, after learning the simple rules by reading the original paper published by the IOTA group [8]. In addition, they had no knowledge of the pathological or clinical information of the patients during evaluation. Only at this time they were encouraged to use diagnosis 1 as a reference. Diagnosis 2 and diagnosis 4 were made by an experienced sonographer before and after referencing the simple rule diagnosis. Diagnosis 3 and diagnosis 5 were made by a less-experienced sonographer before and after referencing the simple rule diagnosis.

Reference standard

Pathological examinations were considered as the golden standard. An experienced pathologist was invited to examine the pathological specimens and to provide a final diagnosis, according to the criteria recommended by the International Federation of Gynecology and Obstetrics [14]. The pathologists had no knowledge of the ultrasonic diagnosis. The borderline masses and masses with low malignant potential were classified into the malignant group too. In benign cases which have no pathological specimens, intraoperative findings made by the surgeons were used as the final diagnoses.

Statistical analysis

For the subjective assessments, the "benign" and "possible benign" results were considered to be negative, while "malignant" and "possible malignant" were considered to be positive. Diagnostic performance was expressed as the sensitivity (Se), specificity (Sp), positive predictive value (PPV), negative predictive value (NPV), and accuracy (Ac). We

compared the diagnostic efficiency of the simple rules with subjective assessments made by the experienced and less-experienced sonographers. We also assessed the performance when the simple rules were used as a second diagnosis by comparing the efficiency of the diagnoses made by the two sonographers, with and without using the simple rules as a reference.

Both SPSS (version 18.0, SPSS Inc., Chicago, IL) and MedCalc were used in the statistical analyses. Student's t test was used to examine the differences between the numeric parameters, which were expressed as the mean $\pm$ standard deviation. The Se, Sp, PPV, NPV, and Ac were calculated for each set of diagnoses. Receiver operating characteristic (ROC) curves were established, and the area under the ROC curves (Az) was compared according to the method proposed by DeLong et al. [15]. McNemar's test was used to check for the statistically significant differences in a paired binomial proportion. A $p < 0.01$ was considered as significantly different.

Results

During the study period, there were 373 eligible patients. A total of 174 were excluded for the following reasons: pregnancy ($n = 11$), patients refused both transvaginal and transrectal ultrasound examinations ($n = 34$), patients accepted surgeries 30 days later than the ultrasound scan ($n = 46$), patients accepted chemotherapy or radiotherapy before the surgery ($n = 28$), and masses were surgically removed in other medical centers ($n = 55$). Ultimately, 199 patients (mean age 45.1 $\pm$ 13.7, range 17~89 years) were included in this study, 59 of whom were postmenopausal.

Pathological examinations confirmed that there were 75 malignant (37.7%) and 124 benign lesions (62.3%), and the ratio of benign to malignant tumors was 1.65:1. The malignant percentage was much higher (66.1%) in postmenopausal patients than that in the premenopausal population (25.7%) ($p < 0.0001$). Detailed pathological types were listed in Table 2. The mean diameter of the masses was 7.7 $\pm$ 4.2 cm (range, 1.0~23.2 cm); the mean diameter of the benign tumors was obviously smaller than that of the malignant ones (6.8 $\pm$ 3.4 cm vs. 9.3 $\pm$ 4.9 cm, $p < 0.01$; power, 0.999).

The performances of the five sets of diagnoses are listed in Tables 3 and 4. The ROC curves for the five sets of diagnoses are shown in Fig. 1. The simple rules yielded a conclusive result for 79.4% (158/199) of the masses. Among the masses with conclusive results, the sensitivity was 98.4% and the specificity was 73.9%. Compared with the subjective assessments performed by the experienced sonographer, the Az of diagnosis 1 was significantly lower (0.85 vs. 0.96, $p < 0.0001$, power = 0.981). However, the difference between the simple rule diagnosis and the diagnosis made by the less-experienced sonographer was not significant (0.85 vs. 0.86, $p = 0.9776$, power = 0.124).

Table 2 Detail pathological types of the enrolled masses

Classifications	Pathological results	Number	Proportion (%)
Benign	Total	124	62.3
	Teratoma	43	21.6
	Chocolate cyst	31	15.6
	Ovarian cystadenoma	19	9.55
	Ectopic gestational mass	8	4.02
	Para-ovarian cyst	7	3.52
	Ovarian thecofibroma	6	3.02
	Thecoma	5	2.51
	Ovarian torsion	1	0.50
	Accessory spleen	1	0.50
	Abscess	2	1.00
	Isolated torsion of the fallopian tube	1	0.50
Malignant	Total	75	37.7
	Cystadenocarcinoma	42	21.1
	Ovarian borderline tumor	15	7.54
	Endometrial cancer	3	1.51
	Metastatic carcinoma	2	1.00
	Yolk sac tumor	2	1.00
	Granulosa cell carcinoma	1	0.50
	Dysgerminoma	1	0.50
	Immature teratoma	7	3.52
	Carcinosarcoma	2	1.00

For the experienced sonographer, the conclusive ratio was 81.4% (162/199). Among the concluded cases, the primary diagnosis missed two malignant masses and yielded four false-positive diagnoses. With the help of the simple rules, 21 more cases were classified as conclusive. However, the diagnostic performance was similar (0.96 vs. 0.97, $p = 0.2055$, power = 0.241) before and after using the simple rules as a reference. Comparison of the sensitivity and specificity of the two diagnoses (diagnoses 2 and 4) yielded no significant difference (sensitivity, 96.2% vs. 100%; specificity, 96.3% vs. 94.0%, $p > 0.05$). Az of the diagnosis made by the experienced sonographer was obviously higher than that of the less-experienced sonographer (Az, 0.96 vs. 0.86, $p < 0.0001$, power = 0.966).

For the less-experienced sonographer, 137 of the 199 cases were correctly diagnosed, with moderate sensitivity and specificity (72.4% and 88.8%). Using the simple rules as a reference, the diagnostic performance of the less-experienced sonographer increased (from 0.86 to 0.92, $p = 0.012$, power = 0.659); however, it remained lower than that of the experienced sonographer (Az, 96% vs. 92%, $p = 0.0241$, power = 0.728). The conclusive ratio showed no significant change (82.9% vs. 81.4%, $p = 0.795$) before and after using the simple rule diagnosis as a reference. The sensitivity of diagnosis 5 (made by the less-experienced sonographer with the help of the simple rules) was obviously higher than that of diagnosis 3 (96.7% vs. 72.4%, $p = 0.012$).

Discussion

Adnexal masses are frequently found in both symptomatic and asymptomatic women at most ages. Benign and malignant masses may be found in adnexal structures. Once a mass has been detected, the physician is faced with the dilemma of how to manage the patient. Appropriate management should be based on the correct preoperative diagnosis. Ultrasound, particularly transvaginal ultrasound, remains the leading established tool to predict the nature of the adnexal masses [16].

In this study, we enrolled 199 adnexal masses detected over 3 years, including 11 types of benign masses and 9 types of malignant masses. We found that the malignant percentage in postmenopausal patients was higher than that in the premenopausal population, and the malignant masses were significantly larger than the benign masses. Thus, it is reasonable to pay more attention to older patients with large adnexal masses.

The simple rules were established by comparing the diagnostic performance with two logic regression models [8]. Up to now, plenty of studies [17, 18] have proved that the simple rules were suitable for about 76–89.3% adnexal tumors. In our study, the conclusive ratio of the simple diagnosis was 79.4%. The ratio increased to 92.0% and 81.4% in experienced and less-experienced examiners, respectively. Therefore, we believe that the simple rules are a user-friendly tool for both experienced and less-experienced examiners. For the masses with conclusive results, the sensitivity in this study was lower

Table 3 Detail results of the five sets diagnoses

Pathological diagnosis	Diagnosis 1		Diagnosis 2		Diagnosis 3		Diagnosis 4		Diagnosis 5	
	−	+	−	+	−	+	−	+	−	+
−	71	25	105	4	95	12	109	7	89	13
+	1	61	2	51	16	42	0	67	2	58
Inconclusive	28	13	15	22	17	17	8	8	22	15

Diagnosis 1 was made by a trainee according to the simple rules. Diagnoses 2 and 3 were made by an experienced and a less-experienced sonographer, respectively, according to their clinical experiences. Diagnoses 4 and 5 were made by the experienced and less-experienced sonographer, respectively, according to their experiences, with diagnosis 1 as a reference. "−" means "benign," "+" means "malignant"

Table 4 Diagnostic performance of the five diagnoses

Diagnoses	Conclusive ratio (%)	Sensitivity (%)	Specificity (%)	PPV (%)	NPV (%)	+LR	−LR	Correct ratio (%)	Az	95% CI
Diagnosis 1	79.4	98.4	73.9	70.9	98.6	3.77	0.02	83.5%	0.85	0.797~0.900
Diagnosis 2	81.4	96.2	96.3	92.7	98.1	26	0.04	96.3	0.96*	0.923~0.983
Diagnosis 3	82.9	72.4	88.8	77.8	85.6	6.46	0.31	83.0	0.86#	0.798~0.901
Diagnosis 4	92.0	100	94.0	90.5	100	16.7	0	96.2	0.97*△	0.934~0.988
Diagnosis 5	81.4	96.7	87.3	81.7	97.8	7.61	0.04	90.7	0.92*#△▲	0.870~0.952

Diagnosis 1 was made by a trainee of ultrasound according to the simple rules. Diagnoses 2 and 3 were made by an experienced and a less-experienced sonographer, respectively, according to their experiences. Diagnoses 4 and 5 were made by the experienced and less-experienced sonographer, respectively, according to their experiences, with diagnosis 1 as a reference

Az area under the ROC curve, *CI* confidence interval, *PPV* positive predictive ratio, *NPV* negative predictive ratio, *+LR* positive likelihood ratio, *−LR* negative likelihood ratio

*Compared with diagnosis 1, $p < 0.01$

#Compared with diagnosis 2, $p < 0.01$

△Compared with diagnosis 3, $p < 0.01$

▲Compared with diagnosis 4, $p < 0.01$

than that in Nunes [19] reported in their meta-analysis, while the specificity was higher. This difference may be partly explained by the fact that this study was performed in a tertiary care university-affiliated hospital, which was considered to be the best hospital in Qingdao, and partly because the simple rule diagnosis was conducted by a trainee with little clinical experience.

The diagnostic performance of the experienced sonographer improved while the sensitivity and specificity remained unchanged when the simple rule diagnosis was used as a reference. The experienced sonographer missed two malignant masses and provided four false-positive diagnoses during the first round of diagnosis. With the help of the simple rules, there were seven false-positive diagnoses and no malignant masses were missed. The three new misdiagnosed cases eventually proved to be inflammatory masses. They were irregular solid masses with abundant blood supplies, and one of the patients had a small amount of ascite, which were diagnosed as malignant according to the simple rules. For the less-experienced sonographer, the sensitivity and specificity, as well as the Az, improved significantly with the help of the simple rule diagnosis. Consequently,

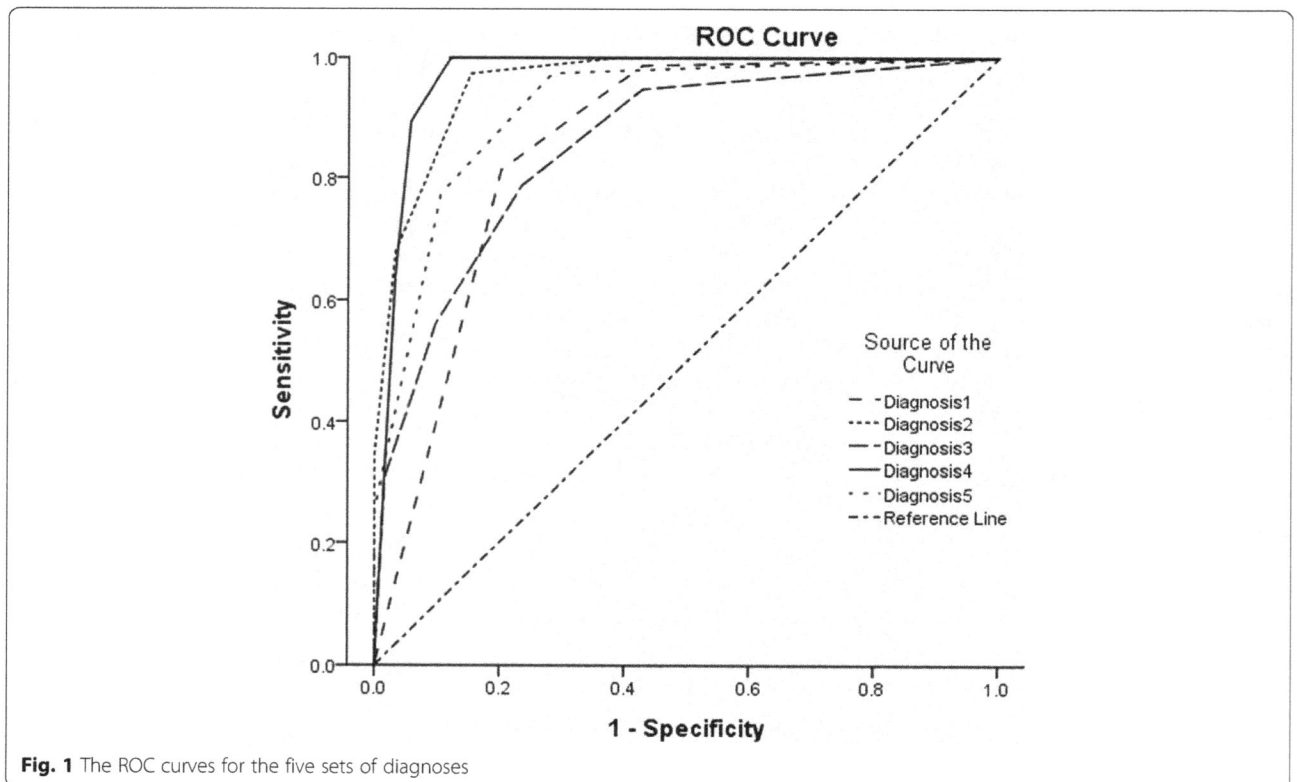

Fig. 1 The ROC curves for the five sets of diagnoses

we believe that the simple rules may be more helpful for less-experienced examiners. However, the Az of diagnosis 4 (made by the less-experienced sonographer with the help of the simple rules) was still significantly lower than that of the experienced sonographer, implying that the clinical experience is crucial for the efficient diagnosis of adnexal masses.

This study has two disadvantages. First, the clinical information and laboratory results were not provided when the masses were assessed. Some of the masses, for example, ectopic pregnancy, could be correctly diagnosed if the results of HCG were provided. In clinical practices, such information could be obtained from inquisitions at the time of scanning. Second, only two sonographers were invited to participate in this study, one with 11 years of experience and the other with 3 years of experience. Examiners with various experience levels should be evaluated in further research.

Conclusions

In conclusion, this study was performed to demonstrate the differences in how the simple rules affect the diagnoses made by the sonographers with different experience levels. We found that the simple rules was more useful for the less-experienced sonographers. When the diagnosis is still inconclusive, it is wise to seek help from the experienced sonographers.

Acknowledgements
We want to express our gratitude to the American Journal Experts for the professional editing of the manuscript.

Funding
This study was partially funded by the National Natural Science Foundation of China (No. 81501477). This funding helped the design and collection of the manuscript. It will also support the publication of the article. This study was also partially funded by the post-doctoral application project of Qingdao.

Authors' contributions
CPN contributed to the protocol/project development, data analysis, and manuscript writing/editing. XLJ contributed to the data analysis and statistics and revised the manuscript. HQW contributed to the data management and analysis. XYD contributed to the data collection and manuscript writing. HTN contributed to the supervision, statistical analysis, and manuscript editing. SBF contributed to the protocol/project development and supervision. All authors read and approved the final manuscript.

Competing interests
The authors declare that they have no competing interests.

Author details
[1]Ultrasound Department, Affiliated Hospital of Qingdao University, Qingdao, Shandong, China. [2]Ultrasound Department, Qingdao Women and Children Hospital, Qingdao, Shandong, China. [3]Urology Department, Affiliated Hospital of Qingdao University, No. 16 of Jiangsu Road, Qingdao, Shandong, China.

References
1. Van Calster B, Timmerman D, Bourne T, Testa AC, Van Holsbeke C, Domali E, Jurkovic D, Neven P, Van Huffel S, Valentin L. Discrimination between benign and malignant adnexal masses by specialist ultrasound examination versus serum CA-125. J Natl Cancer Inst. 2007;99:1706–14.
2. Valentin L, Jurkovic D, Van Calster B, Testa A, Van Holsbeke C, Bourne T, Vergote I, Van Huffel S, Timmerman D. Adding a single CA 125 measurement to ultrasound imaging performed by an experienced examiner does not improve preoperative discrimination between benign and malignant adnexal masses. Ultrasound Obstet Gynecol. 2009;34:345–54.
3. Van Holsbeke C, Daemen A, Yazbek J, Holland TK, Bourne T, Mesens T, Lannoo L, Boes AS, Joos A, Van De Vijver A, et al. Ultrasound experience substantially impacts on diagnostic performance and confidence when adnexal masses are classified using pattern recognition. Gynecol Obstet Investig. 2010;69:160–8.
4. Sladkevicius P, Valentin L. Interobserver agreement in describing the ultrasound appearance of adnexal masses and in calculating the risk of malignancy using logistic regression models. Clin Cancer Res. 2015;21: 594–601.
5. Tailor A, Jurkovic D, Bourne TH, Collins WP, Campbell S. Sonographic prediction of malignancy in adnexal masses using an artificial neural network. Br J Obstet Gynaecol. 1999;106:21–30.
6. Ferrazzi E, Zanetta G, Dordoni D, Berlanda N, Mezzopane R, Lissoni AA. Transvaginal ultrasonographic characterization of ovarian masses: comparison of five scoring systems in a multicenter study. Ultrasound Obstet Gynecol. 1997;10:192–7.
7. Kaijser J, Sayasneh A, Van Hoorde K, Ghaem-Maghami S, Bourne T, Timmerman D, Van Calster B. Presurgical diagnosis of adnexal tumours using mathematical models and scoring systems: a systematic review and meta-analysis. Hum Reprod Update. 2014;20:449–62.
8. Timmerman D, Testa AC, Bourne T, Ameye L, Jurkovic D, Van Holsbeke C, Paladini D, Van Calster B, Vergote I, Van Huffel S, Valentin L. Simple ultrasound-based rules for the diagnosis of ovarian cancer. Ultrasound Obstet Gynecol. 2008;31:681–90.
9. Di Legge A, Testa AC, Ameye L, Van Calster B, Lissoni AA, Leone FP, Savelli L, Franchi D, Czekierdowski A, Trio D, et al. Lesion size affects diagnostic performance of IOTA logistic regression models, IOTA simple rules and risk of malignancy index in discriminating between benign and malignant adnexal masses. Ultrasound Obstet Gynecol. 2012;40:345–54.
10. Alcazar JL, Pascual MA, Olartecoechea B, Graupera B, Auba M, Ajossa S, Hereter L, Julve R, Gaston B, Peddes C, et al. IOTA simple rules for discriminating between benign and malignant adnexal masses: prospective external validation. Ultrasound Obstet Gynecol. 2013;42:467–71.
11. Tinnangwattana D, Vichak-Ururote L, Tontivuthikul P, Charoenratana C, Lerthiranwong T, Tongsong T. IOTA simple rules in differentiating between benign and malignant adnexal masses by non-expert examiners. Asian Pac J Cancer Prev. 2015;16:3835–8.
12. Alcazar JL, Pascual MA, Graupera B, Auba M, Errasti T, Olartecoechea B, Ruiz-Zambrana A, Hereter L, Ajossa S, Guerriero S. External validation of IOTA simple descriptors and simple rules for classifying adnexal masses. Ultrasound Obstet Gynecol. 2016;48:397–402.
13. Timmerman D, Valentin L, Bourne TH, Collins WP, Verrelst H, Vergote I, International Ovarian Tumor Analysis G. Terms, definitions and measurements to describe the sonographic features of adnexal tumors: a consensus opinion from the International Ovarian Tumor Analysis (IOTA) Group. Ultrasound Obstet Gynecol. 2000;16:500–5.
14. Heintz AP, Odicino F, Maisonneuve P, Quinn MA, Benedet JL, Creasman WT, Ngan HY, Pecorelli S, Beller U. Carcinoma of the ovary. FIGO 26th annual report on the results of treatment in gynecological cancer. Int J Gynaecol Obstet. 2006;95(Suppl 1):S161–92.
15. DeLong ER, DeLong DM, Clarke-Pearson DL. Comparing the areas under two or more correlated receiver operating characteristic curves: a nonparametric approach. Biometrics. 1988;44:837–45.
16. Meys EM, Rutten IJ, Kruitwagen RF, Slangen BF, Bergmans MG, Mertens HJ, Nolting E, Boskamp D, Beets-Tan RG, van Gorp T. Investigating the performance and cost-effectiveness of the simple ultrasound-based rules compared to the risk of malignancy index in the diagnosis of ovarian cancer (SUBSONiC-study): protocol of a prospective multicenter cohort study in the Netherlands. BMC Cancer. 2015;15:482.

23

Combined surgical treatment of esophageal cancer and coronary heart diseases in elderly patients

Weiran Zhang[1†], Ban Liu[2†], Yue Zhou[3†], Feng Wang[4†], Chang Gu[5], Qi Wang[6], Xiaofang Wang[7] and Yangyang Zhang[7*] (iD)

Abstract

Objective: The co-incidence of esophageal cancer and coronary heart disease (CHD) is increasing in elderly patients. This study was carried out to analyze the efficiency and safety of simultaneous esophagectomy and cardiac surgery in a selected group of elderly patients.

Methods: Prospective database for coexistency of severe CHD and esophageal or esophageal-gastric junction cancer was firstly reviewed. Twenty-two patients undergoing combined surgical interventions, including first beating-heart coronary artery bypass grafting (off-pump CABG) and then esophagectomy, were involved as group A. Then, 44 patients undergoing isolated esophagectomy were selected as group B using the propensity score matching method. Data including clinic pathological characteristics and postoperative outcomes were investigated. Kaplan–Meier analysis was used.

Results: The surgical procedure was performed through left lateral thoracotomy in all patients, except one patient in group A who received median sternotomy and left lateral thoracotomy. The operation time and blood loss were both more in group A, as a result of two operations performed at one session. Patients in both groups were followed up from 1.3 to 78.3 months. No significant between-group was found in overall survival or relapse-free survival.

Conclusion: The risk of simultaneous esophagectomy and cardiac surgery is not high. Despite certain differences in clinical indicators between groups, the safety of simultaneous procedures in group A is evident.

Keywords: Simultaneous procedures, Esophagectomy, Off-pump, Coronary artery bypass grafting, The elderly

Introduction

China has begun to enter an aging society, while age is the main risk factor for coronary heart disease (CHD) and cancers. CHD is the leading cause of death in the world, accounting for almost one third of all global deaths, and is the secondary cause of death in China [1, 2]. Esophageal cancer, a most common cancer worldwide, is the leading cause of death among all cancers and mostly (over 80%) attacks developing countries [3]. In China, the incidence of esophageal cancer is about twofold higher than that in the world [4].

Since early-staged esophageal cancer is asymptomatic, most patients were diagnosed at the advanced stage, leading to poor survival [4]. Despite significant development in multimodality treatment of esophageal cancer, including chemotherapy, radiation, and targeted therapies, surgical resection is still the most effective means to achieve long-term disease-free survival in patients with early-staged esophageal cancer. Coexistence of malignant disease (e.g., esophageal cancer) and CHD is common and is expected to increase due to diagnostic improvement and the aging population. However, it is very difficult to decide how to treat CHD patients who need a noncardiac surgical treatment simultaneously. Performing both procedures during a

* Correspondence: zhangyangyang_wy@vip.sina.com
†Weiran Zhang, Ban Liu, Yue Zhou and Feng Wang contributed equally to this work.
7Department of Cardiovascular Surgery, Shanghai East Hospital, Tongji University School of Medicine, 150 Jimo Road, Shanghai 200120, China
Full list of author information is available at the end of the article

single operation may eliminate unnecessary delay in cancer treatment [5], but was only reported in a few patients. Our cardiothoracic center has performed simultaneous cardiac and noncardiac surgery since 2010. In this study, we analyzed the outcomes of simultaneous coronary artery bypass grafting (CABG) and esophagectomy in a selected group of patients and demonstrated the possibility and feasibility of this simultaneous session.

Materials and methods

Patients

This retrospective study was approved by the Ethics Committee of Shanghai East hospital (certificate number: 2017-049). Between September 2010 and August 2016, 22 patients diagnosed with a concomitant heart disease and esophageal or esophageal-gastric junction (EGJ) cancer and requiring surgical treatment in our center were enrolled as group A. Patients who underwent isolated esophagectomy during the same time period were selected as group B for comparison of long-term safety of the combined procedures. The propensity score matching method was used to balance the potential confounders between groups. The two groups were matched using a one-to-two nearest-neighbor matching in terms of age, gender, cardio-vascular co-morbidities, and especially the histology (including tumor type and tumor staging) of esophageal cancer. Cancer was staged according to the seventh edition of American Joint Committee on Cancer (AJCC) staging manual [6]. Patients undergoing neoadjuvant therapy were excluded.

The following clinical data were obtained from all patients: age, sex, pathological tumor characteristics, operation time, total estimated blood loss, time of intensive care unit (ICU) stay, time of hospital stay, incidence of complications and recurrence, and survival (Additional file 1). The clinical characteristics of both groups are shown in Table 1. All patients received routine clinical examination, blood serum biochemical examination, electrocardiogram, chest computed tomography (CT), and abdominal ultrasound.

Simultaneous operation types

All patients were operated by the same group of surgeons and underwent double-lumen tracheal intubation under general anesthesia. Posterolateral thoracotomy incision was

Table 1 Clinical characteristic of the patients

Characteristics of patients	Group A	Group B	P value
Sample quantity	22	44	
Female (n, %)	3 (13.64%)	6 (13.64%)	1.000
Age (years)	65.64 ± 6.67	63.80 ± 6.63	0.293
NYHA class (n)			0.000
I	0	43	
II	22	1	
III	0	0	
IV	0	0	
EF (%)	64.09 ± 3.12	65.22 ± 2.95	0.159
CAD classification (n)	22	3	0.000
Stable angina (n, %)	18 (81.82%)	3 (100.00%)	
Unstable angina (n, %)	4 (18.18%)	0	
Number of disease vessels (n)	2.05 ± 0.79		
Tumor location			1.000
Esophagus (n, %)	13 (59.09%)	26 (59.09%)	
EGJ (n, %)	9 (40.91%)	18 (40.91%)	
Hypertension (n, %)	12 (54.55%)	15 (34.09%)	0.111
Diabetes mellitus (n, %)	4 (18.18%)	4 (9.09%)	0.286
Cerebrovascular disease (n, %)	10 (45.45%)	3 (6.82%)	0.000
Smoking (n, %)	9 (40.91%)	21 (47.73%)	0.600
Tumor stage (n)			0.928
I	6 (27.27%)	13 (29.55%)	
II	7 (31.82%)	12 (27.27%)	
III	9 (40.91%)	19 (43.18%)	

Abbreviations: NYHA New York Heart Association, LVEF left ventricular ejection factor, CAD coronary artery disease, EGJ esophageal-gastric junction

performed along the left sixth or seventh intercostal space according to the tumor location. In group A, off-pump beating-heart coronary artery grafting was operated firstly, followed by esophagectomy. The left internal mammary arteries (LIMA) and/or the saphenous veins were taken as the bypass grafts. Proximal anastomosis was at the descending aorta. Patients in both groups received esophagectomy. Lymph nodes around the esophagus, along the descending aorta and inferior pulmonary ligaments, and below the aortic arch and above the diaphragm were completely dissected. The abdominal lymph nodes were cleared via the transdiaphragmatic approach. The anastomosis was constructed by stapling.

Anticoagulant therapy was done in group A, and low-molecular-weight heparin (LMWH) was given according to body weight and blood loss until the discharge from hospital. Brilinta or Plavix was commenced after LMWH was stopped.

Follow-up

All patients were followed up in clinic visits: firstly at 1 month after discharge, secondly at 3 months, and then at 6-month interval. All patients received clinical examination, electrocardiogram, cardiac echo, and chest X-rays at each visit.

Statistical analysis

Survival curves were obtained using the Kaplan–Meier method (Fig. 1). Statistical analyses were performed on SPSS 16.0 (SPSS Inc., Chicago, IL, USA). Data were presented as mean ± standard deviation (SD) for continuous variables. Demographic and clinical data between groups were compared via chi-square test or Fisher exact test. $P < 0.05$ was considered to be statistically significant.

Results

Patient characteristics

The clinical characteristics of patients are summarized in Table 1. Group A consisted of 19 men and 3 women, while group B involved 6 women and 38 men. The average ages were 65.64 ± 6.67 and 63.80 ± 6.63 years, respectively. As for co-morbidities, remarkable differences between groups were found in diabetes mellitus, hypertension, and smoking as the main risk factors of CHD. As for cardiac function, no significant differences between groups were found in left ventricular ejection fraction (LVEF). The pairing method successfully ranked

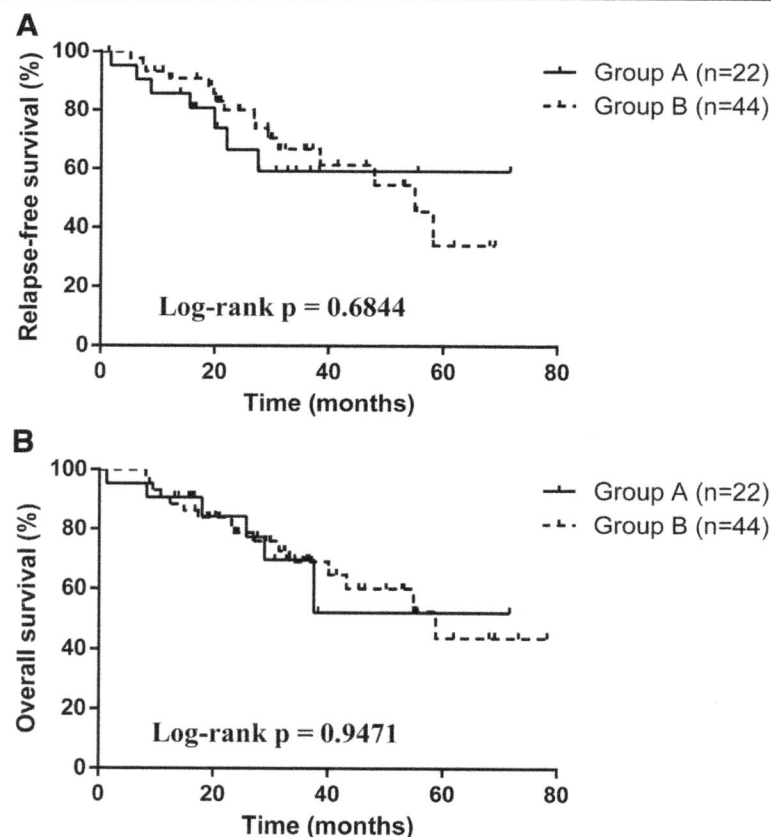

Fig. 1 Kaplan–Meier survival curves for relapse-451 free survival (**a**) and 452 overall survival (**b**) according to matched patients in our study

Table 2 Comparison of surgical outcomes

Variables	Group A	Group B	P value
Operation time	404.73 ± 74.22	212.91 ± 48.97	0.000
Blood loss (ml)	606.82 ± 304.84	223.86 ± 122.23	0.000
Surgery plasma transfusion (ml)	312.73 ± 314.25	50.91 ± 116.00	0.000
Red blood cell transfusion (unit)	1.39 ± 1.42	0.38 ± 0.87	0.001
Bypass graft number (n)	2.36 ± 1.00	0	/
Mechanical ventilation time (min)	862.27 ± 252.09	0	/
ICU stay (min)	1887.05 ± 931.07	2236.82 ± 4124.66	0.697
Postoperative hospital stay (day)	19.59 ± 6.18	12.77 ± 4.62	0.000
24-h drainage after operation (ml)	216.59 ± 170.11	217.16 ± 155.50	0.989
Postoperative total drainage (ml)	2006.59 ± 976.71	760.91 ± 610.15	0.000
Tumor size (cm)	3.49 ± 1.83	3.08 ± 1.52	0.342
Surgical approach (n, %)			0.333
Single incision approach	21 (95.45%)	44 (100%)	
Two-incision approach	1 (4.55%)	0 (0.00%)	
Tumor pathological type			0.236
Adenocarcinoma (n, %)	8 (36.37%)	21 (47.73%)	
Squamous cell carcinoma (n, %)	10 (45.45%)	21 (47.73%)	
Others (n, %)	4 (18.18%)	2 (4.54%)	

Abbreviations: *ICU* intensive care unit

patients into group B with similar tumor location and staging.

Surgical outcomes

Surgical outcomes are summarized in Table 2. There was no recurrent myocardial ischemia or death in the perioperative period in either group. The mean operation time and the length of postoperative hospitalization were longer, and the blood loss and postoperative total drainage were more in group A, as a result of two operations performed at one session. Postoperative mechanical ventilation was used in group A, but not in group B. Only one patient in group A was operated by the mid-sternal incision for CABG and the left approach for esophageal cancer. A single incision from left thoracotomy was employed for the remaining patients from both groups. The ICU stay was shorter in group A, but not significantly. The total postoperative hospital stay was significantly longer in group A, considering the greater trauma of the combined surgeries.

Pathological outcomes are summarized in Table 2. All patients were histologically diagnosed. Ten patients were diagnosed as squamous cell carcinoma, 8 as adenocarcinoma, 2 as gland squamous cell carcinoma, 1 as endocrine cell carcinoma, and 1 as small cell carcinoma in group A. Positive lymph node metastasis was identified in 10 (45.5%) of the 22 patients. The postoperative complications, mainly respiratory complications, are minor and curable in both groups (not listed here).

Follow-up

All the patients from group A were followed up for 1.3 to 71.7 months. Seven patients experienced relapse; finally, five of them died of tumor recurrence or metastasis (8.3, 18.0, 25.7, 28.9, 37.5 months after surgery, respectively), while one patient died of pneumonia after 1.3 months postoperatively, but no patient died of major cardiovascular events during the follow-up. The remaining 16 patients survived for 13.2 to 71.7 months during the follow-up.

All patients in group B were followed up from 8.1 to 78.3 months. Sixteen patients experienced relapse, and finally, 12 patients died. Moreover, other four died of non-cancer-related factors during radio (chemo)-therapy after operation. No patient died of major cardiovascular events during the follow-up. The remaining 28 patients survived from 16.8 to 78.3 months during the follow-up.

The 5-year survival rate was 52.2% in group A and 43.8% in group B (P > 0.05).

Discussion

Our experience shows simultaneous esophagectomy and off-pump CABG can be performed safely and efficiently at a tertiary care center. The path toward the optimal outcome will necessarily take fairly long time, even for operators already skilled in thoracic and cardiac operations. Despite certain differences in clinical indicators between simultaneous operations and single esophagectomy, the simultaneous operations were evidently safe, enabled earlier esophageal cancer resection, and avoided the eventual complications from further surgical procedure.

Esophageal cancer is a leading cause of cancer-related mortality in China [4]. The combination of CHD and malignancy is expected to increase due to an aging population in China and diagnostic technique improvements. Surgery is still the first choice for patients with resectable malignant diseases. The high difficulty in treating cancers accompanied with severe CHD significantly increases operation-related morbidity and mortality [7]. Radiotherapy and chemotherapy are very important cancer treatment techniques, but directly impact the heart. When patients refer to noncardiac operation under general anesthesia, preoperative treatment of CHD is commonly accepted in practice, which may reduce perioperative mortality and morbidity [8].

Cardiac revascularization includes percutaneous coronary intervention (PCI) and CABG. Coronary stents have dramatically improved immediate angiographic results by reducing the incidence of emergent bypass grafting. Consequently, stents are now used in more than 50% of all percutaneous transluminal coronary angioplasty procedures. For patients with coronary stents, intensive anticoagulation treatment greatly increases risk of hemorrhagic complications among those undergoing noncardiac operations. Stent is thrombogenic and requires combined antiplatelet (clopidogrel and aspirin) therapy till endothelialization is completed, which takes 1 month to 1 year according to stent type [9]. During this period, combined antiplatelet therapy must be continued to avoid stent thrombosis. The incidence of fatal perioperative complications is extraordinarily high in patients who undergo noncardiac surgery soon after coronary stent implantation. Hence, when a patient is considered for noncardiac surgery soon after coronary stenting, efforts should be made to avoid PCI if possible [10]. Longer delay in cancer operation may result in cancer progression [11]. As reported, the incidence and mortality of myocardial infarction are lower among patients receiving CABG, compared with the results of noncardiac surgery after either PCI or CABG [10].

Surgical treatment of malignant diseases can be either simultaneously performed with CABG or via a staged approach a few weeks later. However, whether to select either one-stage or two-stage operation remains controversial [12, 13]. A two-stage procedure is two surgical traumas, which may delay the tumor resection and doubles postoperative pains and treatment costs. One method to improve intraoperative and potentially postoperative factors is to utilize a simultaneous surgery for patients with combined cardiac and noncardiac diseases. On the contrary, the one-stage procedure needs double expertise for this complex operation. This procedure

first described in 1990 can improve operative time and is at least as safe as conventional surgery. The simultaneous procedure has gradually been adopted to perform various cardiac and noncardiac operations, including pulmonary lobectomy, esophagectomy, gastrectomy, and colectomy [14, 15]. This approach has been mainly performed in thoracic carcinoma patients and may solve two problems through a single incision [12, 15]. However, in China which has a large population, there are few reports of combined esophagectomy and off-pump CABG. By extensively reviewing relevant literature [12, 16], we present the largest single-center report in China so far. The simultaneous surgeries may prolong the anesthesia time and surgical time and increase the postoperative heparinization-related bleeding risks. Nevertheless, the one-stage procedure provides the immediate solution of two intrathoracic operations and minimizes the risk of intraoperative bleeding. Off-pump CABG compared with on-pump coronary revascularization may improve long-term survival and minimize the incidence of bleeding or tumor dissemination secondary to extracorporeal circulation-induced immunosuppression and coagulopathy [15, 17]. Simultaneous off-pump CABG and tumor resection has been performed to treat several cancer diseases [13, 15]. Although our report suggests its safety and efficiency, this combined operation is not suitable for all patients. The patients to undergo this operation should be well selected and prepared in advance. According to our experience, the simultaneous operation indications are (1) Preoperative estimation of esophageal cancer is able to be radical resection, without distant metastasis; (2) Patients suffer from CHD with CABG indication, without emergency operation; (3) Patients should be able to tolerate combined surgery, so patients with EF < 45% or with heart failure are not recommended; (4) Patients having a history of chest or heart operation or with pleural adhesions are not recommended.

The left transthoracic approach performed here is commonly used for middle third or lower third esophageal tumors in China and is outstanding with shorter hospital stay and lower incidence of postoperative complications [18, 19]. Meanwhile, the left lateral thoracotomy incision enables the off-pump CABG. The use of LIMA in CABG graft is considered the best choice for myocardial revascularization. The 10-year patency rate of saphenous vein graft is 40–60%. Here, the CABG grafts were selected depending on the operative incision, malignant degree of cancer, coronary artery conditions, and life expectancy. The saphenous vein graft can supply blood to heart muscles and help to avoid cardiovascular events during the life expectancy, when the internal mammary artery cannot be easily harvested as a graft. In group A, 4 patients underwent internal mammary arteries grafting and 18 patients underwent saphenous vein grafting, and the mean number of anastomosed coronary vessels was 2.36.

Esophageal cancer is extremely aggressive, as its 5-year survival rate is about 23–46% [20, 21]. Because of the high mortality, all efforts should be made to limit operation-related mortality and morbidity of esophageal cancer. Since surgeon-related factors can contribute to morbidity [22, 23], all operations in our study were conducted by the same team of surgeons. In our center, we performed almost ten thousand esophagectomy or three thousand off-pump CABG in recent decades, which proved our experience and skills were particularly important in achieving good outcomes of combined operations. These surgeons had both thoracic and cardiac skills, which is rare under the current highly professional background. In addition, the preoperative patient selection and the postoperative professional care and nursing also guaranteed patient recovery. After the thoracic operations we have accomplished so far, few patients have complications following esophageal surgery. Patients from both groups had no recurrent myocardial ischemia or death during the perioperative period. Patients from group A had longer mean operation time and more blood loss, as a result of the two operations performed at one session. Only one patient in group A was operated by the mid-sternal incision for CABG and the left approach for esophageal cancer, because his condition was worsened during the surgery and two separated incisions would shorten the revascularization time. The remaining 21 patients were operated by one surgical incision. The 5-year survival rates and relapse-free survival rates were both similar between groups, indicating cardiac surgeries add no risk of complications or mortality to those patients undergoing surgical treatment of malignancy.

This study has several limitations. Firstly, it is a retrospective study. Secondly, the sample size is relatively small, and it is difficult to reach significant power when accessing the results between groups. Thirdly, the oncological outcomes of this series are not confirmed by long-term study, which should be done in the future. Finally, the technical modifications are in part positively influenced by the ongoing gained experience.

Despite these limitations, we believe this is a useful work in guiding surgeons who want to establish a simultaneous approach at their institutions. Our experiences hopefully may provide them some advice when they consider this simultaneous operation for the first time.

In conclusion, the simultaneous approach can be performed effectively and safely by experienced surgeons and is safe and beneficial for the selected group of patients. Sub-optimal outcomes may occur perioperatively, which can be solved through dedication, experience, and progressive technical development. The off-pump CABG adds no negative effect on the life expectancy of patients.

Conclusions

The risk of simultaneous esophagectomy and coronary artery surgery is not high. Despite the certain differences in clinical indicators between groups, the simultaneous procedures are evidently safe, enable earlier esophagectomy, and can avoid the eventual complications from further surgical procedure.

Abbreviations
AJCC: American Joint Committee on Cancer; CABG: Coronary artery bypass grafting; CHD: Coronary heart disease; CT: Computed tomography; EGJ: Esophageal-gastric junction; ICU: Intensive care unit; LIMA: Left internal mammary arteries; LMWH: Low-molecular-weight heparin; LVEF: Left ventricular ejection fraction; PCI: Percutaneous coronary intervention; SD: Standard deviation

Acknowledgements
We wish to thank the help in this study given by Prof. Yongfeng Shao, Prof. Xiaowei Wang, Dr. Jianwei Qin, Dr. Yanhu Wu, Dr. Lei Wei, Dr. Weidong Gu, Dr. Xiaohu Lu, Dr. Xiangxiang Zheng, Dr. Haoliang Sun, Dr. Luyao Ma, and Dr. Wei Zhang.

Funding
This study was funded by Six major talent Summit of Jiangsu Province (2015-WSW-019) and Shanghai Municipal Commission of Health and Family Planning Fund (201640053).

Authors' contributions
YZ designed the study; WZ, BL, YZ, and FW collected the data; CG, QW, and XW performed the statistical analysis; YZ and BL drafted the manuscript; and YZ revised and proofread the manuscript. All authors read and approved the final manuscript.

Competing interests
The authors declare that they have no competing interests.

Author details
Department of Cardiothoracic Surgery, BenQ Hospital, Affiliated Hospital of Nanjing Medical University, Nanjing, China. ²Department of Cardiology, Shanghai Tenth People's Hospital, Tongji University School of Medicine, Shanghai, China. ³Department of Cardiothoracic Surgery, First Affiliated Hospital of Nanjing Medical University, Nanjing, China. ⁴Department of Gastroenterology, Shanghai Tenth People's Hospital, Tongji University School of Medicine, Shanghai, China. ⁵Department of Thoracic Surgery, Shanghai Chest Hospital, Shanghai Jiao Tong University, Shanghai, China. ⁶The Clinical Medical Department of Nanjing Medical University, Nanjing, China. ⁷Department of Cardiovascular Surgery, Shanghai East Hospital, Tongji University School of Medicine, 150 Jimo Road, Shanghai 200120, China.

References
1. GBD 2015 Mortality and Causes of Death Collaborators. Global, regional, and national life expectancy, all-cause mortality, and cause-specific mortality for 249 causes of death, 1980–2015: a systematic analysis for the Global Burden of Disease Study 2015. Lancet. 2016;388:1459–544. https://doi.org/10.1016/S0140-6736(16)31012-1.
2. Zhang XH, Lu ZL, Liu L. Coronary heart disease in China. Heart. 2008; 94:1126–31.
3. Ferlay J, Soerjomataram I, Dikshit R, Eser S, Mathers C, Rebelo M, Parkin DM, Forman D, Bray F. Cancer incidence and mortality worldwide: sources, methods and major patterns in GLOBOCAN 2012. Int J Cancer. 2015;136: E359–86.

4. Chen WQ, Zheng RS, Zhang SW, Li N, Zhao P, Li GL, Wu LY, He J. Report of incidence and mortality in China cancer registries, 2008. Chin J Cancer Res. 2012;24:171–80.

5. Chassot PG, Delabays A, Spahn DR. Preoperative evaluation of patients with, or at risk of, coronary artery disease undergoing non-cardiac surgery. Br J Anaesth. 2002;89:747–59.

6. Edge SB, Compton CC. The American Joint Committee on Cancer: the 7th edition of the AJCC cancer staging manual and the future of TNM. Ann Surg Oncol. 2010;17:1471–4. https://doi.org/10.1245/s10434-010-0985-4.

7. Stephan F, Boucheseiche S, Hollande J, Flahault A, Cheffi A, Bazelly B, Bonnet F. Pulmonary complications following lung resection: a comprehensive analysis of incidence and possible risk factors. Chest. 2000; 118:1263–70.

8. Fleisher LA, Fleischmann KE, Auerbach AD, Barnason SA, Beckman JA, Bozkurt B, Davila-Roman VG, Gerhard-Herman MD, Holly TA, Kane GC, Marine JE, Nelson MT, Spencer CC, Thompson A, Ting HH, Uretsky BF, Wijeysundera DN. 2014 ACC/AHA guideline on perioperative cardiovascular evaluation and management of patients undergoing noncardiac surgery: executive summary: a report of the American College of Cardiology/ American Heart Association Task Force on Practice Guidelines. Circulation. 2014;130:2215–45.

9. King SB 3rd, Smith SC Jr, Hirshfeld JW Jr, Jacobs AK, Morrison DA, Williams DO, Feldman TE, Kern MJ, O'Neill WW, Schaff HV, Whitlow PL, Acc/Aha/Scai, Adams CD, Anderson JL, Buller CE, Creager MA, Ettinger SM, Halperin JL, Hunt SA, Krumholz HM, Kushner FG, Lytle BW, Nishimura R, Page RL, Riegel B, Tarkington LG, Yancy CW. 2007 focused update of the ACC/AHA/SCAI 2005 guideline update for percutaneous coronary intervention: a report of the American College of Cardiology/American Heart Association Task Force on Practice guidelines. J Am Coll Cardiol. 2008;51:172–209.

10. Kaluza GL, Joseph J, Lee JR, Raizner ME, Raizner AE. Catastrophic outcomes of noncardiac surgery soon after coronary stenting. J Am Coll Cardiol. 2000; 35:1288–94.

11. Suzuki S, Usui A, Yoshida K, Matsuura A, Ichihara T, Ueda Y. Effect of cardiopulmonary bypass on cancer prognosis. Asian Cardiovasc Thorac Ann. 2010;18:536–40.

12. Zhao J, Han Y, Lei J, Zhou Y, Lu Q, Tian F, Yang E, Wang X, Li X. Simultaneous esophagectomy and off-pump coronary artery bypass grafting: a practicable approach with good survival. Dis Esophagus. 2017; 30(1):1–5. https://doi.org/10.1111/dote.12465.

13. Chan J, Rosenfeldt F, Chaudhuri K, Marasco S. Cardiac surgery in patients with a history of malignancy: increased complication rate but similar mortality. Heart Lung Circ. 2012;21:255–9.

14. Canver CC, Bhayana JN, Lajos TZ, Raza ST, Lewin AN, Bergsland J, Mentzer RM Jr. Pulmonary resection combined with cardiac operations. Ann Thorac Surg. 1990;50:796–9.

15. Elami A, Korach A, Rudis E. Lung cancer resection or aortic graft replacement with simultaneous myocardial revascularization without cardiopulmonary bypass. Chest. 2001;119:1941–3.

16. Yang Y, Xiao F, Wang J, Song B, Li XH, Li J, He ZS, Zhang H, Yin L. Simultaneous surgery in patients with both cardiac and noncardiac diseases. Patient Prefer Adherence. 2016;10:1251–8.

17. Chaudhry UA, Harling L, Rao C, Ashrafian H, Ibrahim M, Kokotsakis J, Casula R, Athanasiou T. Off-pump versus on-pump coronary revascularization: meta-analysis of mid- and long-term outcomes. Ann Thorac Surg. 2014;98: 563–72.

18. Nozoe T, Kakeji Y, Baba H, Maehara Y. Two-field lymph-node dissection may be enough to treat patients with submucosal squamous cell carcinoma of the thoracic esophagus. Dis Esophagus. 2005;18:226–9.

19. Ma J, Zhan C, Wang L, Jiang W, Zhang Y, Shi Y, Wang Q. The sweet approach is still worthwhile in modern esophagectomy. Ann Thorac Surg. 2014;97:1728–33.

20. Mariette C, Taillier G, Van Seuningen I, Triboulet JP. Factors affecting postoperative course and survival after en bloc resection for esophageal carcinoma. Ann Thorac Surg. 2004;78:1177–83.

21. Chang AC, Ji H, Birkmeyer NJ, Orringer MB, Birkmeyer JD. Outcomes after transhiatal and transthoracic esophagectomy for cancer. Ann Thorac Surg. 2008;85:424–9.

22. Birkmeyer JD, Siewers AE, Finlayson EV, Stukel TA, Lucas FL, Batista I, Welch HG, Wennberg DE. Hospital volume and surgical mortality in the United States. N Engl J Med. 2002;346:1128–37.

23. Dimick JB, Goodney PP, Orringer MB, Birkmeyer JD. Specialty training and mortality after esophageal cancer resection. Ann Thorac Surg. 2005;80:282–6.

24

Robotic versus laparoscopic surgery for rectal cancer in male urogenital function preservation

Xiaoli Tang[1], Zheng Wang[2], Xiaoqing Wu[2], Meiyuan Yang[1] and Daorong Wang[3*]

Abstract

Background: Urogenital dysfunction after rectal cancer surgery can largely affect patients' postoperative quality of life. Whether robotic surgery can be a better option when comparing with laparoscopic surgery is still not well-known.

Methods: Comprehensive search in PubMed, Embase, Cochrane Library, and Clinical Trials was conducted to identify relevant studies in March 2018. Studies comparing robotic surgery with laparoscopic surgery were included. Measurement of urogenital function was through the International Prostate Symptom Score and International Index of Erectile Function.

Results: Six studies with 386 patients in robotic group and 421 patients in laparoscopic group were finally included. Pooled analysis indicated that bladder function was better at 12 months in the robotic group after the procedures (mean difference, − 0.30, 95% CI, − 0.52 to − 0.08). No significant difference was found at 3 and 6 months postoperatively (mean difference, − 0.37, 95% CI, − 1.48 to 0.73; mean difference, − 1.21, 95% CI, − 2.69 to 0.28). Sexual function was better at 3 months in the robotic group after surgery (mean difference, − 3.28, 95% CI, − 6.08 to − 0.49) and not significantly different at 6 and 12 months. (mean difference, 3.78, 95% CI, − 7.37 to 14.93; mean difference, − 2.82, 95% CI, − 8.43 to 2.80).

Conclusion: Robotic surgery may offer faster recovery in urogenital function compared to laparoscopic surgery for rectal cancer.

Background

Rectal cancer is one of the most common malignant neoplasm worldwide [1, 2]. Great improvement in management of rectal cancer has been made over the past few decades, such as recommendation for early screening in high-risk population and use of adjuvant and neoadjuvant chemotherapy [3–5]. However, even with lots of newly invented treatments, surgery is still the only curative treatment for rectal cancer to achieve radical resection so the patient can gain oncological safety. In the past two decades, minimal invasive surgery like laparoscopy has been accepted worldwide. Existed randomized control trials have proved the certain superiority of laparoscopy over conventional open surgery with equal oncological safety [6–8]. Robotic surgery was first used in colorectal disease in 2001 [9], since then, it has gained great popularity around the world as it overcomes some technical limitations compared to laparoscopic surgery. Although the main goals of rectal surgery are accomplishing adequate distal and circumferential margins, postoperative function outcomes like sexual and urological functions greatly influence postoperative psychological well-being and account for a large part of patients' quality of life [10–13]. Previous studies have illustrated urogenital impairment after rectal surgery with approximately 5% of patients suffer permanent bladder dysfunction or impotence problem [14, 15]. When compared to laparoscopy, whether robotic surgery can be a better option regarding recovery of sexual and urological function is still under great debate. The present study aimed at answering this question with current available evidence by conducting a meta-analysis.

Methods

A comprehensive search was conducted in March 2018 within PubMed, Embase, Cochrane Library, and Clinical Trials. The searching terms were "Colorectal Neoplasms" [Mesh] + "Laparoscopy" [Mesh] + "Robotic Surgical

* Correspondence: wdaorong666@sina.com
[3]Department of General Surgery, The northern Jiangsu people's Hospital, Nantong Road No.98, Yangzhou 225001, China
Full list of author information is available at the end of the article

Procedures" [Mesh] + "sexual dysfunction" or "sexual impairment" + "urological dysfunction" or "urological impairment." Clinical studies from January 2001 till the search day which compared robotic surgery with laparoscopic surgery with sexual or urological outcomes as primary or secondary endpoints were identified for further screening, as well as studies containing a subgroup of participants whose urogenital functions were recorded. We included studies both designed as randomized control trials or observational studies. Non-human papers, comment, letter, correspondence, review, expert opinions, and case reports were excluded. Studies with irrelevant topics and studies with no records regarding sexual and urological function were excluded as well. The screening process was shown in Fig. 1. Two researchers independently screened the articles without any consult. If any disagreement occurred, the article was brought into discussion to decide whether it will be included. Data extraction from each enrolled study mainly included author, year, study design, information feasible for quality evaluation, patients baseline date, tumor-related information, operative procedure, and functional outcomes both preoperatively and postoperatively.

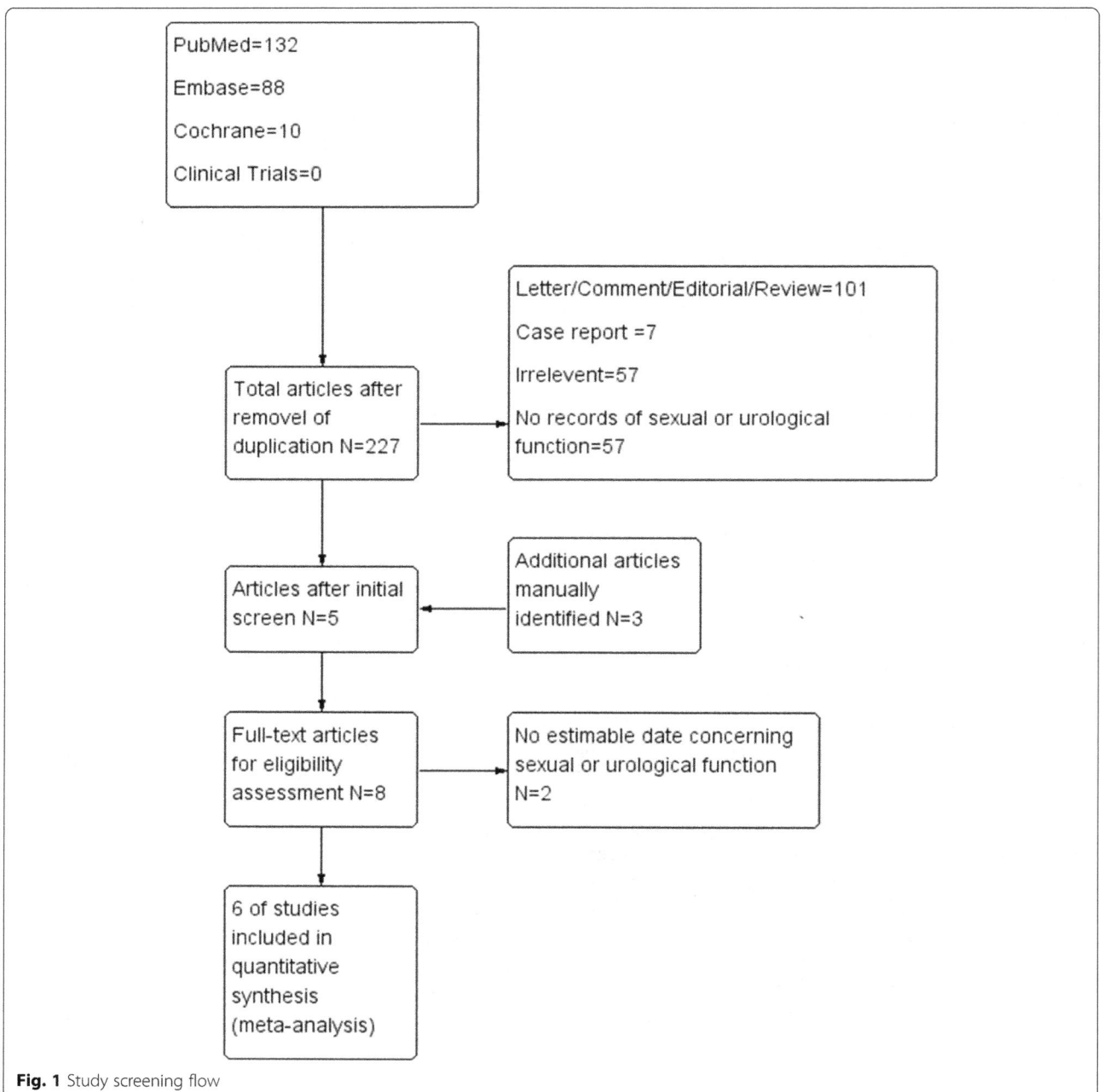

Fig. 1 Study screening flow

Table 1 NOS scale for observational studies

Study	Selection				Comparability	Outcome assessment			Score
	1	2	3	4	5, 6	7	8	9	
D' Annibale 2013	*	*	*	*	*, *	*	*	*	9
Panteleimonitis 2016	*	*	*	*	*, 0	*	*	*	8
Park 2014	*	*	*	*	*, *	*	*	*	9
Kim 2012	*	*	*	*	*, *	*	*	*	9

Explanation
1: Adequate definition of the cases, study-enrolled cases with independent validation. (yes, *; no or not reported, 0)
2: Representative of the cases, consecutive or obviously representative cases. (yes, *; no or not reported, 0)
3: Selection of controls, community controls. (yes, *; no or not reported, 0)
4: Clear definition of the controls, no previous history of the same procedure. (yes, *; no or not reported, 0)
5: Comparability of cases and controls on the basis of the design or analysis, the patients baseline characteristics were similar between different groups. (yes, *; no or not reported, 0)
6: Comparability of cases and controls for other factors, the same type of procedure, the same surgical team to perform the procedure. (yes, *; no or not reported, 0)
7: Ascertainment of exposure, complete surgical records. (yes, *; no or not reported, 0)
8: Same method of ascertainment for cases and controls. (yes, *; no or not reported, 0)
9: Adequacy of follow up of cohorts (yes, *; no or not reported, 0)

The Review Manager software (version 5.3) from Cochrane was used to analyze the extracted data under the instruction of Cochrane handbook.

Results

After screening, six studies [16–21] were included in this meta-analysis. Three hundred and eighty-six patients in total underwent robotic surgery and 421 patients underwent laparoscopic surgery. Among six studies, four of them were retrospectively designed [16–19] and the other two were randomized control trials (RCT) [20, 21]. We used the Newcastle–Ottawa scale to evaluate the quality of observational studies (shown in Table 1) and the risks of bias system from Cochrane to assess the quality of RCTs. Basic characteristics of the studies were summarized in Table 2.

Urological function

All studies used the International Prostate Symptom Score (IPSS) to evaluate the patients urological function mainly concerning seven aspects as bladder emptying, frequency, intermittency, nocturia, urgency, straining, and weak stream. Each aspect of the scale ranges from 0 to 6 points with higher scores indicate worse function. All studies recorded IPSS preoperatively as baseline

status. To minimize heterogeneity among different religions regarding sexual and urological functions, we used the change in the scores from baseline to analyze the difference. Two studies reported IPSSs 3 months after surgery. The pooled estimate indicated that there was no significant difference between the two groups. (mean difference, − 1.21, 95% CI, − 2.69 to 28, $p = 0.11$). No heterogeneity was found among studies. Four studies recorded IPSSs 6 months after the surgery, and the result showed no significant difference between laparoscopy and robotic procedure (mean difference, − 0.37 95% CI − 1.47 to 0.73, $p = 0.51$). Moderate heterogeneity was found among studies with $I^2 = 60\%$, so the random effect model was used and publication bias was detected by conducting the funnel plot (Fig. 5). Four studies reported IPSSs of 12 months after the surgery, and the result favored robotic surgery (mean difference, − 0.30 95% CI, − 0.52 to − 0.08 $p = 0.007$). Almost no heterogeneity was found among studies with $I^2 = 1\%$. Forest plots and funnel plots were shown in Figs. 2, 3, 4, 5, 6, and 7.

Sexual function

All studies used the International Index of Erectile Function (IIEF) score to assess patients' sexual function. The IIEF is a well-recognized self-report questionnaire scale

Table 2 Characteristics of the included studies

Author	Year	Country	Study design	No. of robotic procedures	No. of laparoscopic procedures	Methods of function assessment
Wang	2016	China	RCT	71	66	IPSS, IEFF
Jayne	2017	UK	RCT	175	176	IPSS, IEFF
Panteleimonitis	2016	UK	Retrospective	48	78	IPSS,IEFF
Park	2014	Korea	Retrospective	32	32	IPSS, IEFF
Kim	2012	Korea	Retrospective	30	39	IPSS, IEFF
D'Annibale	2013	Italy	Retrospective	30	30	IPSS, IEFF

Abbreviation: *UK*, United Kingdom; *RCT*, randomized controlled trial; *IPSS*, International Prostate Symptom Score; *IEFF*, International Index of Erectile Function

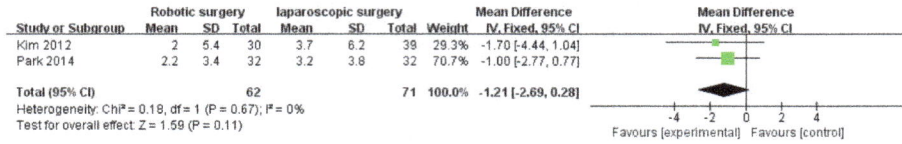

	Robotic surgery			laparoscopic surgery				Mean Difference	Mean Difference
Study or Subgroup	Mean	SD	Total	Mean	SD	Total	Weight	IV, Fixed, 95% CI	IV, Fixed, 95% CI
Kim 2012	2	5.4	30	3.7	6.2	39	29.3%	-1.70 [-4.44, 1.04]	
Park 2014	2.2	3.4	32	3.2	3.8	32	70.7%	-1.00 [-2.77, 0.77]	
Total (95% CI)			62			71	100.0%	-1.21 [-2.69, 0.28]	

Heterogeneity: Chi² = 0.18, df = 1 (P = 0.67); I² = 0%
Test for overall effect: Z = 1.59 (P = 0.11)

Favours [experimental] Favours [control]

Fig. 2 IPSS change from baseline at 3 months postoperatively

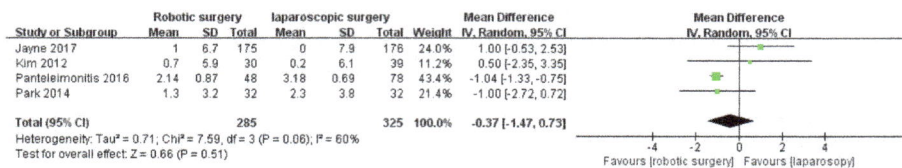

	Robotic surgery			laparoscopic surgery				Mean Difference	Mean Difference
Study or Subgroup	Mean	SD	Total	Mean	SD	Total	Weight	IV, Random, 95% CI	IV, Random, 95% CI
Jayne 2017	1	6.7	175	0	7.9	176	24.0%	1.00 [-0.53, 2.53]	
Kim 2012	0.7	5.9	30	0.2	6.1	39	11.2%	0.50 [-2.35, 3.35]	
Panteleimonitis 2016	2.14	0.87	48	3.18	0.69	78	43.4%	-1.04 [-1.33, -0.75]	
Park 2014	1.3	3.2	32	2.3	3.8	32	21.4%	-1.00 [-2.72, 0.72]	
Total (95% CI)			285			325	100.0%	-0.37 [-1.47, 0.73]	

Heterogeneity: Tau² = 0.71; Chi² = 7.59, df = 3 (P = 0.06); I² = 60%
Test for overall effect: Z = 0.66 (P = 0.51)

Favours [robotic surgery] Favours [laparosopy]

Fig. 3 IPSS change from baseline at 6 months postoperatively

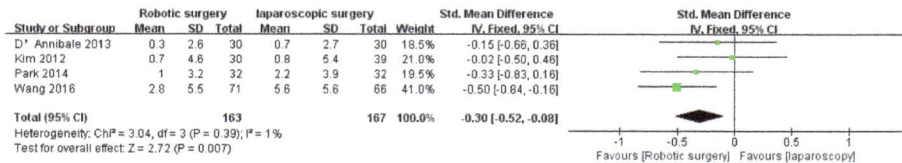

	Robotic surgery			laparoscopic surgery				Std. Mean Difference	Std. Mean Difference
Study or Subgroup	Mean	SD	Total	Mean	SD	Total	Weight	IV, Fixed, 95% CI	IV, Fixed, 95% CI
D' Annibale 2013	0.3	2.6	30	0.7	2.7	30	18.5%	-0.15 [-0.66, 0.36]	
Kim 2012	0.7	4.6	30	0.8	5.4	39	21.0%	-0.02 [-0.50, 0.46]	
Park 2014	1	3.2	32	2.2	3.9	32	19.5%	-0.33 [-0.83, 0.16]	
Wang 2016	2.8	5.5	71	5.6	5.6	66	41.0%	-0.50 [-0.84, -0.16]	
Total (95% CI)			163			167	100.0%	-0.30 [-0.52, -0.08]	

Heterogeneity: Chi² = 3.04, df = 3 (P = 0.39); I² = 1%
Test for overall effect: Z = 2.72 (P = 0.007)

Favours [Robotic surgery] Favours [laparoscopy]

Fig. 4 IPSS change from baseline at 12 months postoperatively

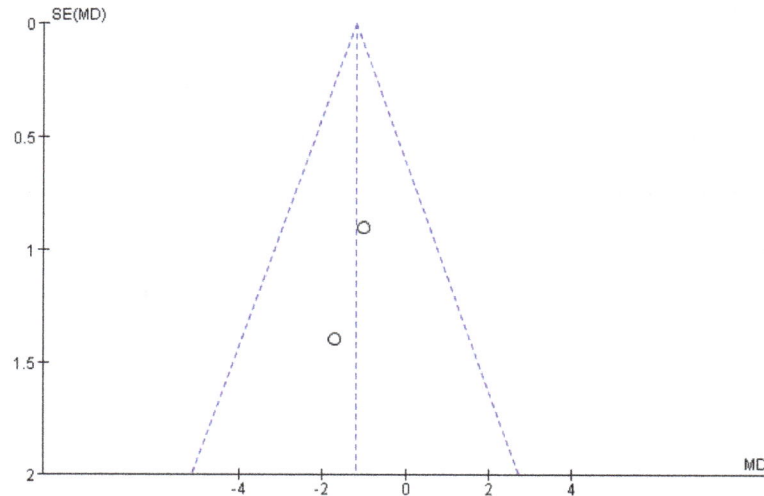

Fig. 5 Funnel plot for IPSS at 3 months

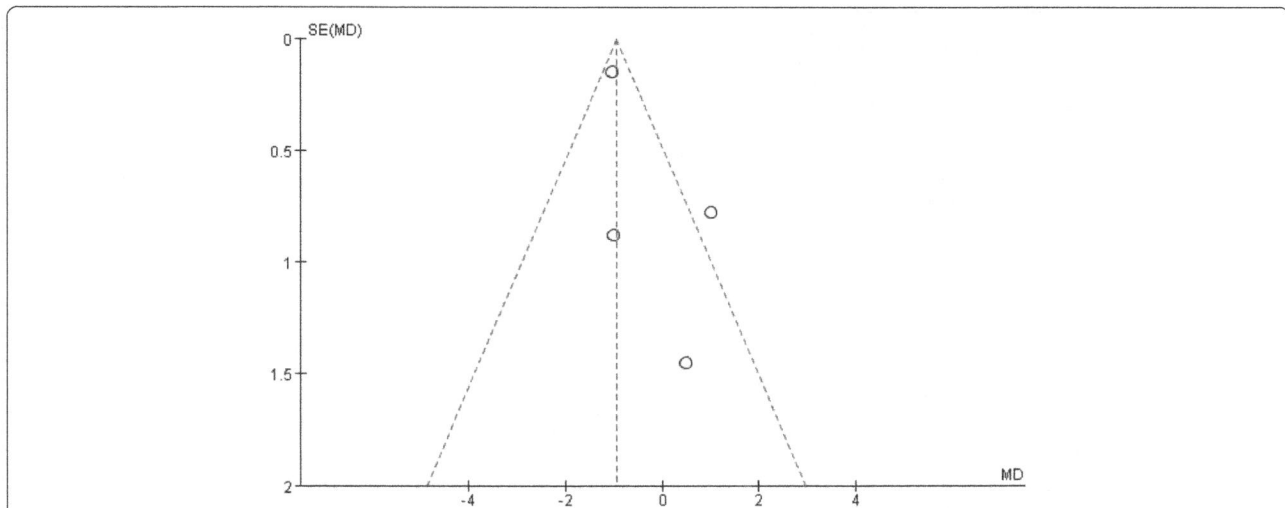

Fig. 6 Funnel plot for IPSS at 6 months

which contains five factors as erectile function, orgasmic function, libido, intercourse satisfaction, and overall satisfaction [22]. The higher scores also indicated better sexual function. To minimize the impact of heterogeneity among different studies, we used the change from baseline date of each study to analyze. Only two studies reported IIEF at 3 months after surgery, and the result favored robotic surgery (mean difference – 3.28, 95% CI – 6.08 to – 0.49, $p = 0.02$). Four studies recorded IIEF scores at 6 months after surgery, and the result showed no significant difference between the two groups (mean difference, 3.78 95% CI – 7.37 to 14.93, $p = 0.51$). Great heterogeneity was found among studies with $I^2 = 99\%$. Two studies reported IIEF scores at 12 months after surgery, and the result showed no significant difference among the two groups (mean difference, – 2.82, 95% CI,

– 8.43 to 2.80). Moderate heterogeneity was found with $I^2 = 42\%$. The forest plots and funnel plots of IIEF were shown in Figs. 8, 9, 10, 11, 12 and 13.

Discussion

Robotic surgery for colorectal cancer has been widely accepted over the past decade. High-quality evidence such as RCTs and meta-analysis has suggested that robotic surgery can achieve oncological safety compared to laparoscopy with lower conversion rate and faster recovery [23, 24]. However, it is still not well explored whether the advantages of robotic surgery can translate into better urogenital function after the procedure. Few previously published meta-analyses have tried to answer this question with available evidence. For the specific topic of urogenital function outcomes, Malene Broholm

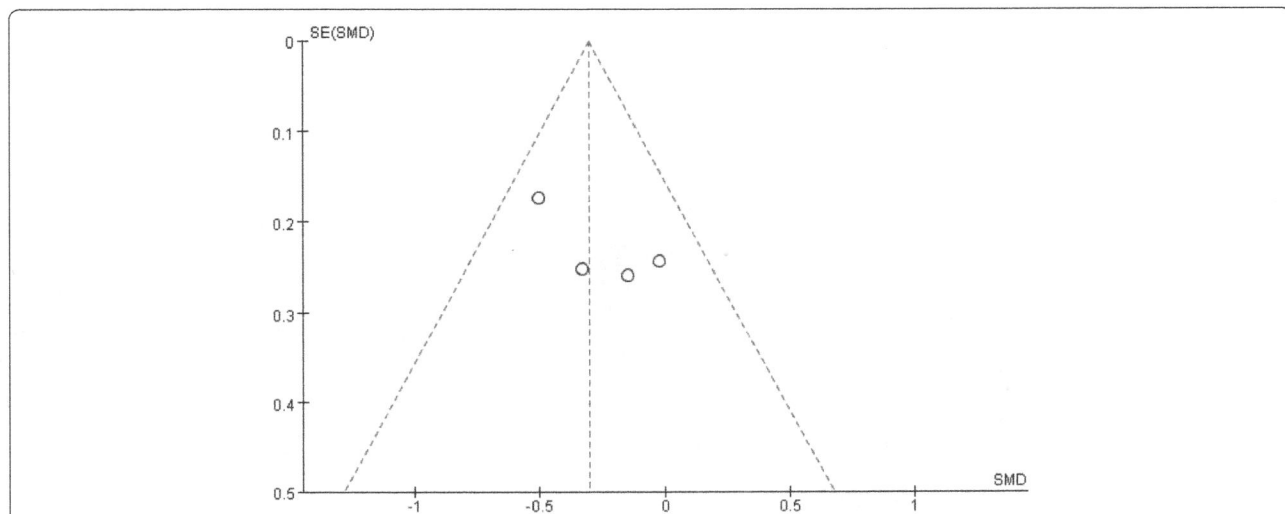

Fig. 7 Funnel plot for IPSS at 12 months

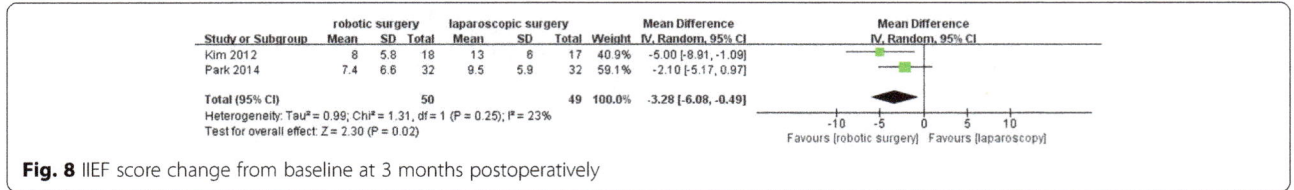

Fig. 8 IIEF score change from baseline at 3 months postoperatively

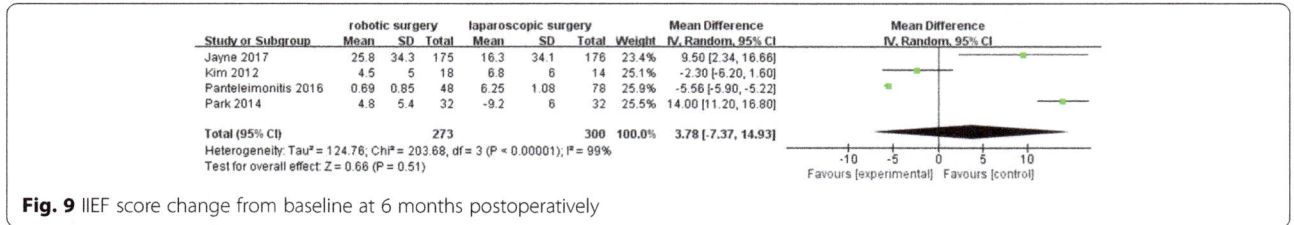

Fig. 9 IIEF score change from baseline at 6 months postoperatively

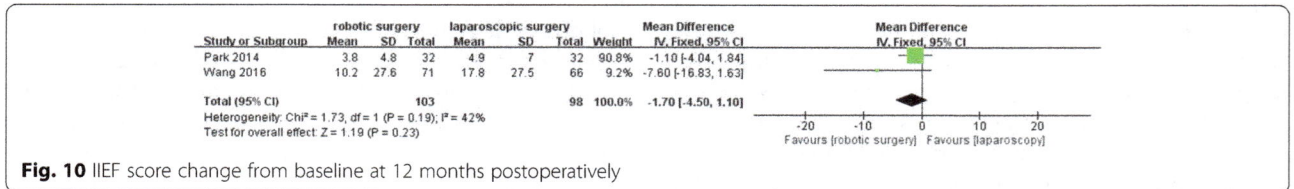

Fig. 10 IIEF score change from baseline at 12 months postoperatively

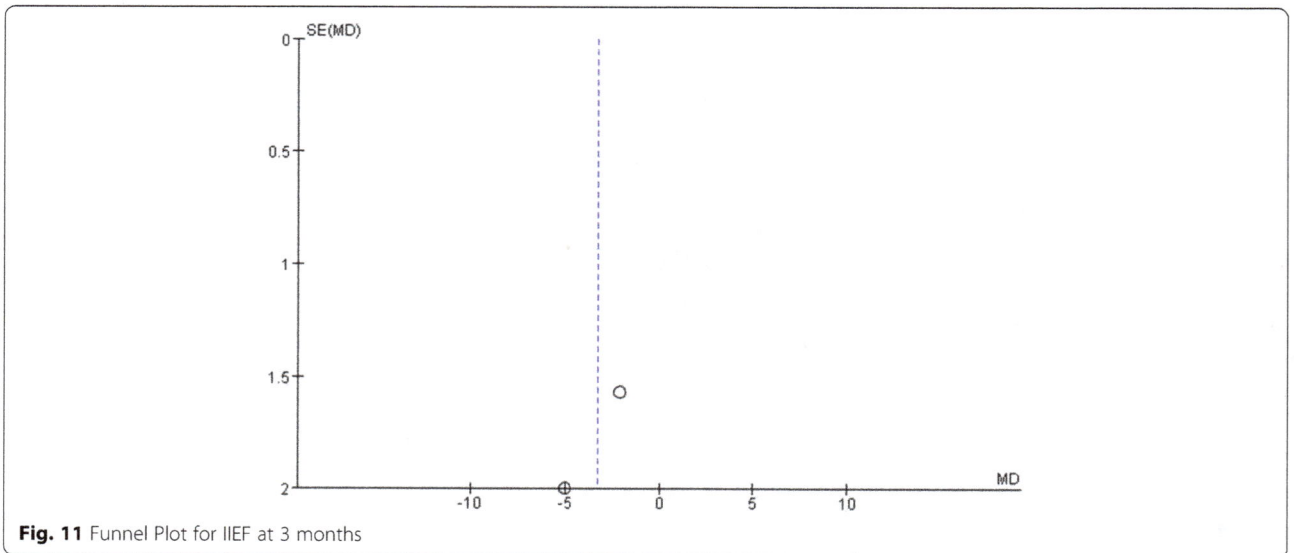

Fig. 11 Funnel Plot for IIEF at 3 months

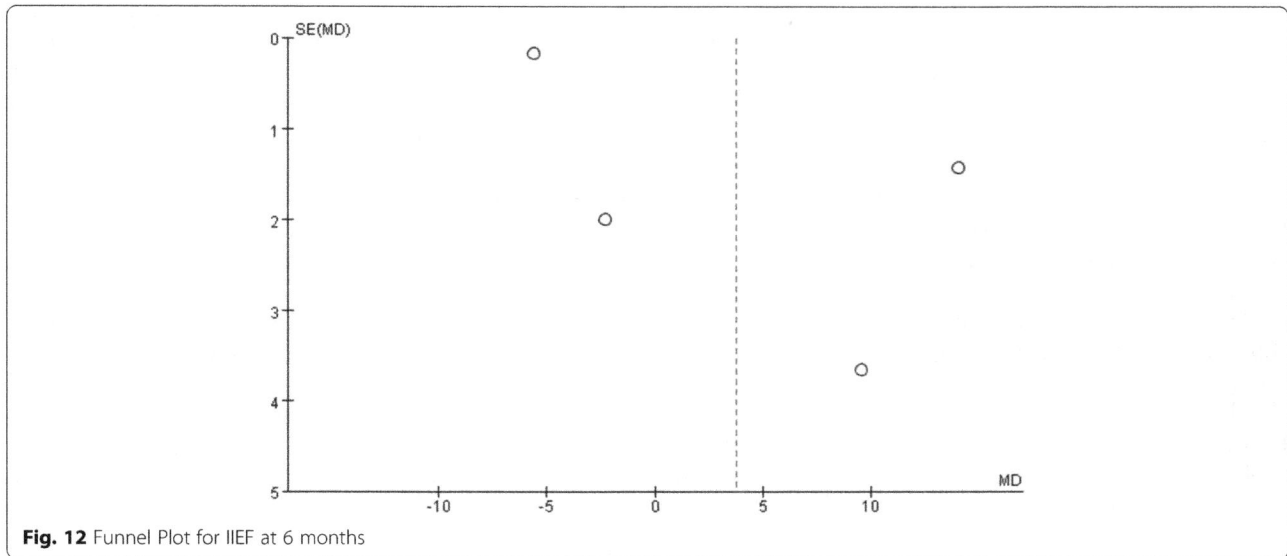

Fig. 12 Funnel Plot for IIEF at 6 months

et al. conducted a meta-analysis with 10 studies enrolled [25]. They suggested that IPSS was better at 3 months and 12 months after surgery in robotic surgery group. As for IIEF score, they found better results in robotic group at both 3 and 6 months after surgery. However, they found that the feasible data from these 10 studies were scarce; thus the results should be interpreted cautiously. Another meta-analysis conducted by Lee et al. found that robotic patients had a better IPSS at 3 months after surgery, but this superiority did not present at 6 months and 12 months [23]. As for sexual function, researchers found that patients in robotic surgery had

better IIEF scores at both 3 and 6 months postoperatively. However, they also claimed limitations in their study, like limited data and vague information about follow-ups. They were also concerned about the impact of equipment learning curve on postoperative outcomes because all the procedures were not performed by the same surgical team. Panteleimonitis et al. did a critical analysis of currently available evidence of urogenital function following robotic surgery for rectal cancer [26]. They searched the literature for studies of robotic surgery without conducting a meta-analysis due to great heterogeneity. They concluded that there seemed to be a

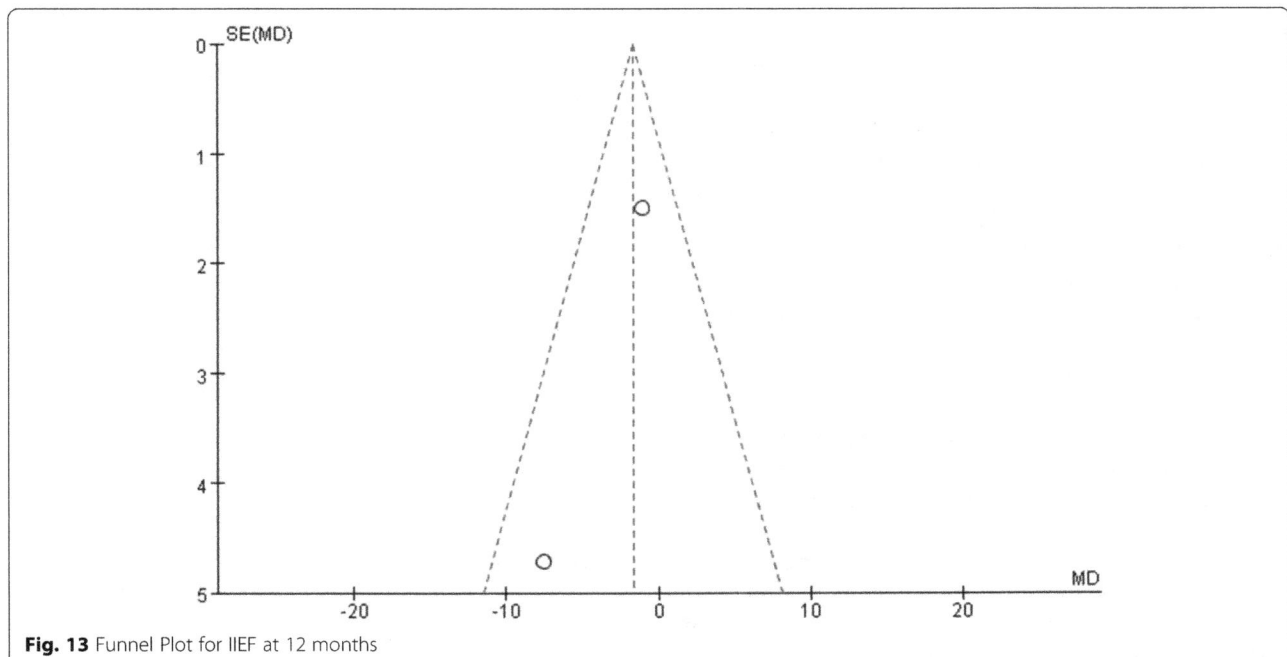

Fig. 13 Funnel Plot for IIEF at 12 months

trend towards better urogenital function following robotic surgery when comparing with laparoscopic surgery. However, they found that many identified studies were not well-designed, so that it was not feasible to form a high-quality evidence based on the situation.

The present study found that IPSSs at 12 months were better after robotic surgery. No significant difference was found between laparoscopic and robotic procedures at 3 and 6 months. However, previous studies have indicated that the minimum perceptible differences detected by IPSS should be more than 3 points [27]. Our result showed that the pooled difference between the two groups was only 0.3. Therefore, this significant difference should be interpreted cautiously. Further evidence with larger samples and more comprehensive investigation of urological function is needed to form a more solid conclusion. As for sexual function recovery, the study found that at 3 months after the procedure, patients that underwent robotic surgery scored better at IIEF. This difference was not found at 6 months and 12 months.

Normal bladder and sexual function were regulated by intact supply of parasympathetic and sympathetic nerve. These regulation nerves usually lie among the pelvic side-walls which make them susceptible to be injured during rectal resection [28]. Although the appearance of urogenital dysfunction is polyfactorial, iatrogenic damage during surgery is thought to be the main cause [29–31]. In addition, urogenital dysfunction after the procedures largely depends on perioperative damage to the autonomic nerve and the site of anastomosis [11, 32]. In conventional laparoscopic surgery, the leading surgeon had to dissect the rectum in a narrow pelvic space with stiff equipment. In these cases, the autonomic nerve lying among the pelvic walls are easily damaged especially when the tumor is bulky [33]. Robotic surgery is supposed to conquer these technical limitations due to its flexible-wristed tremor-free instruments which mimic the surgeon's hands. In addition, based on a stable platform, the camera, which can provide a high-definition 3D image, is easier to control. These advantages should theoretically benefit patients with better nerve preservation, thus better postoperative functional outcomes.

The present meta-analysis has certain limitations. The most important one is that many detail information concerning the height of anastomosis and type of surgery, whether the patients were sexually active before the procedures, are not mentioned in the original studies. We figured that it is one of the reasons for great heterogeneity among studies. In addition, lack of detailed information can also bring great confounding factors which made the result less reliable. Another limitation is scarce data. Although we included newly published studies, the estimable data for each result is still not abundant enough to establish a solid conclusion. However, we did find it crucial to provide necessary education and counseling about possible urogenital dysfunction after rectal surgery to help patients facilitate realistic expectation and psychological preparation, especially in preoperative sexually active patients [34, 35].

Conclusion

Our study formed a primary result that rectal cancer patients underwent robotic surgery may recover faster in urological functions 12 months postoperatively. As for sexual function recovery, patients gained better sexual function at 3 months postoperatively in robotic group while no significant difference was found between robotic surgery and laparoscopic surgery at 6 and 12 months. Future well-designed, larger enrolled participant studies are needed to further address this question for rectal cancer patients.

Abbreviations
CI: Confidence interval; IIEF: International Index of Erectile Function; IPSS: International Prostate Symptom Score; RCT: Randomized control trials

Funding information
The authors received funding from Jiangsu Provincial Science and Technology Department, grant number BE2015664.

Authors' contributions
The paper was written by XT and MY. Study search and screening were done by ZW and XW. Date analysis was done by XT. The whole process was instructed by DW. All authors read and approved the final manuscript.

Competing interests
Xiaoli Tang, Zheng Wang, Xiaoqing Wu, Meiyuan Yang, and Daorong Wang declared that they have no conflict of interest.

Author details
[1]Department of General Surgery, The Second Xiangya Hospital of Central South University, Renmin Road No.139, Changsha 410001, China. [2]Department of General Surgery, Medical College of Yangzhou University, Huaihai Road No.7, Yangzhou 225001, China. [3]Department of General Surgery, The northern Jiangsu people's Hospital, Nantong Road No.98, Yangzhou 225001, China.

Reference
1. Ferlay J, Soerjomataram I, Dikshit R, Eser S, Mathers C, Rebelo M, et al. Cancer incidence and mortality worldwide: sources, methods and major patterns in GLOBOCAN 2012. Int J Cancer. 2015;136(5):E359–86.
2. Siegel R, Desantis C, Jemal A. Colorectal cancer statistics, 2014. CA Cancer J Clin. 2014;64(2):104–17.
3. van de Velde CJ, Boelens PG, Borras JM, Coebergh JW, Cervantes A, Blomqvist L, et al. EURECCA colorectal: multidisciplinary management: European consensus conference colon & rectum. Eur J Cancer. 2014;50(1):1.e–e34.
4. Heald RJ, Ryall RD. Recurrence and survival after total mesorectal excision for rectal cancer. Lancet. 1986;1(8496):1479–82.
5. Heald RJ, Husband EM, Ryall RD. The mesorectum in rectal cancer surgery-- the clue to pelvic recurrence? Br J Surg. 1982;69(10):613–6.
6. Green BL, Marshall HC, Collinson F, Quirke P, Guillou P, Jayne DG, et al. Long-term follow-up of the Medical Research Council CLASICC trial of

conventional versus laparoscopically assisted resection in colorectal cancer. Br J Surg. 2013;100(1):75–82.

7. Jayne DG, Thorpe HC, Copeland J, Quirke P, Brown JM, Guillou PJ. Five-year follow-up of the Medical Research Council CLASICC trial of laparoscopically assisted versus open surgery for colorectal cancer. Br J Surg. 2010;97(11):1638–45.

8. Kuhry E, Schwenk WF, Gaupset R, Romild U, Bonjer HJ. Long-term results of laparoscopic colorectal cancer resection. Cochrane Database Syst Rev. 2008;(2):Cd003432.

9. Weber PA, Merola S, Wasielewski A, Ballantyne GH. Telerobotic-assisted laparoscopic right and sigmoid colectomies for benign disease. Dis Colon Rectum. 2002;45(12):1689–94 discussion 95-6.

10. Traa MJ, De Vries J, Roukema JA, Den Oudsten BL. Sexual (dys)function and the quality of sexual life in patients with colorectal cancer: a systematic review. Ann Oncol. 2012;23(1):19–27.

11. Engel J, Kerr J, Schlesinger-Raab A, Eckel R, Sauer H, Holzel D. Quality of life in rectal cancer patients: a four-year prospective study. Ann Surg. 2003;238(2):203–13.

12. Hassan I, Cima RR. Quality of life after rectal resection and multimodality therapy. J Surg Oncol. 2007;96(8):684–92.

13. Hendren SK, O'Connor BI, Liu M, Asano T, Cohen Z, Swallow CJ, et al. Prevalence of male and female sexual dysfunction is high following surgery for rectal cancer. Ann Surg. 2005;242(2):212–23.

14. Gogenur I, Wittendorff HE, Colstrup H, Rosenberg J, Fischer A. Complications after treatment of colorectal cancer, with special focus on stomas, urological conditions and sexual dysfunction. Ugeskr Laeger. 2005;167(45):4272–5.

15. Donovan KA, Thompson LM, Hoffe SE. Sexual function in colorectal cancer survivors. Cancer Control. 2010;17(1):44–51.

16. Kim JY, Kim NK, Lee KY, Hur H, Min BS, Kim JH. A comparative study of voiding and sexual function after total mesorectal excision with autonomic nerve preservation for rectal cancer: laparoscopic versus robotic surgery. Ann Surg Oncol. 2012;19(8):2485–93.

17. Panteleimonitis S, Ahmed J, Ramachandra M, Farooq M, Harper M, Parvaiz A. Urogenital function in robotic vs laparoscopic rectal cancer surgery: a comparative study. Int J Color Dis. 2017;32(2):241–8.

18. D'Annibale A, Pernazza G, Monsellato I, Pende V, Lucandri G, Mazzocchi P, et al. Total mesorectal excision: a comparison of oncological and functional outcomes between robotic and laparoscopic surgery for rectal cancer. Surg Endosc. 2013;27(6):1887–95.

19. Park SY, Choi GS, Park JS, Kim HJ, Ryuk JP, Yun SH. Urinary and erectile function in men after total mesorectal excision by laparoscopic or robot-assisted methods for the treatment of rectal cancer: a case-matched comparison. World J Surg. 2014;38(7):1834–42.

20. Wang G, Wang Z, Jiang Z, Liu J, Zhao J, Li J. Male urinary and sexual function after robotic pelvic autonomic nerve-preserving surgery for rectal cancer. Int J Med Robot. 2017;13(1).

21. Jayne D, Pigazzi A, Marshall H, Croft J, Corrigan N, Copeland J, et al. Effect of robotic-assisted vs conventional laparoscopic surgery on risk of conversion to open laparotomy among patients undergoing resection for rectal cancer: the ROLARR randomized clinical trial. JAMA. 2017;318(16):1569–80.

22. Rosen RC, Riley A, Wagner G, Osterloh IH, Kirkpatrick J, Mishra A. The international index of erectile function (IIEF): a multidimensional scale for assessment of erectile dysfunction. Urology. 1997;49(6):822–30.

23. Lee SH, Lim S, Kim JH, Lee KY. Robotic versus conventional laparoscopic surgery for rectal cancer: systematic review and meta-analysis. Ann Surg Treat Res. 2015;89(4):190–201.

24. Zhang X, Wei Z, Bie M, Peng X, Chen C. Robot-assisted versus laparoscopic-assisted surgery for colorectal cancer: a meta-analysis. Surg Endosc. 2016;30(12):5601–14.

25. Broholm M, Pommergaard HC, Gogenur I. Possible benefits of robot-assisted rectal cancer surgery regarding urological and sexual dysfunction: a systematic review and meta-analysis. Color Dis. 2015;17(5):375–81.

26. Panteleimonitis S, Ahmed J, Harper M, Parvaiz A. Critical analysis of the literature investigating urogenital function preservation following robotic rectal cancer surgery. World J Gastrointest Surg. 2016;8(11):744–54.

27. Barry MJ. Evaluation of symptoms and quality of life in men with benign prostatic hyperplasia. Urology 2001;58(6 1):25–32; discussion.

28. Leung ALH, Chan WH, Cheung HYS, Lui GKL, Fung JTK, Li MKW. Initial experience on the urogenital outcomes after robotic rectal cancer surgery. Surg Pract. 2013;17(1):13–7.

29. Lange MM, van de Velde CJ. Urinary and sexual dysfunction after rectal cancer treatment. Nat Rev Urol. 2011;8(1):51–7.

30. Havenga K, Enker WE. Autonomic nerve preserving total mesorectal excision. Surg Clin North Am. 2002;82(5):1009–18.

31. Masui H, Ike H, Yamaguchi S, Oki S, Shimada H. Male sexual function after autonomic nerve-preserving operation for rectal cancer. Dis Colon Rectum. 1996;39(10):1140–5.

32. Moriya Y. Function preservation in rectal cancer surgery. Int J Clin Oncol. 2006;11(5):339–43.

33. Quah HM, Jayne DG, Eu KW, Seow-Choen F. Bladder and sexual dysfunction following laparoscopically assisted and conventional open mesorectal resection for cancer. Br J Surg. 2002;89(12):1551–6.

34. Ness RM, Holmes A, Klein R, Greene J, Dittus R. Outcome states of colorectal cancer: identification and description using patient focus groups. Am J Gastroenterol. 1998;93(9):1491–7.

35. Holzer B, Gyasi A, Schiessel R, Rosen HR. Patients' expectations of colorectal surgery for cancer. Color Dis. 2006;8(3):186–91.

25

Clinicopathological characteristics and prognosis of primary appendiceal stromal tumors

Bao Zhang[1†], Guo Liang Zheng[2†] ⓘ, Hai Tao Zhu[2], Yan Zhao[2] and Zhi Chao Zheng[2*]

Abstract

Background: Gastrointestinal stromal tumors (GISTs) account for less than 1% of all gastrointestinal tumors. The biological behaviors of GISTs vary from benign to malignant. GISTs are common in the stomach (55.6%) and small intestine (31.8%), but rarely in the rectum, colon (6%), and other sites (5.5%). Currently, the majority of published reports of primary appendiceal stromal tumors (PASTs) are case reports or case series.

Methods: The PASTs described in this study were identified from a literature review (23 cases) and our center (one case). The relationship between PAST gross types and clinicopathological factors was analyzed and summarized. At the same time, the study also analyzed the related risk factors and survival of PASTs and GISTs.

Results: Twenty-four cases of PASTs were compared with 254 cases of GISTs from our center. The results showed that there was a significant difference between the two groups in tumor size ($P < 0.001$), histological type ($P = 0.013$), CD34 expression ($P < 0.001$), and DOG-1 expression ($P < 0.001$). Disease-free survival (DFS) analysis of 11 cases of PASTs and 227 cases of GISTs found that a comparison of 3-year and 5-year DFS was not statistically significant ($P = 0.894$ and $P = 0.846$, respectively). In the DFS multivariate analysis, tumor mucosal ulceration, tumor size, and NIH risk classification were independent prognostic factors in 3-year and 5-year DFS.

Conclusion: In this study, there was no significance in the survival of patients with appendix and gastric stromal tumors, which we hypothesized to be associated with the low sample size and incomplete follow-up records. Based on this, we conclude that the prognosis of primary appendiceal stromal tumors may be better than gastric tumors, but this needs to be confirmed in further prospective studies.

Keywords: Clinicopathological, Characteristics, Prognosis, PASTs, GISTs

Background

Gastrointestinal stromal tumors (GISTs) account for less than 1% of all gastrointestinal tumors and are generally considered to emanate from the interstitial cells of Cajal (ICCs) [1–3]. GISTs were first termed in 1983 by Mazur and Clark [4], who, using immunohistochemistry (IHC), discovered that the majority of gastric wall tumors are not derived from smooth muscle but instead are of nerve sheath origin. GISTs are classified into spindle

cells (70%), epithelial cells (20%), and mixed cells (10%) by IHC and observation of histological characteristics under light microscopy [5].

The biological behaviors of GISTs vary from benign to malignant. CD117, CD34, and DOG1 expression is usually positive in IHC staining, and thus these proteins are useful when confirming diagnosis [2]. GISTs are common in the stomach (55.6%) and small intestine (31.8%), but rarely in the rectum, colon (6%), and other sites (5.5%) [6]. According to literature reports, PASTs are extremely rare [7] and without specific clinical symptoms. PASTs are often identified because of other diseases of the appendix (such as appendicitis or other tumors) or ileocecal tumor surgery [8]. Therefore, correct diagnoses

* Correspondence: drzhengzhichao1@163.com
†Bao Zhang and Guo Liang Zheng contributed equally to this work.
²Department of Gastric Surgery, Cancer Hospital of China Medical University, Liaoning Cancer Hospital & Institute, No.44 Xiaoheyan Road, Dadong District, Shenyang 110042, Liaoning Province, People's Republic of China
Full list of author information is available at the end of the article

of PASTs are very difficult to obtain prior to surgery. Currently, the majority of published reports of PASTs are case reports or case series. Therefore, this study aimed to assess the clinicopathological features and prognosis of PASTs.

Materials and methods

The cases used in this study were identified through a review of databases and from our center. Cases were retrieved from Chinese and foreign databases. The Chinese databases were China National Knowledge Infrastructure (CNKI) (seven cases), VIP (eight cases), WANFANG DATA (13 cases), while the foreign databases included PubMed (12 cases) and EMBASE (four cases). After data synthesis, 20 reports were filtered [8–27], which included a total of 24 cases. One case of PAST that was identified during autopsy was excluded. From January 2009 to October 2017, our center reported only one case of PAST, a 59-year-old female patient, who received an exploratory laparotomy following the identification of a mass in the right lower quadrant upon CT examination for cervical cancer. During the exploration, a 10-cm-sized tumor was found on the appendix, with the ileocecal valve violated, and the patient received a right hemicolectomy and appendectomy. According to the National Institutes of Health (NIH) primary GIST standard [2, 28], this case was diagnosed as a high-risk appendiceal stromal tumor. Modified NIH risk classification is divided into categories according to tumor size and mitotic phase, as follows: very low risk, low risk, intermediate risk, and high risk [29].

The clinicopathological data of PASTs in this study included age, sex, tumor size, gross type, rupture, local ulceration, histological type, mitotic phase, NIH risk classification, gene mutation types, clinical symptoms, and survival data. For survival analysis, the exclusion criteria were as follows [30]: (1) stromal tumors with other sites, (2) the presence of other malignancies, (3) preoperative chemotherapy with imatinib, (4) no follow-up data, and (5) tumor rupture or metastasis before surgery. And inclusion criteria including (1) postoperative pathological diagnosis were PASTs and (2) R0 excision.

Statistical analysis was performed using SPSS 19.0 (SPSS Inc., USA). In this study, numerical variables were expressed as the mean ± SD. The χ^2-test and Fisher exact test were applied to identify differences in clinicopathological parameters between GISTs and PASTs. Risk factors for survival were identified by univariate analysis and multivariate analysis using the Cox proportional hazards regression model. Estimations for disease-free survival (DFS: defined as the time from surgery to disease recurrence/death (months)) were obtained using the Kaplan-Meier method, and differences between Kaplan-Meier curves were investigated by log-rank test. P values of < 0.05 were considered to be statistically significant.

Results

The clinicopathological features of the PASTs are shown in Table 1. A total of 24 cases of PASTs were included in this study. The patients' age ranged from 7 to 88 years old (median, 59.17 years old) and tumor size ranged from 10 to 100 mm in maximum diameter; 11 cases exhibited tumors of less than 2 cm in diameter (45.8%) and only four cases (16.7%) were larger than 100 mm. Twenty tumors were solid (83.3%), and others were cystic (16.7%). Intraoperative exploration found that two cases of PASTs were ruptured, and appendix ulceration occurred in one case. The pathological results of the cases were spindle type (21/24, 87.5%), epithelial type (2/24, 8.3%), and mixed type (1/24, 4.2%). Only 17 of the 24 patients reported a mitotic index, with ≤ 5/50 HPF (high power field) in 14 cases (82.4%) and > 5/50 HPF in three cases (17.6%). Immunohistochemistry showed that 23 cases were CD117-positive (23/24, 95.8%), 15 were CD34-positive (15/20, 75%), and three were DOG-1-positive (3/5, 60%). There were only three cases with a mutation in exon 11 of gene encoding *KIT* and two wild-type mutations in all of the studies. According to the modified NIH risk classification and literature reports, 11 patients were at very low risk (45.8%), two patients were low-risk (8.3%), four patients were at intermediate risk (16.7%), and seven patients were at high risk (29.2%).

The relationship between PAST gross types and clinicopathological factors were analyzed and are summarized in Table 2. According to the results of the analysis, there is no statistical significance ($P > 0.05$). We suspect that this may be related to the low sample size. The clinicopathological factors of 24 cases of PASTs such as age, sex, tumor size, histological type, mitotic index, CD117 expression, CD34 expression, DOG-1 expression, ulceration, and NIH risk classification were compared with 254 cases of GISTs from our center (Table 3). The results showed that there were significant differences between the two groups in tumor size ($P < 0.001$), histological type ($P = 0.013$), CD34 expression ($P < 0.001$), and DOG-1 expression ($P < 0.001$).

Finally, the survival data of 11 cases were selected for analysis according to the exclusion criteria. These patients had a DFS ranging from 4 to 96 months and a median DFS of 29 months (mean, 37.23 ± 34.10 months). The 3-year and 5-year DFS rates were 45.5% and 18.2%, respectively. The DFS of PAST patients was analyzed using Kaplan-Meier survival analysis and is shown in Fig. 1. Analysis of 11 cases of PASTs and 227 cases of GISTs

Table 1 Clinicopathological characteristics of 24 cases of PASTs

Characteristics	N(%)
Age (year)/($\Sigma = 24$)	
<59	11(45.8)
≥59	13(54.2)
Sex ($\Sigma = 24$)	
Male	14(58.3)
Female	10(41.7)
Tumor size (cm)/($\Sigma = 24$)	
≤2	11(45.8)
2.1–5.0	1(4.2)
5.1–10	8(33.3)
>10	4(16.7)
Gross type ($\Sigma = 24$)	
Solid	20(83.3)
Mixed	4(16.7)
Cystic	0(0.0)
Histologic type ($\Sigma = 24$)	
Spindle	21(87.5)
Epithelioid	2(8.3)
Mixed	1(4.2)
Lymph node metastasis ($\Sigma = 24$)	
Yes	1(4.2)
No	23(95.8)
Mitotic index(%)/($\Sigma = 17$)	
≤5	14(82.4)
>5	3(17.6)
Ki-67(%)/($\Sigma = 6$)	
<5	4(66.7)
≥5	2(33.3)
Immunohistochemistry ($\Sigma = 24$)	
CD117 ($\Sigma = 24$)	23(95.8)
CD34 ($\Sigma = 20$)	15(75.0)
DOG-1 ($\Sigma = 5$)	3(60.0)
SMA ($\Sigma = 17$)	4(23.5)
S-100 ($\Sigma = 24$)	7(29.2)
Mutational status ($\Sigma = 5$)	
Kit	3(60.0)
PDGFRA	0(0.0)
Wild type	2(40.0)
SDHB	0(0.0)
NIH risk category ($\Sigma = 24$)	
Very low risk	11(45.8)
Low risk	2(8.3)
Intermediate risk	4(16.7)
High risk	7(29.2)

Table 1 Clinicopathological characteristics of 24 cases of PASTs (Continued)

Characteristics	N(%)
Rupture ($\Sigma = 24$)	
Yes	2(8.3)
No	22(91.7)
Ulceration ($\Sigma = 24$)	
Yes	1(4.2)
No	23(95.8)
Symptoms ($\Sigma = 24$)	
Appendicitis	14(58.3)
Abdominal distension or pain or mass	17(70.8)
Hematochezia or anemia	3(12.5)
Nausea or emesis	3(12.5)
Others	6(25.0)

PASTs primary appendiceal stromal tumors, *NIH* National Institute of Health

found that the two groups of 3-year and 5-year DFS were not statistically significant ($P = 0.894$ and $P = 0.846$, respectively) (Fig. 2). In the DFS multivariate analysis (Table 4), tumor mucosal ulceration, tumor size, and NIH risk classification were independent prognostic factors in both groups.

Discussion

This study represented the largest number of PAST cases analyzed thus far. The clinicopathological features and prognosis of PASTs were statistically analyzed, and the survival rate of appendiceal stromal tumors was compared with that of gastric stromal tumors treated at our center; no difference was found between the two groups.

PASTs are extremely rare, constituting approximately 0.1% of all cancer diagnoses [7]. Other tumors also identified in the appendix include leiomyosarcoma, gastrointestinal stromal tumor, Kaposi's sarcoma, granular cell tumor, gangliocytic paraganglioma, schwannoma, lipoma, hemangioma, and neural tumors. While PASTs are infrequently diagnosed, they cannot be neglected.

GISTs are generally considered to emanate from the interstitial cells of Cajal (ICC), which are pacemaker cells that regulate gut motility [31]. At present, there is no report about the origin of appendix stromal tumors. However, the appendix is part of the digestive tract, and thus gastrointestinal tumor data may have been combined with previously confirmed cases of appendix stromal tumors. We speculate that ICCs or ICC-like cells and multipotential mesenchymal stem cells also exist in the appendix. Of course, this conjecture requires further relative research to corroborate it.

PASTs usually present with nonspecific or appendicitis-like symptoms and lack of corresponding hematology detection

Table 2 The relationship between gross type and clinicopathologic characteristics of PASTs

Characteristics	Solid	Cystic	Mixed	P
Age (year)/($\Sigma = 24$)				0.637
<59	9	0	2	
≥ 59	11	0	2	
Sex ($\Sigma = 24$)				0.094
Male	10	0	4	
Female	10	0	0	
Tumor size (cm)/($\Sigma = 24$)				0.112
≤ 2	11	0	0	
2.1–5.0	1	0	0	
5.1–10	6	0	2	
>10	2	0	2	
Histologic type ($\Sigma = 24$)				0.064
Spindle	18	0	3	
Epithelioid	0	0	1	
Mixed	2	0	0	
Mitotic index (%)/($\Sigma = 24$)				0.115
≤ 5	18	0	2	
>5	2	0	2	
Ki-67(%)/($\Sigma = 6$)				0.445
<5	4	0	0	
≥ 5	2	0	0	
NIH risk category ($\Sigma = 24$)				0.089
VLR	11	0	0	
VL	2	0	0	
IR	2	0	2	
HR	5	0	2	
Ulceration ($\Sigma = 24$)				0.167
Yes	0	0	1	
No	20	0	3	

Table 3 Comparison of clinicopathologic parameters between GISTs and PASTs

Characteristics	Appendix ($N = 24$)	Gastric ($N = 254$)	P
Age (year)			0.697
< 59	11.00	106	
≥ 59	13.00	148	
Sex			0.335
Male	14.00	122	
Female	10.00	132	
Tumor size (cm)			0.000
≤ 2	11.00	31	
2.1–5.0	1.00	90	
5.1–10	8.00	88	
> 10	4.00	43	
Censored	0.00	2	
Histologic type			0.013
Spindle	21.00	232	
Epithelioid	2.00	20	
Mixed	1.00	0	
Censored	0.00	2	
Mitotic index (%)			0.111
≤ 5	20.00	158	
> 5	4.00	89	
Censored	0.00	7	
CD117			0.556
+	23.00	226	
−	1.00	24	
Undetected	0.00	4	
CD34			
+	15.00	236	
−	4.00	12	0.000
Undetected	5.00	6	
DOG-1			0.000
+	3.00	182	
−	2.00	29	
Undetected	19.00	43	
Ulceration			0.008
Yes	1.00	74	
No	23.00	164	
Censored	0.00	16	
NIH risk category			0.000
VLR	11.00	24	
VL	2.00	66	
IR	4.00	75	
HR	7.00	88	
Censored	0.00	1	

marker. Therefore, correct diagnoses of PASTs are very difficult to obtain prior to surgery. In general, CT and magnetic resonance imaging (MRI) are the first choice to study tumor location and extension [32]. If the tumor is small, it is more difficult to find using CT or MRI, and because of their special anatomical structure, current endoscopy approaches are not yet suitable for this tumor type. The appendiceal small stromal tumors identified in our cases resulted from other diseases of the appendix (such as appendicitis or other tumors) or ileocecal tumor surgery. When tumor volume is large, it is not difficult to identify them using CT or MRI. Ultrasound or CT-guided fine needle aspiration (US/CT-FNA) may be helpful for the diagnosis of PASTs.

Immunohistochemical staining is useful to confirm the diagnosis of stromal tumors [33–35]. In GISTs, the

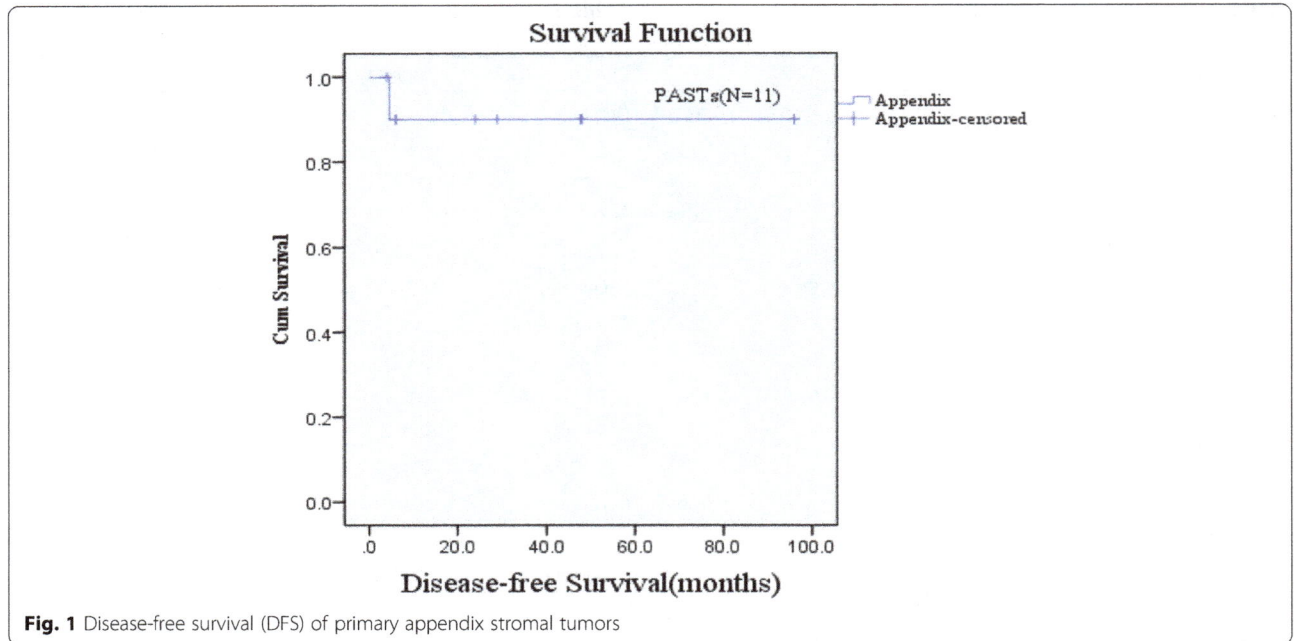

Fig. 1 Disease-free survival (DFS) of primary appendix stromal tumors

positive rate of CD34 is about 50–80% and that of CD117 is 80–100% [36, 37]. The results of this study are similar, with 75% of cases CD34-positive and 95.8% CD117-positive. It has been shown that DOG-1 protein is characterized by high sensitivity (89%) and specificity (94.8%) relative to stromal tumor cell GISTs [33, 38], which is quite different to the results of our study,

probably because of the low detection rate of DOG-1 (only five cases were tested). It was reported that *KIT* and *PDGFRA* gene mutations occurred in approximately 78.5% and 5–8% of GISTs, respectively [39]. In this study, there were only five cases of mutations (three cases of exon 11 mutations and two cases of wild type); thus, we did not study the gene mutation types further.

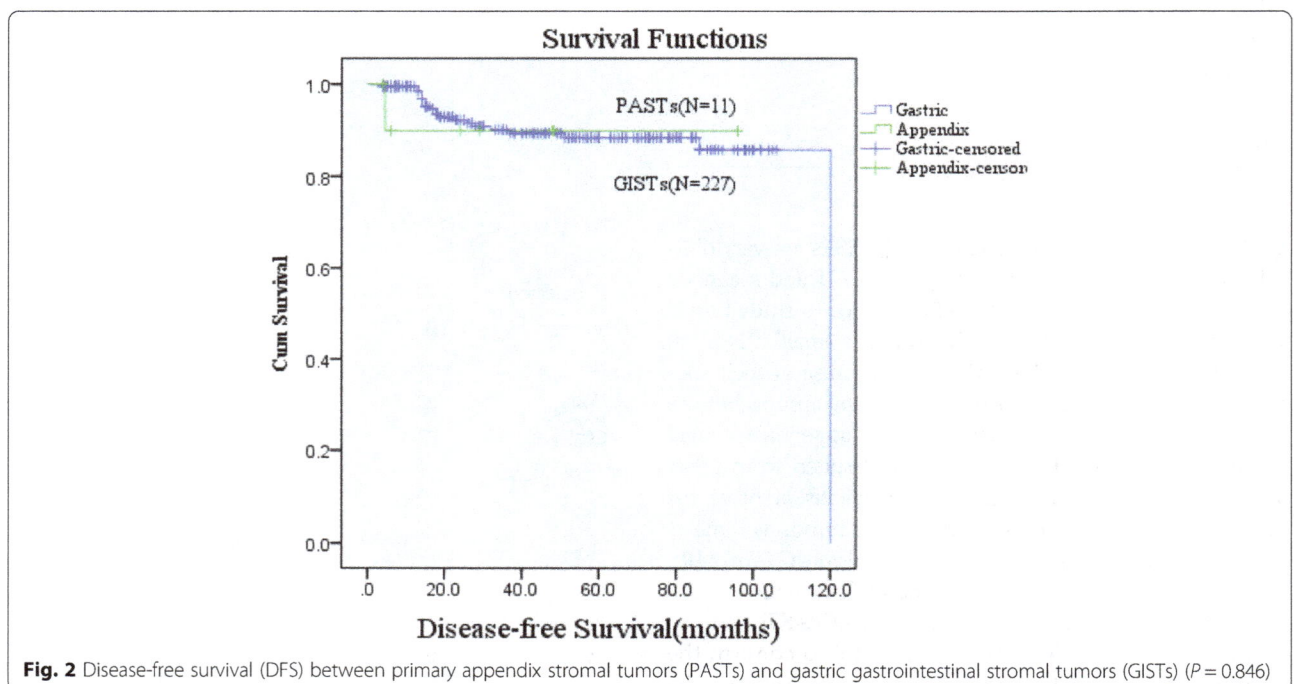

Fig. 2 Disease-free survival (DFS) between primary appendix stromal tumors (PASTs) and gastric gastrointestinal stromal tumors (GISTs) (*P* = 0.846)

Table 4 Univariate and multivariate analyses of prognostic factors for PASTs and GISTs

Prognostic factors	Univariate analysis			Multivariate analysis		
	β	HR(95%CI)	P	β	HR(95%CI)	P
DFS						
Age	0.633	1.883(0.730–4.860)	0.191			
Sex	−1.008	0.365(0.142–0.941)	0.037			
Location	0.192	1.210(0.162–9.030)	0.852			
Ulceration	−0.842	0.431(0.247–0.751)	0.003	−0.697	0.498(0.271–0.915)	0.025
Tumor size	−1.731	0.177(0.059–0.529)	0.002	1.054	2.868(1.166–7.054)	0.022
Mitotic index	1.569	4.802(1.952–11.814)	0.001			
Histologic type	1.249	3.488(1.380–8.816)	0.008			
NIH risk category	1.129	3.093(1.649–5.801)	0.000	0.955	2.598(1.402–4.815)	0.002

DFS disease-free survival

Complete surgical resection with negative microscopic margins is the standard treatment for GISTs [30, 40].Vassos et al [8] found that simple appendectomy was the standard treatment for most cases that were located in the body or tail of the appendix. In some cases, resection of adjacent tissue and organs or the base of the cecum may be necessary for complete removal of the tumor to minimize the risk of local recurrence. Chinese guidelines for the diagnosis and treatment of gastrointestinal stromal tumors indicate that lesions of less than 5 cm in diameter located in favorable anatomic sites, such as the greater curvature or anterior wall of gastric body and fundus, can be considered by laparoscopic method [41]. Considering the pathological features of cases in this study, 11 were small stromal tumors (45.8%) and more than half (54.2%) were located in the body or tail; thus, laparoscopic appendectomy may be feasible. However, relevant prospective clinical studies are needed to further confirm the feasibility and safety of laparoscopic surgery of PASTs. Since tumor rupture is an independent adverse prognostic factor [2, 28], surgery should follow the principle of "no touch, less compression." Endoscopic application of an "extract bag" to avoid tumor rupture and spillage should be performed [41–43], and open surgery for resectable and over-sized stromal tumors is necessary.

It has been reported that tumor size, mitotic index, and tumor location are the best prognostic indicators for determining the malignant potential of GISTs [44], but the prognosis of appendix stromal tumors has not been described. The results of the multivariate analysis performed in this study showed that tumor ulcers, tumor size, and NIH grading were independent prognostic factors, and we compared the survival of appendix and gastric stromal tumors as well. However, since there are minimal overall survival (OS) data on appendix stromal tumors in these cases, we only performed a DFS analysis. There was no statistically significant difference in DFS between PASTs and GISTs. At present, because of the low numbers of appendix stromal tumor cases and incomplete follow-up records, the survival analysis of the present study may be different from the real clinical situation.

The current study has some limitations. This is a retrospective study with a short follow-up time, so the data integrity is limited. The sample size is not large enough, and some appendix stromal tumors are less than 1 cm in diameter, which will lead to sampling errors. Because the number of stromal tumor cases identified in other locations were limited at our center (particularly lower gastrointestinal stromal tumors), they could not be compared with appendix clinical pathology and survival characteristics.

Conclusions

In this study, most of the PASTs were solid (20/24, 83.3%); there were no cystic cases, and most of the pathological diagnosis of PASTs were spindle cells (21/24, 87.5%). According to the NIH classification criteria, the median risk was more than 50% (13/24, 54.2%). By analyzing the data of PASTs and GISTs from our center, we found that there was a significant statistical difference between tumor size, histological type, CD34 expression, DOG-1 expression, ulceration, and NIH grade. Only one patient died of postoperative lymph node metastases in all selected cases. Rutkowski et al. [45] reported that the location of the primary tumor is an independent prognostic factor that affects the prognosis of GISTs. However, in this study, there was no significance in the survival of patients with appendix and gastric stromal tumors, which we hypothesized to be associated with the low sample size and incomplete follow-up records. Based on this, we conclude that the prognosis of primary appendiceal stromal tumors may be better than gastric tumors, but this needs to be confirmed in further prospective studies.

Acknowledgements
We thank the Liaoning Cancer Hospital & Institute, the Dept. of Gastric Surgery (Zhichao Zheng, PhD) for kind permission to use clinical data.

Funding
None.

Authors' contributions
BZ and GLZ contributed equally to the study. BZ planned the study, oversaw the study data collection and analysis, and wrote the manuscript. GLZ provided input into the data collection and analysis and helped write the manuscript. HTZ, YZ, and ZCZ modified and edited the manuscript. All authors approved the final manuscript.

Competing interests
The authors declare that they have no competing interests.

Author details
[1]China Medical University, No.77 Puhe Road, Shenbei New District, Shenyang 110013, Liaoning Province, People's Republic of China. [2]Department of Gastric Surgery, Cancer Hospital of China Medical University, Liaoning Cancer Hospital & Institute, No.44 Xiaoheyan Road, Dadong District, Shenyang 110042, Liaoning Province, People's Republic of China.

References

1. Sircar K, Hewlett BR, Huizinga JD, Chorneyko K, Berezin I, Riddell RH. Interstitial cells of Cajal as precursors of gastrointestinal stromal tumors. Am J Surg Pathol. 1999;23(4):377.
2. Lim KT, Tan KY. Current research and treatment for gastrointestinal stromal tumors. World J Gastroenterol. 2017;23(27):4856–66.
3. Kindblom LG, Remotti HE, Aldenborg F, Meis-Kindblom JM. Gastrointestinal pacemaker cell tumor (GIPACT): gastrointestinal stromal tumors show phenotypic characteristics of the interstitial cells of Cajal. Am J Pathol. 1998; 152:1259–69.
4. Mazur MT, Clark HB. Gastric stromal tumors. Reappraisal of histogenesis. Am J Surg Pathol. 1983;7(6):507–19.
5. Corless CL, Fletcher JA, Heinrich MC. Biology of gastrointestinal stromal tumors. Journal of Clinical Oncology. Proc Am Soc Clin Oncol. 2004;22(18): 3813.
6. Søreide K, Sandvik OM, Søreide JA, Giljaca V, Jureckova A, Bulusu VR. Global epidemiology of gastrointestinal stromal tumours (GIST): a systematic review of population-based cohort studies. Cancer Epidemiol. 2016;40:39–46.
7. Misdraji J, Graemecook FM. Miscellaneous conditions of the appendix. Semin Diagn Pathol. 2004;21(2):151–63.
8. Vassos N, Agaimy A, Günther K, Hohenberger W, Schneider-Stock R, Croner RS. A novel complex KIT mutation in a gastrointestinal stromal tumor of the vermiform appendix. Hum Pathol. 2013;44(4):651–5.
9. Guo ALWZQ, Wang W. A case of low grade appendix malignant stromal tumor. Chin J Pathol. 2001;03:29.
10. Miettinen M, Sobin LH. Gastrointestinal stromal tumors in the appendix: a clinicopathologic and immunohistochemical study of four cases. Am J Surg Pathol. 2001;25(11):1433–7.
11. He JFLSL. A case of malignant tumor of appendix. Chin J Pathol. 2002;02:31.
12. Wu YQWY. A case of misdiagnosis of malignant stromal tumors in the ileocecal region. Chin J Misdiagnostics. 2004;04:639.
13. Yap WM, Tan HW, Goh SG, Chuah KL. Appendiceal gastrointestinal stromal tumor. Am J Surg Pathol. 2005;29(11):1545–7.
14. Guo HNLXM, Huang JYWJX. One case of giant low grade gastrointestinal stromal tumor of appendix. J Diag PAthol. 2006;1:48.
15. Kyu-Jong K, Park S, Park S, Hyun B, Kwon C. Gastrointestinal stromal tumor of appendix incidentally diagnosed by appendiceal hemorrhage. World J Gastroenterol. 2007;13(23):3265 7.
16. Agaimy A, Pelz AF, Wieacker P, Roessner A, Wünsch PH, Schneider-Stock R. Gastrointestinal stromal tumors of the vermiform appendix: clinicopathologic, immunohistochemical, and molecular study of 2 cases with literature review. Hum Pathol. 2008;39(8):1252–7.
17. Agaimy A, Wünsch PH, Dirnhofer S, Bihl MP, Terracciano LM, Tornillo L. Microscopic gastrointestinal stromal tumors in esophageal and intestinal surgical resection specimens: a clinicopathologic, immunohistochemical, and molecular study of 19 lesions. Am J Surg Pathol. 2008;32(6):867–73.
18. Elazary R, Schlager A, Khalaileh A, Appelbaum L, Bala M, Abu-Gazala M, Khatib A, Neuman T, Rivkind AI, Almogy G. Malignant appendiceal GIST: case report and review of the literature. J Gastrointest Cancer. 2010; 41(1):9–12.
19. Yang F. A case of Appendiceal stromal tumor. Chin Health Care Nutrition. 2012;22(14):2647.
20. Tran S, Dingeldein M, Mengshol SC, Kay S, Chin AC. Incidental GIST after appendectomy in a pediatric patient: a first instance and review of pediatric patients with CD117 confirmed GISTs. Pediatr Surg Int. 2014;30(4):457–66.
21. Back J, Jeanty J, Landas S. Gastrointestinal stromal tumor of the appendix: case report and review of the literature. Human Pathology Case Reports. 2015;2(4):94–8.
22. Luo WXZHH, Cui XHLDN, et al. Misdiagnosis of stromal tumors of gynecological tumors in 2 cases and literature review. Chin J Clin Obstet Gynecol. 2015;16(01):75–6.
23. Pan YLXY. A case of low grade appendix malignant stromal tumor. Chin J Postgrad Med (z1). 2015:193–4.
24. Zhu CY, Zhu YM. Gastrointestinal stromal tumor of the vermiform appendix: a case report and literature review. World Chin J Digestol. 2015;23(1):176.
25. Rahimi K, Gologan A, Haliotis T, Lamoureux E, Chetty R. Gastrointestinal stromal tumor with autonomic nerve differentiation and coexistent mantle cell lymphoma involving the appendix. Int J Clin Exp Pathol. 2009;2(6):608–13.
26. Chung JC, Song OP. Gastrointestinal stromal tumor of the appendix. Turk J Gastroenterol. 2012;23:303–4.
27. Bouassida M, Chtourou MF, Chalbi E, Chebbi F, Hamzaoui L, Sassi S, et al. Appendiceal GIST: report of an exceptional case and review of the literature. Pan Afr Med J. 2013;15:85.
28. Fletcher CD, Berman JJ, Corless C, Gorstein F, Lasota J, Longley BJ, Miettinen M, O'Leary TJ, Remotti H, Rubin BP. Diagnosis of gastrointestinal stromal tumors: a consensus approach. Hum Pathol. 2002;33(5):459–65.
29. Joensuu H. Risk stratification of patients diagnosed with gastrointestinal stromal tumor. Hum Pathol. 2008;39:1411–9.
30. Liu Z, Tian Y, Xu G, Liu S, Guo M, Lian X, et al. Pancreatic gastrointestinal stromal tumor: clinicopathologic features and prognosis. J Clin Gastroenterol. 2017;51:850–6.
31. Miettinen M, Lasota J. Gastrointestinal stromal tumors: pathology and prognosis at different sites. Semin Diagn Pathol. 2006;23(2):70–83.
32. Demetri GD, Von MM, Antonescu CR, Dematteo RP, Ganjoo KN, Maki RG, Pisters PW, Raut CP, Riedel RF, Schuetze S. NCCN task force report: update on the management of patients with gastrointestinal stromal tumors. J Natl Compr Canc Netw Jnccn 8 Suppl. 2010;2(4):S1.
33. Lopes LF, West RB, Bacchi LM, Van dRM, Bacchi CE. DOG1 for the diagnosis of gastrointestinal stromal tumor (GIST): comparison between 2 different antibodies. Appl Immunohistochem Mol Morphol. 2010;18(4):333–7.
34. Miettinen M, Lasota J. Gastrointestinal stromal tumors: review on morphology, molecular pathology, prognosis, and differential diagnosis. Arch Pathol Lab Med. 2006;130:1466–78.
35. Rubin BP, Cooper K, Fletcher CD, Folpe AL, Gannon FH, Hunt JL, et al. Protocol for the examination of specimens from patients with tumors of soft tissue. Arch Pathol Lab Med. 2010;134:e31–9.
36. Hirota S, Isozaki K, Moriyama Y, Hashimoto K, Nishida T, Ishiguro S, Kawano K, Hanada M, Kurata A, Takeda M. Gain-of-function mutations of c-kit in human gastrointestinal stromal tumors. Science. 1998;279(5350):577.
37. Sarlomo-Rikala M, Kovatich AJ, Barusevicius A, Miettinen M. CD117: a sensitive marker for gastrointestinal stromal tumors that is more specific than CD34. Mod Pathol. 1998;11:728–34.
38. Miettinen M, Wang ZF, Lasota J. DOG1 antibody in the differential diagnosis of gastrointestinal stromal tumors: a study of 1840 cases. Am J Surg Pathol. 2009;33(9):1401–8.

39. Li K, Cheng H, Li Z, Pang Y, Jia X, Xie F, et al. Genetic progression in gastrointestinal stromal tumors: mechanisms and molecular interventions. Oncotarget. 2017;8:60589–604.

40. Valsangkar N, Sehdev A, Misra S, Zimmers TA, O'Neil BH, Koniaris LG. Current management of gastrointestinal stromal tumors: surgery, current biomarkers, mutations, and therapy. Surgery. 2015;158(5):1149–64.

41. Jian Y, Jian W, Zhang S, Yingqiang Y, Xiaobo L. Chinese consensus guidelines for diagnosis and management of gastrointestinal stromal tumor. Chin J Cancer Res. 2017;29(4):281–93.

42. Ford SJ, Gronchi A. Indications for surgery in advanced/metastatic GIST. Eur J Cancer. 2016;63:154–67.

43. Huang CM, Chen QF, Lin JX, Lin M, Zheng CH, Li P, Xie JW, Wang JB, Lu J, Chen QY. Can laparoscopic surgery be applied in gastric gastrointestinal stromal tumors located in unfavorable sites?: a study based on the NCCN guidelines. Medicine (Abingdon). 2017;96(14):e6535.

44. Dematteo RP, Gold JS, Saran L, Gönen M, Liau KH, Maki RG, Singer S, Besmer P, Brennan MF, Antonescu CR. Tumor mitotic rate, size, and location independently predict recurrence after resection of primary gastrointestinal stromal tumor (GIST). Cancer. 2008;112(3):608.

45. Rutkowski P, Nowecki ZI, Michej W, Debiecrychter M, Woźniak A, Limon J, Siedlecki J, Grzesiakowska U, Kakol M, Osuch C. Risk criteria and prognostic factors for predicting recurrences after resection of primary gastrointestinal stromal tumor. Ann Surg Oncol. 2007;14(7):2018–27.

26

Early decrease in postoperative serum albumin predicts severe complications in patients with colorectal cancer after curative laparoscopic surgery

Yong Wang[†], Honggang Wang[†], Jianguo Jiang[†], Xiaofei Cao[*] and Qinghong Liu[*]

Abstract

Background: Postoperative severe complications are always associated with prolonged hospital stays, increased economic burdens, and poor prognoses in patients with colorectal cancer (CRC). This present study aimed to investigate potential risk factors including serum albumin (Alb) for severe complications in CRC patients.

Methods: Eligible patients with primary CRC undergoing elective laparoscopic colectomy from July 2015 to July 2017 were included. Postoperative severe complications were defined as grade III and IV according to the Clavien–Dindo classification. ΔAlb was defined as (preoperative Alb – nadir Alb within POD2)/preoperative Alb × 100%. The baseline characteristics, intraoperative data, and laboratory data were obtained from the database for the analysis. Univariate and multivariate logistic regression analyses were utilized for the assessment of the association between risk factors and postoperative severe complications. The predictive value of ΔAlb for postoperative severe complications was evaluated by receiver operating characteristic (ROC) curve analysis.

Results: A total of 193 patients were finally included in the analysis data set, of which 38 (19.7%) patients had postoperative severe complications. In the final multivariate logistic regression analysis, ΔAlb was the only independent factor associated with postoperative severe complications (OR 1.66, 95%CI 1.18–2.33, $p = 0.003$). The area under the curve (AUC) of ΔAlb was 0.916, with the sensitivity and specificity of 0.842 and 0.858 ($p < 0.001$).

Conclusions: The ΔAlb was an independent risk factor for severe complications in CRC patients after curative laparoscopic surgery.

Keywords: Colorectal cancer, Postoperative complications, Predictor, Albumin

Background

Colorectal cancer (CRC) has been widely accepted as the third most common malignant neoplasm worldwide with an increasing incidence in recent years [1]. Surgical resection remains the cornerstone curative treatment for CRC, and laparoscopic colorectal surgery is developing constantly in the recent decades. Despite the great improvements in surgical procedures, perioperative managements, and multidisciplinary therapies, postoperative severe complications persist to some extent [2]. As illustrated by the previous data, the incidence of postoperative severe complication can reach as high as approximately 25% [3]. The severe complications are always associated with prolonged hospital stays, increased economic burdens, and poor prognoses [4]. Therefore, to investigate potential factors for postoperative severe complications can help to stratify complication risks and improve clinical decision-making.

After surgery, circulating acute phase proteins, such as interleukin-6 (IL-6) and C-reactive protein (CRP), usually increase because of the surgical stress and proinflammatory cytokines [5, 6]. Previous data has widely considered these two proteins as potential predictors for

* Correspondence: 2856029308@qq.com; drliuqinghong@126.com
[†]Yong Wang, Honggang Wang and Jianguo Jiang contributed equally to this work.
Department of General Surgery, Taizhou People's Hospital, Taizhou Clinical Medical College of Nanjing Medical University, Medical School of Nantong University, No.366 Taihu Road, Taizhou 225300, Jiangsu, China

postoperative complications after elective colorectal surgery [7]. Albumin (Alb), as a negative acute phase protein and nutritional marker, decreases immediately after operation in response to surgical stress. Previous literature has suggested the prognostic role of preoperative hypoalbuminemia in patients undergoing colorectal surgery [8]. However, few studies have focused on the effect of the change of serum Alb on postoperative complications. This present study aimed to investigate potential risk factors including proinflammatory cytokines and nutritional markers for severe complications in CRC patients.

Methods

Patients

This retrospective study protocol was approved by the Medical Institutional Ethics Committee of Jiangsu province. Eligible patients with primary CRC undergoing elective laparoscopic colectomy at the Department of General surgery, Taizhou People's Hospital from July 2015 to July 2017 were included. The inclusion criteria were as follows: (1) adult patients aged over 18, (2) first pathologically diagnosed with primary CRC supported by operative and pathological results, and (3) patients who underwent a curative laparoscopic resection of primary tumors for the first time. The exclusion criteria were as follows: (1) with tumor metastasis found either pre-operatively or intra-operatively, (2) with emergency operation due to complications (bowel obstruction, perforation, etc.), (3) with neo-adjuvant treatment, (4) accompanied by other malignancies; (5) and with laparotomy or laparoscopic conversion to laparotomy.

Study design

The surgical procedures, including the extent of both colectomy and lymph node dissection, were conducted according to the Colorectal Cancer Treatment Guidelines [9]. All the enrolled patients received the same perioperative managements. The diet was not resumed until the patients passed flatus. No patients died within postoperative day (POD) 30 in this present study.

The baseline characteristics (age, gender, etc.), intraoperative data (duration of operation, intraoperative blood transfusion, etc.), and laboratory data (CRP, Alb, etc.) were obtained from the database for the analysis. The pathological classifications were evaluated following the guidance of the 7th edition of American Joint Committee on Cancer (AJCC) TNM Classification.

Definitions and outcomes

The primary outcome was the occurrence of postoperative complications within postoperative 30 days [10]. Postoperative severe complications were defined as grade III and IV according to the Clavien–Dindo classification [11].

Enrolled patients were initially grouped according to the presence of severe complications.

As reported by previous studies [12], the relative change of the serum Alb (ΔAlb) was defined as (preoperative Alb – nadir Alb within POD2)/preoperative Alb $\times$ 100%. The relative changes of the hemoglobin (Hb) and hematocrit (Hct) were with the same definitions. The median ΔAlb level was accepted as the cutoff value for the discrimination of high versus low value [7].

Statistical analysis

Data were analyzed by the SPSS 23.0 (SPSS, Inc., IA, USA) and GraphPad Prism 5.0 (GraphPad Inc., CA, USA), and a $p < 0.05$ was considered statistically significant. Before the study, we performed a sample size estimation of 150 patients. According to our clinical experience and previously published reports [7], the estimated incidence of postoperative severe complications was used as a basis for the minimum sample size estimation. Categorical data are presented as a number with percentage, whereas quantitative data is presented as median (range) or mean $\pm$ standard error (SE) respectively. Mann–Whitney U test or Student t test was used for continuous variables analysis, whereas chi-square test or Fisher's exact test was used for categorical variables analysis as appropriate. Only those potential risk factors ($p < 0.05$) on univariate analysis were enclosed into the final multivariate logistic regression analysis. Binary multivariate stepwise logistic regression model was used in this study. The continuous data used in the logistic model was divided into two groups (high vs low, using the median value as the cutoff value). The predictive value of ΔAlb for postoperative severe complications was evaluated by receiver operating characteristic (ROC) curve analysis.

Results

Patient characteristics

Of 218 consecutive patients, 25 patients were excluded according to the exclusion criteria (6 tumor metastases found intra-operatively, 7 emergency operations, 4 with neo-adjuvant treatment, 3 laparoscopic conversions to laparotomy, and 5 lack of albumin values within postoperative 2 days), which is shown in Fig. 1. A total of 193 patients were finally included in the multivariate analysis dataset, of which 60.1% (116/193) were male patients, as shown in Table 1. Eventually, 38 patients had postoperative severe complications according to the Clavien–Dindo grade, with an incidence of 19.7%. Postoperative severe complications included 6 severe bleedings, 9 anastomotic leakages, 18 severe infections, 4 bowel obstructions, and 1 severe cardiopulmonary failure. The mean age and BMI of the total cohort were 53.4 years and 20.8 kg/m^2 respectively. Patients with severe complications had an older age

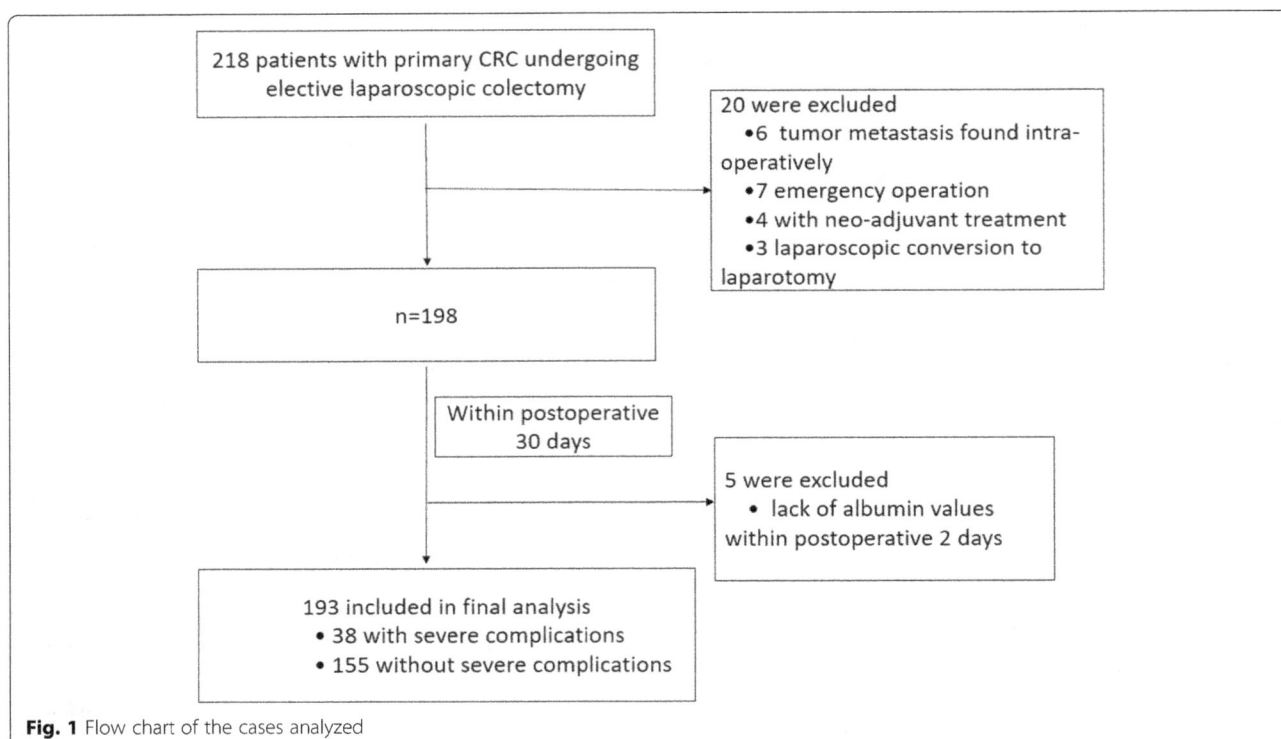

Fig. 1 Flow chart of the cases analyzed

than those without severe complications (52.5 ± 11.7 vs 57.2 ± 12.1, $p = 0.029$). Patients with the comorbidity of hypertension were at an increased risk of postoperative severe complications ($p = 0.029$). The history of previous abdominal surgery was also significantly associated with increased severe complications ($p = 0.030$). In addition, patients with severe complications had a longer duration of operation ($p = 0.043$) and more estimated intraoperative blood loss ($p = 0.032$). Those patients with perioperative blood transfusion were also frequent in the patients with severe complications ($p = 0.026$). No significant differences were found in gender, BMI, smoking habits, ASA class, tumor location, AJCC stage, intraoperative fluid utilization, number of lymph nodes resection, and time to first flatus between the patients with or without severe complications (all $p > 0.05$).

Laboratory tests

As summarized in Table 2, the patients with severe complications had a significantly higher ΔAlb value than those without severe complications (13.3 ± 2.9 vs 19.0 ± 3.5, $p < 0.001$). In addition, higher ΔHb ($p = 0.034$) and peak CRP level within POD3 ($p = 0.005$) were also significantly associated with postoperative severe complications.

Risk factors associated with postoperative severe complications

Subsequently, univariate and multivariate analyses were performed to investigate potential risk factors for

postoperative severe complications. These nine potential risk factors mentioned above (Tables 1 and 2) were enclosed into the univariate analysis. Of the nine factors, five (duration of operation, perioperative blood transfusion, ΔHb, ΔAlb, and peak CRP within POD3) were significantly associated with postoperative severe complications. In the final multivariate logistic regression analysis, ΔAlb was the only independent factor associated with postoperative severe complications (OR 1.66, 95%CI 1.18–2.33, $p = 0.003$, see Table 3).

Predictive value of ΔAlb for postoperative severe complications

The receiver operator characteristic (ROC) curve analysis was applied to establish the predictive power of ΔAlb for postoperative severe complications. As illustrated in Fig. 2, the area under the curve (AUC) of ΔAlb was 0.916, with the cutoff value of 17.3%. The sensitivity and specificity were 0.842 and 0.858, respectively ($p < 0.001$).

Discussion

In this current study, we focused on the potential association between serum Alb, an acute phase protein, and postoperative severe complications within POD 30. Our results revealed that a greater change in the serum Alb within POD 2 was an independent risk factor associated with postoperative severe complications. Postoperative severe complications were with a rate of 19.7% in this

Table 1 Clinicopathological characteristics of CRC patients with severe complications or not

Parameters	Postoperative severe complications		p value
	No (n = 155)	Yes (n = 38)	
Age (year)	52.5 ± 11.7	57.2 ± 12.1	0.029*
Gender, n (%)			
Male	92 (59.4)	24 (63.2)	
Female	63 (40.6)	14 (36.8)	0.67
BMI (kg/m^2)	20.9 ± 1.3	20.6 ± 1.5	0.218
Comorbidities, n (%)			
Hypertension	28 (18.1)	13 (34.2)	0.029*
Diabetes mellitus	18 (11.6)	6 (15.8)	0.48
Smoking status, n (%)			
Current smoker	17 (11.0)	7 (18.4)	
History of smoking	14 (9.0)	5 (13.2)	
Never	124 (80.0)	26 (68.4)	0.30
ASA class, n (%)			
II	121 (78.1)	28 (73.7)	
III	34 (21.9)	10 (26.3)	0.56
Previous abdominal surgery, n (%)	38 (24.5)	16 (42.1)	0.030*
Tumor location, n (%)			
Colon	90 (58.1)	20 (52.6)	
Rectum	65 (41.9)	18 (47.4)	0.54
AJCC stage, n (%)			
I–II	88 (56.8)	18 (47.4)	
III	67 (43.2)	20 (52.6)	0.30
Duration of operation (min)	203.4 ± 30.1	215.4 ± 41.2	0.043*
Estimated blood loss (mL)	180 (60–710)	240 (80–850)	0.032*
Intraoperative fluid utilization (mL)	1800 (1300–3100)	1900 (1400–2900)	0.28
Number of lymph nodes resection	10.7 ± 5.2	10.9 ± 5.8	0.836
Perioperative blood transfusion, n (%)	34 (21.9)	15 (39.5)	0.026*
Time to first flatus (d)	3.0 ± 0.6	3.1 ± 0.9	0.410

CRC colorectal cancer, BMI body mass index, ASA American Society of Anesthesiologists, AJCC American Joint Committee on Cancer. p values were calculated by chi-square test, Fisher's exact test, Mann–Whitney U, or t test. *p value < 0.05

present study, which was relatively similar to previous reports [13].

As reported by previous data, preoperative or early postoperative hypoalbuminemia is accepted as a risk factor for postoperative complications after a gastrointestinal operation, especially surgical site infections [8, 14]. However, whether the relative change in perioperative serum Alb closely correlates with postoperative complications remains unclear. As widely proved, decreased Alb expression after the surgery is always observed due to the systemic inflammatory response syndrome [15]. As illustrated by a recent pilot study, postoperative albumin concentration is significantly decreased and it is suggested as a response biomarker for

operation stress [16], which is quite in accordance with our results. In addition, perioperative hemodilution and fluid overload are also important explanations for decreased serum Alb after operation [17]. As summarized by previous studies, the decreased Alb level is ascribed to various factors, including Alb redistribution, perioperative blood loss, catabolism, and hemodilution [17]. A recent study has revealed increased postoperative CRP level as an independent factor associated with Alb reduction [7], which strongly suggests the close association between Alb and inflammatory response. Accumulating evidence has suggested CRP as a predictor for postoperative complications and prognosis after abdominal surgery [18]. Our univariate analysis showed

Table 2 Laboratory tests in CRC patients with severe complications or not

Laboratory tests	Postoperative severe complications		p value
	No (n = 155)	Yes (n = 38)	
Preoperative Hb	117.5 ± 7.5	116.4 ± 8.4	0.43
Preoperative Alb	39.2 ± 4.6	37.8 ± 5.1	0.10
Preoperative Hct	0.42 ± 0.07	0.43 ± 0.05	0.41
Preoperative CRP	10.8 ± 3.5	11.1 ± 2.7	0.62
ΔHb (%)	14.1 ± 4.2	15.7 ± 3.9	0.034*
ΔAlb (%)	13.3 ± 2.9	19.0 ± 3.5	< 0.001*
ΔHct (%)	− 10.2 ± 12.4	− 11.4 ± 13.6	0.60
Peak CRP within POD3	89.4 ± 6.8	104.4 ± 9.1	0.005*

CRC colorectal cancer, *Hb* hemoglobin, *Alb* albumin, *Hct* hematocrit, *CRP* C-reactive protein, *POD* postoperative day. p values were calculated by Mann–Whitney U or t test. *p value < 0.05

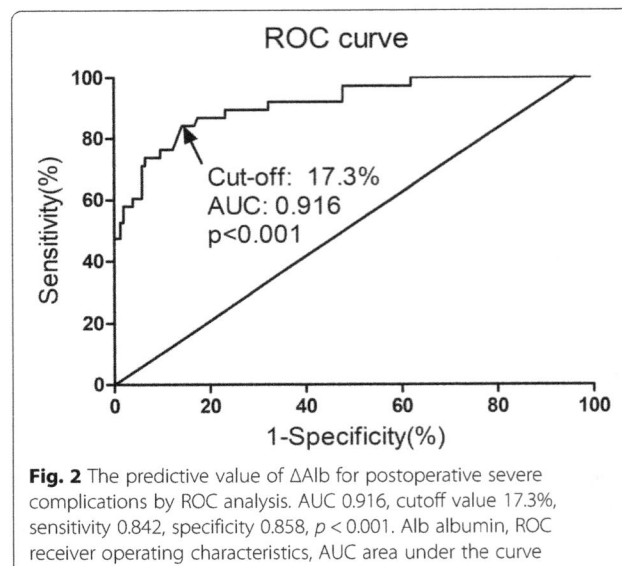

Fig. 2 The predictive value of ΔAlb for postoperative severe complications by ROC analysis. AUC 0.916, cutoff value 17.3%, sensitivity 0.842, specificity 0.858, p < 0.001. Alb albumin, ROC receiver operating characteristics, AUC area under the curve

that peak CRP within POD3 was significantly associated with postoperative severe complications; however, the final multivariate results did not suggest its predictive role.

Previous reports have revealed that malnutrition and inflammatory response strongly correlate with severe postoperative complications [19]. As for those patients with malignancy, the development of inflammatory response is closely associated with decreased Alb and total lymphocyte count [20, 21]. Serum Alb is reported to act various roles, including cell growth stabilization, DNA replication, sex hormone homeostasis maintaining, and systemic inflammation modulation[22].

A recent study in patients with cancer has shown that hypoalbuminemia reflects the condition of malnutrition and immunosuppression, and it is at an increased risk of

disease severity, tumor progression, and poor prognosis [23]. Furthermore, serum Alb level has also been widely used in various prognostic indexes, including a prognostic nutritional index (PNI) [24], a systematic inflammation index (IPI) [25], and Naples prognostic score (NPS) [26]. Serum Alb plays important roles in colloid osmotic pressure maintenance, free radical scavenging, and capillary membrane permeability alteration [27]. The important physiologic functions of serum Alb may be potential explanations for the predictive role of ΔAlb for postoperative severe complications.

This study has some certain limitations. First, our data set came from a retrospective and single-center design, and the sample size was relatively small. Second, this study did not take the impacts of liver function and body fluid volume on serum albumin concentrations into consideration. Nevertheless, to our knowledge, this is the first study that highlighted the significance of ΔAlb for postoperative severe complications. Of course, additional larger-scale prospective studies and basic researches are needed to confirm our results.

Table 3 Univariate and multivariate logistic regression analyses of perioperative factors on postoperative severe complications

Variables	Univariate		Multivariate	
	OR (95% CI)	p value	OR (95% CI)	p value
Age	1.02 (0.98–1.05)	0.75		
Hypertension	1.22 (0.76–1.94)	0.43		
Previous abdominal surgery	1.40 (0.93–2.04)	0.12		
Duration of operation	1.38 (1.03–1.94)	0.043*	0.93 (0.57–1.49)	0.72
Estimated blood loss	0.82 (0.58–1.14)	0.23		
Perioperative blood transfusion	2.46 (1.47–4.02)	0.012*	1.33 (0.62–2.77)	0.43
ΔHb	2.34 (1.29–4.61)	0.009*	1.66 (0.68–3.89)	0.23
ΔAlb	1.68 (1.22–2.32)	0.002*	1.66 (1.18–2.33)	0.003*
Peak CRP within POD3	0.70 (0.48–0.99)	0.032*	1.12 (0.65–1.94)	0.65

Hb hemoglobin, *Alb* albumin, *CRP* C-reactive protein, *POD* postoperative day, *OR* odds ratio, *CI* confidence interval. *p value < 0.05

Conclusions

In conclusion, our results revealed that the ΔAlb was an independent risk factor for severe complications in CRC patients after curative laparoscopic surgery. The surgeon and anesthetist could differentiate the patients according to the reduction trend of serum Alb and treat them accordingly. Predicting the risk of postoperative severe complications with serum Alb detections helps the surgeon in the outcome evaluation. The evaluation of the nutritional status prior to surgery is of great importance and if possible, correcting the deficit is recommended by our results.

Abbreviations

AJCC: American Joint Committee on Cancer; Alb: Albumin; ASA: American Society of Anesthesiologists; BMI: Body mass index; CI: Confidence interval; CRC: Colorectal cancer; CRP: C-reactive protein; Hb: Hemoglobin; Hct: Hematocrit; OR: Odds ratio; POD: Postoperative day; ROC: Receiver operating characteristic; SE: Standard error

Funding

This work was supported partly by funding from the National Natural Science Foundation of China (Grant no. 81600434), Jiangsu Natural Science Foundation (Grant no. BK20160572 and BK20170358), and Jiangsu Provincial Medical Youth Talent (Grant no. QNRC2016514).

Authors' contributions

YW, HGW, and JGJ participated in the conception and design, data collection, statistical analysis, and writing of the manuscript. XFC and QHL participated in the conception and design and data collection. All authors read and approved the final manuscript.

Competing interests

The authors' declare that they have no competing interests.

References

1. Global Burden of Disease Cancer C, Fitzmaurice C, Dicker D, Pain A, Hamavid H, Moradi-Lakeh M, et al. The global burden of cancer 2013. JAMA Oncol. 2015;1(4):505–27.
2. Papamichael D, Audisio RA, Glimelius B, de Gramont A, Glynne-Jones R, Haller D, et al. Treatment of colorectal cancer in older patients: International Society of Geriatric Oncology (SIOG) consensus recommendations 2013. Ann Oncol. 2015;26(3):463–76.
3. Henneman D, Snijders HS, Fiocco M, van Leersum NJ, Kolfschoten NE, Wiggers T, et al. Hospital variation in failure to rescue after colorectal cancer surgery: results of the Dutch Surgical Colorectal Audit. Ann Surg Oncol. 2013;20(7):2117–23.
4. Ortega-Deballon P, Radais F, Facy O, d'Athis P, Masson D, Charles PE, et al. C-reactive protein is an early predictor of septic complications after elective colorectal surgery. World J Surg. 2010;34(4):808–14.
5. Rettig TC, Verwijmeren L, Dijkstra IM, Boerma D, van de Garde EM, Noordzij PG. Postoperative interleukin-6 level and early detection of complications after elective major abdominal surgery. Ann Surg. 2016;263(6):1207–12.
6. Warschkow R, Beutner U, Steffen T, Muller SA, Schmied BM, Guller U, et al. Safe and early discharge after colorectal surgery due to C-reactive protein: a diagnostic meta-analysis of 1832 patients. Ann Surg. 2012;256(2):245–50.
7. Ge X, Dai X, Ding C, Tian H, Yang J, Gong J, et al. Early postoperative decrease of serum albumin predicts surgical outcome in patients undergoing colorectal resection. Dis Colon Rectum. 2017;60(3):326–34.
8. Moghadamyeghaneh Z, Hwang G, Hanna MH, Phelan MJ, Carmichael JC, Mills SD, et al. Even modest hypoalbuminemia affects outcomes of colorectal surgery patients. Am J Surg. 2015;210(2):276–84.
9. Watanabe T, Itabashi M, Shimada Y, Tanaka S, Ito Y, Ajioka Y, et al. Japanese Society for Cancer of the Colon and Rectum (JSCCR) guidelines 2014 for treatment of colorectal cancer. Int J Clin Oncol. 2015;20(2):207–39.
10. Cao X, Zhao G, Yu T, An Q, Yang H, Xiao G. Preoperative prognostic nutritional index correlates with severe complications and poor survival in patients with colorectal cancer undergoing curative laparoscopic surgery: a retrospective study in a single Chinese institution. Nutr Cancer. 2017;69(3): 454–63.
11. Clavien PA, Barkun J, de Oliveira ML, Vauthey JN, Dindo D, Schulick RD, et al. The Clavien-Dindo classification of surgical complications: five-year experience. Ann Surg. 2009;250(2):187–96.
12. Spolverato G, Kim Y, Ejaz A, Frank SM, Pawlik TM. Effect of relative decrease in blood hemoglobin concentrations on postoperative morbidity in patients who undergo major gastrointestinal surgery. JAMA Surg. 2015;150(10):949–56.
13. Boer BC, de Graaff F, Brusse-Keizer M, Bouman DE, Slump CH, Slee-Valentijn M, et al. Skeletal muscle mass and quality as risk factors for postoperative outcome after open colon resection for cancer. Int J Color Dis. 2016;31(6): 1117–24.
14. Lee JI, Kwon M, Roh JL, Choi JW, Choi SH, Nam SY, et al. Postoperative hypoalbuminemia as a risk factor for surgical site infection after oral cancer surgery. Oral Dis. 2015;21(2):178–84.
15. Fleck A, Raines G, Hawker F, Trotter J, Wallace PI, Ledingham IM, et al. Increased vascular permeability: a major cause of hypoalbuminaemia in disease and injury. Lancet. 1985;1(8432):781–4.
16. Hubner M, Mantziari S, Demartines N, Pralong F, Coti-Bertrand P, Schafer M. Postoperative albumin drop is a marker for surgical stress and a predictor for clinical outcome: a pilot study. Gastroenterol Res Pract. 2016;2016: 8743187.
17. Ryan AM, Hearty A, Prichard RS, Cunningham A, Rowley SP, Reynolds JV. Association of hypoalbuminemia on the first postoperative day and complications following esophagectomy. J Gastrointest Surg. 2007;11(10): 1355–60.
18. Watt DG, Horgan PG, McMillan DC. Routine clinical markers of the magnitude of the systemic inflammatory response after elective operation: a systematic review. Surgery. 2015;157(2):362–80.
19. Mohri Y, Inoue Y, Tanaka K, Hiro J, Uchida K, Kusunoki M. Prognostic nutritional index predicts postoperative outcome in colorectal cancer. World J Surg. 2013;37(11):2688–92.
20. Erdman SE, Poutahidis T. Roles for inflammation and regulatory T cells in colon cancer. Toxicol Pathol. 2010;38(1):76–87.
21. Crumley AB, Stuart RC, McKernan M, McMillan DC. Is hypoalbuminemia an independent prognostic factor in patients with gastric cancer? World J Surg. 2010;34(10):2393–8.
22. Gupta D, Lis CG. Pretreatment serum albumin as a predictor of cancer survival: a systematic review of the epidemiological literature. Nutr J. 2010;9:69.
23. Nazha B, Moussaly E, Zaarour M, Weerasinghe C, Azab B. Hypoalbuminemia in colorectal cancer prognosis: nutritional marker or inflammatory surrogate? World J Gastrointest Surg. 2015;7(12):370–7.
24. Tokunaga R, Sakamoto Y, Nakagawa S, Miyamoto Y, Yoshida N, Oki E, et al. Prognostic nutritional index predicts severe complications, recurrence, and poor prognosis in patients with colorectal cancer undergoing primary tumor resection. Dis Colon Rectum. 2015;58(11):1048–57.
25. Hong T, Shen D, Chen X, Cai D, Wu X, Hua D. A novel systematic inflammation related index is prognostic in curatively resected non-metastatic colorectal cancer. Am J Surg. 2018;216(3):450–7.
26. Galizia G, Lieto E, Auricchio A, Cardella F, Mabilia A, Podzemny V, et al. Naples prognostic score, based on nutritional and inflammatory status, is an independent predictor of long-term outcome in patients undergoing surgery for colorectal cancer. Dis Colon Rectum. 2017;60(12):1273–84.
27. Margarson MP, Soni N. Serum albumin: touchstone or totem? Anaesthesia. 1998;53(8):789–803.

Permissions

List of Contributors

Natasa Colakovic and Zlatko Skuric
Department of Surgical Oncology, University Medical Center "Bezanijska Kosa", Bezanijska kosa bb, Belgrade 11080, Serbia

Darko Zdravkovic, Jasna Gacic and Nebojsa Ivanovic
Faculty of Medicine, University of Belgrade, Belgrade, Serbia

Davor Mrda
Department of Radiology, University Medical Center "Bezanijska Kosa", Belgrade, Serbia

Zhou-Feng Chen, Xiu-Li Dong, Qing-Ke Huang, Wang-Dong Hong, Wen-Zhi Wu, Jian-Sheng Wu and Shuang Pan
Department of Gastroenterology, The First Affiliated Hospital of Wenzhou Medical University, Wenzhou 325000, Zhejiang, People's Republic of China

Haiyan Zhou and Xiao Li
Department of Cleft Palate Speech, The First Affiliated Hospital of Harbin Medical University, Harbin 150001, People's Republic of China

Haiyan Zhou, Chuhan Zhang and Xiao Li
Department of Oral and Maxillofacial Surgery, The First Affiliated Hospital of Harbin Medical University, No. 23 Youzheng Road, Nangang District, Harbin 150001, Heilongjiang Province, People's Republic of China

Jing Yang and Yuwei Zhang
Department of Basic Medical Science, Heilongjiang University of Chinese Medicine, Harbin 150040, People's Republic of China

Rui Wang
Department of Pharmacy, Heilongjiang University of Chinese Medicine, Harbin 150040, People's Republic of China

Shuainan Zhang
Department of Pharmacy, Guiyang University of Chinese Medicine, Guiyang 550025, People's Republic of China

Ye Mao, Yan Tie and Jing Du
Cancer Center, West China Hospital, West China Medical School Sichuan University, No. 37, Guoxue Alley, Chengdu 610041, Sichuan Province, China

Christian Galata, Stefan Post and Karoline Horisberger
Department of Surgery, University Hospital Mannheim, Medical Faculty Mannheim, University of Heidelberg, Theodor-Kutzer-Ufer 1-3, 68167 Mannheim, Germany

Kirsten Merx and Ralf-Dieter Hofheinz
Interdisciplinary Tumor Centre, III. Department of Internal Medicine, University Hospital Mannheim, Medical Faculty Mannheim, University of Heidelberg, Mannheim, Germany

Sabine Mai and Frederik Wenz
Institute for Radiotherapy and Radiooncology, University Hospital Mannheim, Medical Faculty Mannheim, University of Heidelberg, Mannheim, Germany

Timo Gaiser
Institute for Pathology, University Hospital Mannheim, Medical Faculty Mannheim, University of Heidelberg, Mannheim, Germany

Karoline Horisberger
Department of Visceral and Transplant Surgery, Universitätsspital Zürich, Zürich, Switzerland

Peter Kienle
Department of Surgery, Theresienkrankenhaus Mannheim, Mannheim, Germany

Wenqi Zhou, Faliang Xu and Xiaohua Zeng
Breast Center, Chongqing University Cancer Hospital and Chongqing Cancer Institute and Chongqing Cancer Hospital, Chongqing 400030, People's Republic of China

Shizhe Chen
Xiehe Affiliated Hospital of Fujian Medical University, Fuzhou 350000, Fujian, People's Republic of China

Zhiqiang Qin, Mei Lin, Jinkun Wu and Ning Wang
Department of Pathology, School of Basic Medicine, Medical College, Qingdao University, No. 308 Ningxia Road, Qingdao 266071, Shandong, People's Republic of China

Xinjuan Yu
Central Laboratories, Qingdao Municipal Hospital, Qingdao 266071, Shandong, People's Republic of China

Shupei Ma
Department of Hematology, Qingdao Municipal Hospital, Qingdao 266011, Shandong, People's Republic of China

Jie Ren, Bingjing Leng, Rongkuan Hu and Guoqin Jiang
Department of General Surgery, The Second Affiliated Hospital of Soochow University, Suzhou 215006, China

Liyan Jin
Department of Thyroid and Breast Surgery, Traditional Chinese Medicine Hospital of Kunshan, Suzhou 215006, China

William F. Morano, Mohammad F. Shaikh, Elizabeth M. Gleeson, Marian Khalili and Wilbur B. Bowne
Division of Surgical Oncology, Department of Surgery, Drexel University College of Medicine, 245 N. 15th Street, Suite 7150, Philadelphia, PA 19102, USA

Alvaro Galvez and Elizabeth P. Renza-Stingone
Division of Minimally Invasive Surgery, Department of Surgery, Drexel University College of Medicine, 245 N. 15th St, Suite 7150, Philadelphia, PA 19102, USA

John Lieb II
Division of Gastroenterology and Hepatology, Department of Medicine, Drexel University College of Medicine, 219 N Broad St, 5th Floor, Philadelphia, PA 19107, USA

Xinghui Song and Xiaoning Zhong
Department of respiration, the First Affiliated Hospital of Guangxi Medical University, N0.6 Shuangyong Road, Nanning 530021, Guangxi, China

Kaijiang Tang and Yin Jiang
Department of rheumatism, Liuzhou Worker's Hospital, Liuzhou 545005, Guangxi, China

Gang Wu
Department of neurosurgery, Liuzhou General Hospital, Liuzhou 545006, Guangxi, China

Xin Liu, Ji-bin Li, Gang Shi, Rui Guo and Rui Zhang
Department of Colorectal Surgery, Cancer Hospital of China Medical University, Liaoning Cancer Hospital and Institute, No 44 Xiaoheyan Road, Dadong District, Shenyang 110042, Liaoning Province, People's Republic of China

Ming-Wei Ma, Xian-Shu Gao, Xiao-Bin Gu, Mu Xie, Ming Cui, Min Zhang and Ling Liu
Department of Radiation Oncology, Peking University First Hospital, No.7 Xishiku Street, Beijing 100034, People's Republic of China

Huan Yin
Department of Medical and Pharmaceutical Science and Technology Strategy Research, Institute of Medical Information, Chinese Academy of Medical Sciences, No. 3 Yabao Road, Beijing, China

Long-Qi Chen
Department of Thoracic Surgery, West China School of Medicine/West China Hospital of Sichuan University, No. 37 Guoxue Alley, Chengdu 610041, Sichuan, People's Republic of China

Youkang Ni, Ping Lu, Zhi Yang, Wenlong Wang, Wei Dai, Zhong-zheng Qi, Weiyi Duan, Zhong-fei Xu, Chang-fu Sun and Fayu Liu
Department of Oromaxillofacial-Head and Neck Surgery, School of Stomatology, China Medical University, No. 117 Nanjing North Street, Heping District, Shenyang 110002, Liaoning, People's Republic of China

Yi-Jian Tsai and Jen-Kou Lin
Division of Colon and Rectal Surgery, Department of Surgery, Taipei-Veterans General Hospital, No 201, Sec 2, Shih-Pai Rd, 11217 Taipei, Taiwan

Sheng-Chieh Huang, Hung-Hsin Lin, Chun-Chi Lin, Yuan-Tzu Lan, Huann-Sheng Wang, Shung-Haur Yang, Jeng-Kai Jiang, Wei-Shone Chen, Tzu-chen Lin and Shih-Ching Chang
Department of Surgery, Faculty of Medicine, National Yang-Ming University, Taipei, Taiwan

Vivienne Keding, Wolf O. Bechstein and Andreas A. Schnitzbauer
Clinic for General and Visceral Surgery, University Hospital Frankfurt, Goethe University Frankfurt/Main, Theodor-Stern-Kai 7, 60590 Frankfurt/Main, Germany

Kai Zacharowski and Patrick Meybohm
Department of Anesthesiology, Intensive Care Medicine, and Pain Therapy, University Hospital Frankfurt, Goethe University Frankfurt, Frankfurt/Main, Germany

Wen Gao
Department of Trauma Surgery, Tianjin Fourth Central Hospital, No.1 Zhongshan Road, Hebei District, Tianjin 300010, China

Ning Guo
Department of Breast Surgery, Tianjin Fourth Central Hospital, No.1 Zhongshan Road, Hebei District, Tianjin 300010, China

Ting Dong
Department of Cardiovascular Medicine, Guizhou Provincial People's Hospital, No. 83 Zhongshandong Road, Guiyang City 550002, Guizhou, China

Chaoran Yu, Pei Xue, Luyang Zhang, Ruijun Pan, Zhenhao Cai, Zirui He, Jing Sun and Minhua Zheng
Department of General Surgery, Ruijin Hospital, Shanghai Jiao Tong University, School of Medicine, Shanghai 200025, People's Republic of China
Shanghai Minimally Invasive Surgery Center, Ruijin Hospital, Shanghai Jiao Tong University, School of Medicine, Shanghai 200025, People's Republic of China

Wangjian Li, Lihong Ye, Yongliang Chen
Department of Urology, Shaoxing Hospital of China Medical University, Zhejiang, China

Peng Chen
Department of Radiation Oncology, Hangzhou Cancer Hospital, Zhejiang, China

Nan Zhang, Qian Fei, Jiajia Gu, Li Yin and Xia He
Department of Radiation Oncology, Jiangsu Cancer Hospital and Jiangsu Institute of Cancer Research and Affiliated Cancer Hospital of Nanjing Medical University, Nanjing Medical University Affiliated Cancer Hospital, 42 Baiziting, Nanjing 210009, Jiangsu, China

Qian Fei, Li Yin and Xia He
The Fourth Clinical School of Nanjing Medical University, Nanjing, China

Ningning Zhang, Zhende Shang, Zhigang Wang, Xianbing Meng, Zheng Li, Hailong Tian, Dezhang Huang and Xin Yin
Department of Neurosurgery, Shandong University Qilu Hospital, Qingdao, Shandong, China

Ningning Zhang, Zhende Shang, Xianbing Meng, Zheng Li, Bin Zheng and Xinhua Zhang
Department of Neurosurgery, Affiliated Hospital of Taishan Medical University, Tai An, Shandong, China

Ze-Qun Zhang, Li Xiong, Jiang-Jiao Zhou, Xiong-Ying Miao, Qing-Long Li, Yu Wen and Heng Zou
Department of General Surgery, The Second Xiangya Hospital, Central South University, Changsha 410011, Hunan, China

Chun-ping Ning, Hong-qiao Wang and Xiao-ying Du
Ultrasound Department, Affiliated Hospital of Qingdao University, Qingdao, Shandong, China

Xiaoli Ji
Ultrasound Department, Qingdao Women and Children Hospital, Qingdao, Shandong, China

Hai-tao Niu and Shi-bao Fang
Urology Department, Affiliated Hospital of Qingdao University, No. 16 of Jiangsu Road, Qingdao, Shandong, China

Weiran Zhang
Department of Cardiothoracic Surgery, BenQ Hospital, Affiliated Hospital of Nanjing Medical University, Nanjing, China

Ban Liu
Department of Cardiology, Shanghai Tenth People's Hospital, Tongji University School of Medicine, Shanghai, China

Yue Zhou
Department of Cardiothoracic Surgery, First Affiliated Hospital of Nanjing Medical University, Nanjing, China

Feng Wang
Department of Gastroenterology, Shanghai Tenth People's Hospital, Tongji University School of Medicine, Shanghai, China

Chang Gu
Department of Thoracic Surgery, Shanghai Chest Hospital, Shanghai Jiao Tong University, Shanghai, China

Qi Wang
The Clinical Medical Department of Nanjing Medical University, Nanjing, China

Xiaofang Wang and Yangyang Zhang
Department of Cardiovascular Surgery, Shanghai East Hospital, Tongji University School of Medicine, 150 Jimo Road, Shanghai 200120, China

Xiaoli Tang and Meiyuan Yang
Department of General Surgery, The Second Xiangya Hospital of Central South University, Renmin Road No.139, Changsha 410001, China

Zheng Wang and Xiaoqing Wu
Department of General Surgery, Medical College of Yangzhou University, Huaihai Road No.7, Yangzhou 225001, China

Daorong Wang
Department of General Surgery, The northern Jiangsu people's Hospital, Nantong Road No.98, Yangzhou 225001, China

Bao Zhang
China Medical University, No.77 Puhe Road, Shenbei New District, Shenyang 110013, Liaoning Province, People's Republic of China

Guo Liang Zheng, Hai Tao Zhu, Yan Zhao and Zhi Chao Zheng
Department of Gastric Surgery, Cancer Hospital of China Medical University, Liaoning Cancer Hospital and Institute, No.44 Xiaoheyan Road, Dadong District, Shenyang 110042, Liaoning Province, People's Republic of China

Yong Wang, Honggang Wang, Jianguo Jiang, Xiaofei Cao and Qinghong Liu
Department of General Surgery, Taizhou People's Hospital, Taizhou Clinical Medical College of Nanjing Medical University, Medical School of Nantong University, No.366 Taihu Road, Taizhou 225300, Jiangsu, China

Index